BOVINE SURGERY AND LAMENESS

T0176523

BOVINE SURGERY AND LAMENESS
Third Edition

A. David Weaver
BSc, Dr med vet, PhD, FRCVS, Dr hc (Warsaw)
Professor emeritus, College of Veterinary Medicine
University of Missouri, USA and Bearsden, Glasgow, Scotland

Owen Atkinson
BVSc, DCHP, MRCVS
Royal College of Veterinary Surgeons Specialist in Cattle Health and Production
Dairy Veterinary Consultancy Ltd, Cheshire, UK

Guy St. Jean
DMV, MS, Dipl ACVS
Professor of Surgery, Former Head, Department of Veterinary
Clinical Sciences, School of Veterinary Medicine
Ross University, St Kitts, West Indies

Adrian Steiner
Dr med vet, FVH, MS, Dr habil, Dipl ECVS, Dipl ECBHM
Professor and Head, Clinic for Ruminants, Vetsuisse-Faculty of Berne
Switzerland

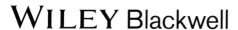

This edition first published 2018
© 2018 John Wiley and Sons Ltd.

Edition History
Blackwell Scientific Publications (1e, 1986); Wiley-Blackwell (2e, 2005)

The right of A. David Weaver, Owen Atkinson, Guy St. Jean, and Adrian Steiner to be identified as the authors of this work has been asserted in accordance with law.

Registered Offices
John Wiley & Sons, Inc., 111 River Street, Hoboken, NJ 07030, USA
John Wiley & Sons Ltd, The Atrium, Southern Gate, Chichester, West Sussex, PO19 8SQ, UK

Editorial Office
9600 Garsington Road, Oxford, OX4 2DQ, UK

For details of our global editorial offices, customer services, and more information about Wiley products visit us at www.wiley.com.

Wiley also publishes its books in a variety of electronic formats and by print-on-demand. Some content that appears in standard print versions of this book may not be available in other formats.

Library of Congress Cataloging-in-Publication Data

Names: Weaver, A. David (Anthony David), author. | Atkinson, Owen, author. |
   St. Jean, Guy, author. | Steiner, Adrian, 1959- author.
Title: Bovine surgery and lameness [electronic resource] / by A. David
   Weaver, Owen Atkinson, Guy St. Jean, Adrian Steiner.
Description: Third edition. | Hoboken, NJ : Wiley, 2018. | Includes
   bibliographical references and index. |
Identifiers: LCCN 2017050346 (print) | LCCN 2017055592 (ebook) | ISBN
   9781119040514 (pdf) | ISBN 9781119040491 (epub) | ISBN 9781119040460 (pbk.)
Subjects: LCSH: Cattle–Surgery. | Lameness in cattle. | MESH: Cattle
   Diseases | Cattle–surgery | Lameness, Animal
Classification: LCC SF961 (ebook) | LCC SF961 .W43 2018 (print) | NLM SF 961
   | DDC 636.2/0897–dc23
LC record available at https://lccn.loc.gov/2017050346

Cover Design: Wiley
Cover Images: Courtesy of Owen Atkinson

Set in 9.5/11.5 pt PhotinaMTStd by Thomson Digital, Noida, India

Printed in Singapore by C.O.S. Printers Pte Ltd

10 9 8 7 6 5 4 3 2 1

Contents

Preface

Having discarded the prefaces of the first two editions of "Bovine Surgery and Lameness", the third edition has some changes in its format. However, the emphasis of this paperback, designed to be available in the car for easy access (rather than gathering dust on the practice bookshelf), has the same aims as its predecessors. It should give the "nuts and bolts" or "how to . . ." of the previous editions. It has an additional author, Owen Atkinson, a dairy consultant veterinarian who has over twenty years experience of intensive dairy cattle practice in England. Owen has completely rewritten the lameness chapter, and has also reorganised the introductory sections to give greater emphasis to supportive therapy and certain selected diagnostic procedures.

Other changes include expansion of the surgical management of abomasal disorders to include laparoscopic techniques introduced into veterinary medicine over the last 15 years. These techniques have been clarified by greater use of line drawings, that were appreciated in the second edition. Three such line drawings illustrate the front cover.

As well as ethical considerations, the problems of the economic viability of any surgical intervention in cattle must be carefully assessed. The importance of sterile surgical packs, effective anaesthesia and asepsis cannot be over-emphasised. Failures in operative procedures in cattle lead to a natural reluctance by farmers to agree to repeat such operations. The attention today (2018) on the worldwide attempts to reduce antibiotic usage is also relevant to bovine surgery, where effective asepsis often makes post-operative antibiotic cover unnecessary.

The quality of veterinarian-farmer communication is particularly relevant at a time when ethical considerations have become more important. The general public is now more conscious of animal welfare and their view, as consumers and customers, should not be ignored. The veterinary profession has an important role here. For example, the need for pain relief should be promoted in routine procedures such as disbudding/dehorning and castration, frequently performed by the unsupervised farmer following instruction by the veterinarian. The relatively recent recognition of the usefulness of NSAIDs to reduce post-operative pain is applauded and their more widespread use is encouraged in this revised edition.

Other challenges in the bovine surgical field cannot be avoided, such as surgery in a suboptimal environment e.g. a dusty dark cowshed late at night, or the ill-lit corner of a field. More hypothetical challenges such as the layperson's question: "is castration justified?" fall outside our remit in this book. However, wherever possible a practical approach has been suggested, including some handy tips often learned the hard way.

Despite this book often describing the surgical correction of conditions once they occur, the reader is encouraged to make efforts to prevent problems, such as an unacceptable incidence of displaced abomasum cases, or of digital dermatitis. Whilst other books, (see further reading section) are able to explore preventive measures in greater depth, we have included in this edition some discussion boxes to promote a preventive approach.

The authors would welcome comments and suggestions for improvements. We have often given only our personal preferred surgical technique, aware that in other hands there can be excellent alternatives.

A. David Weaver, Owen Atkinson, Guy St. Jean and Adrian Steiner
March 2018

Acknowledgements

Permission to reproduce again illustrations from the first and second editions was graciously given by several authors and publishers as below.

Figs. 1.9, 4.5, 5.2, 5.12 Dr. K.M. Dyce, Edinburgh and W.B. Saunders 'Essentials of Bovine Anatomy', 1971 by Dyce and Wensing

Figs. 4.4, 4.9, 5.1, 5.4, 5.5 Professor Claude Pavaux, Toulouse, and Maloine s.a. editeur from 'Colour Atlas of Bovine Anatomy: Splanchnology' 1982

Fig. 5.17, Dr. John Cox, Liverpool, and Liverpool University Press 'Surgery of the Reproductive Tract in Large Animals' 1987

Fig. 3.3, Adapted from Dr. M.E. Smart, Saskatoon and Veterinary Learning Systems, Yardley, PA, USA from 'Compendium of Continuing Education for the Practicing Veterinarian' 7, S327, 1985

Fig. 5.20, Dr. H. Kümper, Giessen and Blackwell Science from 'Innere Medizin und Chirurgie des Rindes' 4e 2002 edited by G. Dirksen, H-D. Gründer and M. Stöber (fig. 6.125)

Fig. 6.6, Dr. R.S. Youngquist, Columbia, Missouri and W.B. Saunders from 'Current Therapy in Large Animal Theriogenology' 1997 (fig. 57.2)

Fig. 9.31, Dr. M. Steenhaut, Gent, and Blackwell Science from 'Innere Medizin und Chirurgie des Rindes' 4e 2002 edited by G. Dirksen, H-D. Gründer and M. Stöber (fig. 9.159)

The authors are grateful to the many practicing vets and colleagues who helped with previous editions, checking for inaccuracies, providing comment or drawing sketches. They include the American Association of Bovine Practitioners (AABP), Dominic Alexander, George Constantinescu, Keith Cutler, Jan Huckin, Lesley Johnson, David Noakes, David Pritchard, David Ramsay, Jonathan Reader, Phil Scott, John Sproat, Eva Steiner, David Taylor and Thomas Wittek. Thanks also to Dr. R.S. Youngquist and Colin D. Penny who reviewed the new Chapter 8.

David Weaver thanks Christina Mclachlan of Milngavie for both her accuracy and patience whilst typing large sections of manuscript.

Guy St. Jean thanks his mentors Bruce Hull, Michael Rings and Glen Hoffsis, not only for their earlier advice and encouragement during his residency, but also for their continuing friendship. He also thanks Kim Carey for secretarial help and his wife Kathleen Yvorchuk-St. Jean for continual support.

Adrian Steiner would like to dedicate the book to Christian.

Owen Atkinson thanks the farmers and many veterinary colleagues who have contributed to his understanding of bovine surgery and lameness. He thanks Laura for her support.

Finally thanks are given to all at Wiley Publishing for their expertise and encouragement through the writing of this third edition. They include Patricia Bateson, Catriona Cooper, Susan Engelken, Jessica Evans, Atiqah Abdul Manaf, Purvi Patel, and Justinia Wood.

A. David Weaver, Owen Atkinson, Guy St. Jean and Adrian Steiner
March 2018

The authors have made every effort to ensure that medicines and their dosage regimes are accurate at the time of publication. Nevertheless, readers should check the product information provided by the manufacturer of each medicine before its use or prescription. In particular, medicine authorisation by regulatory authorities varies from country to country. Some medicines included in the text are not authorised for use for food- producing animals in some countries. The reader should exercise individual judgement in coming to a clinical decision on medicine usage, bearing in mind professional skill and experience, and should at all times remain within the regulatory framework of the country.

Whilst all reasonable care has been taken in the book's preparation, including peer review, no warranty is given as to its accuracy, nor liability accepted for any loss or damage caused by reliance upon any statement in or omission from this publication.

About the Companion Website

This book is accompanied by a companion website:

www.wiley.com/go/weaver/bovine-surgery

The website includes:

- Videos
- Annotated PDF documents of videos

CHAPTER 1

General considerations and anaesthesia

1.1 Pre-operative assessment

Introduction

The bovine patient is a stoical animal and modern crushes and physical restraint options allow many techniques to be carried out in the field. However, this should not excuse a thorough **clinical** and **ethical** assessment prior to any surgical procedure.

Assessment should include numerous factors apart from the physical condition of the subject:

- welfare implications of the procedure
- potential duration of a productive life
- economic situation including insurance status and economic return on the surgery
- surgical risk regarding complete recovery
- future breeding prospects including heritability of the condition being corrected
- pathology of other body systems directly or indirectly related to the primary condition

General physical examination is essential before emergency or elective surgery to assess risks and concurrent disorders.

Bovine Surgery and Lameness, Third Edition. A. David Weaver, Owen Atkinson, Guy St. Jean and Adrian Steiner.
© 2018 John Wiley & Sons Ltd. Published 2018 by John Wiley & Sons Ltd.
Companion website: www.wiley.com/go/weaver/bovine-surgery

Welfare and quality of life

Animal welfare may be judged using a number of criteria. Making these judgements is an essential part of the vet's role. Vets must also lead by example. Decisions to perform surgery, and how it is to be done, are complex. Foremost in the process must be the welfare of the cow or calf. The surgeon should ask themselves:

- How necessary is this procedure: will benefits to the animal outweigh any pain or discomfort?
- What will the animal's quality of life be afterwards? Is the procedure likely to lead to a 'life worth living' or preferably 'a good life' for the animal in question?
- How does this procedure compare with an alternative option of humane slaughter or euthanasia?
- To what extent can pain and discomfort be mitigated during and after the procedure?
- To what extent can fear and distress be mitigated during and after the procedure?
- What can we learn from this situation to make life better for cows and calves in the future?

The last question is vital: sometimes it is easy for the surgeon to focus on the individual animal in question (that is important too) but lose sight of the greater picture. For example: performing surgery on a cow with toe necrosis can greatly improve her quality of life, but what measures can be put in place to prevent further cases? You are asked to dehorn or castrate some yearling cattle: could it be done at a younger age next time?

Warning

Some procedures are deemed to be simply unethical and there is legislation in place preventing them, though there are regional variations. Examples in the UK of illegal procedures include:

- tail docking in calves or adult cattle (except in cases of injury)
- castration over one week by means of an elastrator
- castration without anaesthetic for animals over two months of age

Furthermore, the Veterinary Surgeons Act means that any surgery involving entering a body cavity (e.g. joint spaces; abdomen; thoracic cavity) can only be carried out by a qualified veterinary surgeon in the UK. It is incumbent on the vet to provide suitable anaesthesia and analgesia.

Anaesthesia techniques are described in Section 1.7–1.9. Peri-operative analgesia is discussed in Section 2.11, though there is clearly overlap in these two areas of pharmacology and surgical preparation. The use of a crush/ squeeze chute should never replace adequate analgesia and sedation for surgical procedures.

Tip

Learn and practice good communication techniques. Effective communication between farm vet and producer is vital to ensure that pain and suffering are reduced to a minimum among stock. Vets should be the leaders in animal welfare: this leadership requires exact personal skills, which is in addition to any technical abilities or scientific knowledge required of vets.

Laboratory tests

Under farm practice conditions laboratory tests may not be performed, but major parameters very simply estimated with minimal apparatus are:

- packed cell volume: microcentrifuge, microhaematocrit apparatus
- total protein: refractometer

Normal haematological and biochemical parameters of cattle are listed in Table 1.1.

In some abdominal conditions (abomasal torsion or volvulus, intestinal obstruction) estimation of plasma electrolytes (e.g. chloride) is valuable in assessing prognosis and calculating requirements for fluid replacement. Fluid therapy is discussed in Chapter 2.

Congenital defects

Incidence of congenital defects in cattle is 0.2–3%, with 40–50% born dead. Most defects are visible externally. Congenital defects reduce the value of affected calves and economic losses are most severe when combined with embryonic or foetal mortality, particularly if it results in an extended subsequent calving interval. Close collaboration between the vet, farmer and geneticist is essential and good breeding records are vital.

Tip

'Congenital' is not synonymous with 'heritable' or 'genetic'. Where it is likely that the condition is inherited, steps should be taken (e.g. castration, sterilisation) to avoid breeding from such stock. As it is not always easy to know if a congenital defect is heritable, a precautionary approach is best.

Table 1.1   Reference ranges (haematology and plasma biochemistry) in cattle.

	Units	Average (%)	Range (± 2SD)
Haematology			
Erythrocytes	$\times 10^{12}$/l	7.0	(5–10)
Haemoglobin	g/dl	11.0	(8–15)
PCV (haematocrit)	1/l	35.0	28–38
Fibrinogen	g/l	4.0	(2–7)
Leucocytes	$\times 10^{9}$/l	7.0	(4–12)
Neutrophils (non-segmented bands)	$\times 10^{9}$/l	0.02 (0.5%)	0–1.12 (0–2%)
Neutrophils (segmented mature)	$\times 10^{9}$/l	2.0 (28%)	0.6–4 (25–48%)
Lymphocytes	$\times 10^{9}$/l	4.5 (58%)	2.5–7.5 (45–75%)
Monocytes	$\times 10^{9}$/l	0.4 (4%)	0.02–0.8 (2–7%)
Eosinophils	$\times 10^{9}$/l	0.65 (9%)	0–2.4 (0–20%)
Basophils	$\times 10^{9}$/l	0.05 (0.5%)	0–0.2 (0–2%)
Neutrophil: lymphocyte ratio	—	0.45 : 1	—
Plasma biochemistry			
Urea	mmol/l	4.2	2.0–6.6
Creatinine	μmol/l	100	44–165
Calcium	mmol/l	2.5	2.0–3.4
Inorganic phosphate	mmol/l	1.7	1.2–2.3
Sodium	mmol/l	139	132–150
Potassium	mmol/l	4.3	3.6–5.8
Chloride	mmol/l	102	90–110
Magnesium	mmol/l	1.02	0.7–1.2
Total protein	g/l	67	51–91
Albumin	g/l	34	21–36
Globulin	g/l	43	30–55
Glucose	mmol/l	2.5	2.0–3.2
Alkaline phosphatase	iu/l	24	20–30
AST SGOT	iu/l	40	20–100
ALT SGPT	iu/l	10	4–50
Lactate dehydrogenase (LDH)	iu/l	700	600–850
Bilirubin	μmol/l	4.1	0–6.5
Cholesterol	mmol/l	2.6	1.0–3.0
Creatine phosphokinase	mmol/l	3.0	0–50

The above values refer to healthy adult (> 3 years old) cattle, and have been compiled from various sources. Interpretation of possible deviations from the above ranges should consider variations due to the laboratory technique, breed, lactational and nutritional status, and should always be related to the presenting signs and symptoms of the individual or group. Units are given as SI units

A limited number of conditions can be corrected surgically. Examples of the more common defects of each body system are:

- **skeletal**: single and isolated defects include spinal abnormalities such as scoliosis, kyphosis, tibial hemimelia, polydactyly, syndactyly
- **systemic skeletal defects**: chondrodysplasia (dwarfism), osteopetrosis
- **joint defects**: arthrogryposis and congenital muscle contracture ('ankylosis'), hip dysplasia, bilateral femorotibial osteoarthritis
- **muscular**: arthrogryposis, congenital flexed pastern and/or fetlocks, muscular hypertrophy, spastic paresis
- **CNS**: internal hydrocephalus, spina bifida, Arnold Chiari malformation (herniation of cerebellar tissue through *foramen magnum* into cranial cervical spinal canal), cerebellar hypoplasia, cerebellar ataxia, spastic paresis, spastic syndrome
- **skin**: epitheliogenesis imperfecta, entropion
- **cardiovascular**: ventricular septal defect, patent *ductus arteriosus*
- **digestive**: atresia of ileum, colon, rectum and anus
- **hernias**: umbilical, scrotal/inguinal, schistosomus reflexus
- **reproductive**: testicular hypoplasia, intersex (hermaphrodite and freemartin), ovarian hypoplasia, rectovaginal constriction (Jerseys) and prolonged gestation

Many of the above musculoskeletal defects (e.g. muscular hypertrophy or double muscling in the Belgian Blue) can give rise to dystocia.

Surgical correction of several of these defects is considered elsewhere: umbilical hernia (see Section 5.13), rectal and anal atresia (see Section 5.15) and spastic paresis (see Section 9.27).

1.2 Instrumentation

A good worker needs good tools. Maintain instruments in good condition and store in sterile surgical packs for the common procedures (caesarean section, laparotomy and teat surgery).

Sterilisation

Instrument sterilisation methods include the following (the first two are recommended) (see Tables 1.2. and 1.3):

- **autoclaving** by pressurised steam, 750 mm/Hg at 121 °C for 15 minutes or at 131 °C for three minutes for non-packed instruments, or for a shorter time in high vacuum or high pressure autoclaves; 30 minutes for packs at 121 °C or 18 minutes at 134 °C.
- **gas sterilisation** by ethylene oxide followed by air drying for several days to avoid diffusion of residual gases from the materials into animal tissues.

Table 1.2   Suitability of various surgical materials for sterilisation.

	Dry heat	Autoclave	Boiling water	Ethylene oxide	Liquid chemicals
PVC (e.g. endotracheal tubes)	no	yes	yes	yes	doubtful
Polypropylene (e.g. connectors)	no	yes	yes	yes	yes
Polyethylene (e.g. catheters, packing film)	no	no	yes*, no[†]	yes	yes
Nylon (e.g. i.v. cannulae)	no	yes	yes	no	doubtful
Acrylic (e.g. perspex)	no	no	doubtful	yes	yes
Silicon rubber	yes	yes	yes	yes	doubtful

* high density,
[†] low density

Some acrylic plastic materials, polystyrene and certain lensed instruments may be damaged during this process.

- **cold (chemical) sterilisation** in commercially available solutions (e.g. containing glutaraldehyde). Prolonged immersion is necessary. Most equipment that is safe for immersion in water is safe for immersion in 2% glutaraldehyde. After the proper immersion period, instruments should be rinsed with copious amounts of sterile water.
- **simple boiling** of instruments: a poor, slow and tiresome means of reduction of infectious agents likely to cause damage. The minimal period of boiling is 30 minutes, longer at altitudes over 300 m. Addition of alkali to the steriliser increases bactericidal efficiency and boiling time may be safely reduced to 15 minutes. Corrosion is avoided by the addition of 0.5–1% washing soda (Na_2CO_3). Accumulation of lime in serrations or joints is removed by leaving instruments in 5% acetic acid overnight and then brushing off.

Table 1.3   Efficiency of different methods of sterilisation.

	Bacteria	Dry spores	Moulds	Fungi	Viruses
Autoclaving	+	+	+	+	+
Gas sterilisation	+	+	+	+	+
Chemical antiseptics	+	—	+	(+)	+
Boiling	(+)	—	(+)	(+)	(+)

Abbreviations: + = effective; (+) = limited efficacy; — = not effective

---

Warning

Ethylene oxide and glutaraldehyde are carcinogenic: environmental and safety hazards associated with these chemicals are numerous and severe.

Basic instruments for caesarean section or laparotomy

The following is a suggested list of equipment to cover most eventualities (see Figure 1.1):

- towel clamps (Backhaus) × 4, 8.8 cm
- haemostatic forceps (Spencer Wells) × 4 straight 15.2 cm, (Criles) × 2 curved 14 cm, (Halsted) × 2 mosquito straight 12.7 cm
- scalpel handle (Swann-Morton® or Bard-Parker®) × 2, P (no. 4, blades no. 22, or handle no. 3 and blade no. 10)
- rat tooth dissecting forceps (Lane) 15.2 cm
- plain dissecting forceps (Bendover) 15.2 cm
- straight scissors (Mayo) 16 cm
- needle holder (McPhail's or Gillies), right- or left-handed 16 cm
- Allis tissue forceps × 4, 15 cm
- sterile nylon calving ropes for caesarean section × 4
- embryotomy finger knife (for incision into the uterine wall, which cannot be brought near the body wall)

Also needed are suture needles. Two each of the following types and sizes are recommended (see Figure 1.2):

- 3/8 circle cutting-edged 4.7 cm and 7.0 cm
- 3/8 circle round-bodied (taper cut) 4.5 cm
- 1/2 circle cutting-edged 4.6 cm
- 1/2 curved cutting-edged 6.7 cm
- swaged-on curved round-bodied needle 4.5 cm
- intestinal straight round-bodied (Mayo) 6.2 cm
- straight cutting-edged (Hagedorn) 6.3 cm
- double-curved post-mortem needle 12.5 cm

1.3 Asepsis

Surgery involving regions where adequate skin preparation is feasible (i.e. with avoidable microbial contamination of tissues or sterile materials) should be performed under aseptic conditions. Instruments and cloths should be sterile.

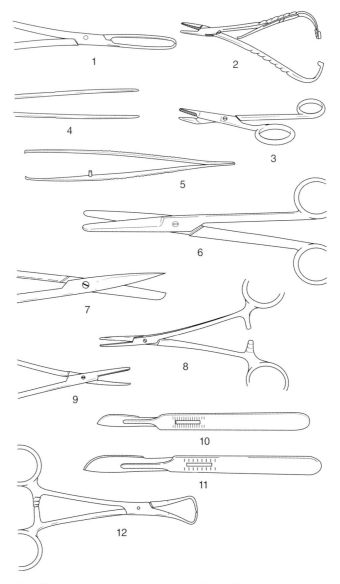

Figure 1.1   Basic instruments for caesarean section or laparotomy.
1. Allis tissue forceps; 2. McPhail's needle holder; 3. Gillies combined scissors and needle holder; 4. plain forceps; 5. rat tooth forceps; 6. Mayo scissors (blunt/blunt), slightly curved; 7. Mayo scissors (pointed/blunt), straight; 8. straight haemostatic forceps; 9. curved haemostatic forceps; 10. scalpel handle no. 4 and no. 22 blade; 11. scalpel handle no. 3 and no. 10 blade; 12. towel clip (Backhaus).

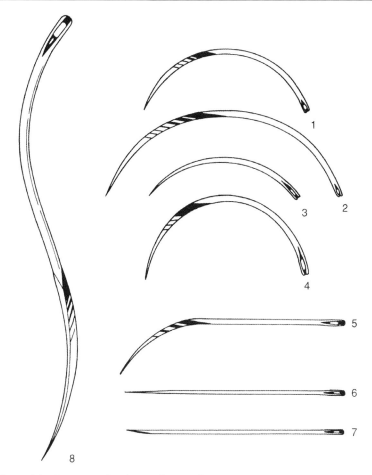

Figure 1.2 Suture needles (shown full scale).
1 and 2. 3/8 circle cutting-edged 4.7 and 7 cm; 3. 3/8 circle round-bodied (taper cut)
4.5 cm; 4. 1/2 circle cutting-edged 4.6 cm; 5. 1/2 curved cutting-edged 6.7 cm; 6.
intestinal straight round-bodied (Mayo) 6.3 cm; 7. straight cutting-edged (Hagedorn)
6.3 cm; 8. double-curved post-mortem needle 12.5 cm.

Preparation of operative field

This example is for the flank:

- close clip wide area, minimum 60 cm cranial-caudal and 90 cm vertically
  (preferable to shaving)
- alternatively shave operative field after application of disinfectant, soap and
  water (Schick razor is suitable)

- wash area with soap and water twice, then scrub with povidone-iodine solution or 4% chlorhexidine gluconate, dry off, wash with 70% alcohol and rescrub
- repeat this procedure three times before respraying with diluted povidone-iodine solution or chlorhexidine solution
- large impervious sterile towels or disposable drapes (rubber or plastic) are useful for placing on the site
- place sterile towel on suitable flat surface for instruments, use sterilised gauze swabs, instruments and suture materials, and sterile gloves

---

Tip

Using sterile isotonic saline instead of alcohol for rinsing after scrubbing with chlorhexidine is preferable as it does not reduce the long-term effect of chlorhexidine. Never mix povidone-iodine with chlorhexidine solution.

Hand disinfection

For 'scrubbing up', effective hand and forearm sterilisation procedures include (see Table 1.4):

- commercial chlorhexidine 'scrubs'
- 0.5% chlorhexidine concentrate in 90% ethyl alcohol with 1% glycerine as emollient (cheapest)
- commercially available povidone-iodine soaps
- hexachlorophane suspension (requires a full rinse-off after a 5 minute scrub)
- 10 ml is first applied to clean dry hands and permitted to dry, before further application and a 5 minute scrub-up. At least five minutes contact time is required for all disinfectants
- sterile surgical gloves should be worn whenever practicable after scrubbing up

1.4 Sutures and suturing

Suture materials are constantly being improved and new products come on to the veterinary market at regular intervals (see Table 1.5). This section selects a limited number of materials and methods of usage, and attempts to justify the selection. In few cases can the cost of the material be considered an important factor in selection.

Table 1.4   Properties of three common antiseptic compounds.

Generic name	Povidone-iodine	Chlorhexidine gluconate or acetate	Benzalkonium chloride
Bactericidal	+	+	(+)
Fungicidal	+	+	+
Virucidal	+	—	—
Dilution for instruments	undiluted (5%, 7.5% or 10%)		10% diluted 1:500
Skin ('scrub')	undiluted (0.75%)	4% or 15 ml of 7.5% solution + 485 ml of 70% alcohol	10% diluted 1:100
Wound lavage	0.1%	0.05%	—
Disadvantages	brown skin when dry	incompatible with soap and anionic detergents	incompatible with soap and anionic detergents; fails to kill spore-bearing organisms
Advantages	not inactivated by organic matter	not inactivated by organic matter	—

Abbreviations: + = active; (+) = limited activity; — = no activity

Suture materials

Non-absorbable suture materials:

- monofilament nylon (e.g. Ethilon®): skin
- monofilament polypropylene (e.g. Prolene®): skin
- pseudomonofilament polyamide polymer (e.g. Supramid®): skin
- mono- or multifilament surgical steel: skin, bone; exceptionally *linea alba*

Absorbable suture materials:

- chromic catgut: subcutis, muscle, peritoneum, bowel, urinary bladder, uterus, penis
- multifilament polyglycolic acid or PGA (e.g. Dexon®): bowel, muscle including teat intermediate layer
- multifilament polyglactin 910 (Vicryl®): subcutis, muscle including teat intermediate layer, bowel, urinary bladder
- monofilament polyglyconate (e.g. Maxon®): subcutis, bowel, teat intermediate layer, urinary bladder, uterus

Table 1.5 Comparative qualities (graded undesirable to desirable, + to +++), of nine selected suture materials for cattle.

Generic name (trade name examples)	Origin	Tensile strength	Knot security	Handling	Tissue reaction	Resistance to infection	Absorption without inflammation after tissue repair	Cost
Absorbable								
Chromic catgut	collagen	(+)	+	++	+++	+	+	low
Coated braided PGA (PGS), (Dexon Plus®)	glycolic acid polymer, coated surfactant	++(+)	++	++(+)	++	++	++	high
Polydioxanone monofilament (PDS)	polymer of paradioxanone	+++	++	++	+	+++	+	high
Coated braided Polyglactin 910 (coated Vicryl®)	glycolic-lactic acid copolymer	++(+)	++	+	++	++	++	high
Monofilament polyglyconate (Maxon)	copolymer of glycolic acid and trimethylene	+++	++		+	+++	+	high
Non-absorbable								
Polypropylene monofilament (Prolene, Surgelene®, Prodek®)	polymerised polyolefin hydrocarbons	+++	(+)	+(+)	(+)	+++	NA	low
Surgical steel	alloy of iron	+++	+++	+	+	+++	NA	low
Monofilament nylon (Dermalon®, Ethilon, Surgidek®)	polyamide filament	++(+)	+	+	+	+	NA	low
Polyfilament polyamide polymer (Supylon®, Vetafil®, Braunamid®)	polyamide polymer	++(+)	++	+++	+	++	NA	low

NA = not applicable

- monofilament polydioxanone (PDS): bowel, muscle, *linea alba*
- 'soft' gut (Softgut®): muscle, bowel, teat intermediate layer

---

Tip

Suture patterns are discussed under the specific procedures. Skin under considerable or potential tension at certain sites, such as the vulval lips and peri-anal region (e.g. following replacement of prolapsed cervix or rectum), is usually sutured with sterile woven nylon tape 3–5 mm in diameter.

Discussion

Selection of suture material should be based on the known biological and physical properties of the suture, wound environment and tissue response to the suture.

- **Monofilament nylon** remains encapsulated in body tissues when buried, but the inflammatory reaction is minimal. It has a great size-to-strength ratio and tensile strength. It is somewhat stiff and is therefore not particularly easily handled, an important point when operating in sub-optimal conditions of poor light and awkward corners. Knot security is only fair.
- **Multifilament polyamide polymer**, encased in an outer tubular sheath (pseudomonofilament), has good strength and provokes little tissue reaction unless the outer sheath is broken, but it loses strength when autoclaved. It is therefore usually drawn from a sterile spool as and when required. It is very easily handled.
- **Surgical steel** has the greatest tensile strength of all sutures and retains strength when implanted. It has the greatest knot security and creates little or no inflammatory reaction. Surgical steel, however, tends to cut tissue, has poor handling and cannot withstand repeated bending without breaking. It is sometimes used in tissues that heal slowly (e.g. infected *linea alba* or bone).
- **Chromic catgut**, of the six absorbable materials listed, is still most commonly used, but synthetic absorbable material does have distinct advantages. Catgut has relatively good handling characteristics, but has disadvantages of relatively rapid loss of strength in well vascularised sites (50% in the first week) and poor knot security (tendency to unwrap and loosen when wet). The potential minute risk of the transfer of infectious prion material into food-producing

animals and hence into the human food chain has led to a ban on the use of chromic catgut in some countries (vCJD risk)

- **Multifilament polyglycolic acid** (PGA) has greater strength that is lost evenly, provoking much less tissue reaction than chromic catgut. PGA is non-antigenic, has a low coefficient of friction and therefore requires multiple throws to improve knot security, but is easily handled.
- **Monofilament polydioxanone** (PDS) is very strong, retaining its strength for many weeks (58% at four weeks), is characterised by its strong memory and has low knot security, but provokes minimal tissue reaction. *Linea alba* is best sutured with PDS.
- **'Soft' catgut** is undoubtedly the most easily handled absorbable material for delicate bowel anastomoses. Plain or soft catgut is absorbed quickly and maintains its strength for a short time.
- PDS and PGA are slowly replacing chromic catgut, which will retain its place as a general purpose material. Vicryl® in its coated form is very easy to handle and has minimal tissue reaction and tissue drag. It is stable in contaminated wounds. Polyglyconate monofilament (Maxon™) has three times the strength of Vicryl® at day 21 of wound healing.

1.5 Restraint

Introduction

Restraint is necessary for:

- administration of drugs for (a) pre-medication and sedation, (b) infiltration of local analgesic drugs and (c) induction of general anaesthesia
- examination and minor procedures carried out without sedation or analgesia/anaesthesia
- prevention of movement during surgery
- safety of operators

Restraint may involve physical manipulation of tail, head or nostrils, or involve application of halter and ropes.

Techniques

Physical restraint by a stock person includes:

- halter
- nose grip (fingers or nose tongs)
- tail elevation

- skin grip of crural fold
- calves in lateral recumbency: lifting bottom fore leg and hind leg with elbow pressure on neck

Rope restraint includes:

- hind limb elevation by a rope above the hock and round an overhead bar
- Reuff's method of casting (see Figure 1.3), employing a rope squeeze of the abdomen

Many forms of cattle crush or squeeze chute are available with an excellent head restraint, which are suitable for surgery of the head and cranial neck (e.g. tracheotomy) and of the perineum. Many are unsuitable for flank laparotomy, caesarean sections or rumenotomy, though an increasing number of manufacturers offer modified crushes to improve access to the paralumbar fossa. A veterinary practice may find it advantageous to have such a crush available for surgery on the practice premises or to be transported to the farm. Some crushes have poor facilities for the elevation and restraint of hind or fore limbs for clinical examination and digital surgery. The Wopa crush is an example of an excellent crush for digital surgery.

Warning

An essential feature of crushes or chutes is the need to release the head rapidly should the animal collapse. Asphyxiation can result, or pressure on the point of the shoulder can cause irreversible radial nerve paralysis and a 'downer cow'.

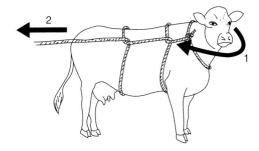

Figure 1.3 Reuffs method of casting a cow with a rope and maintaining in lateral recumbency.
The first operator (1) brings the cow's head round tightly to her right shoulder, using a halter. The second operator (2) pulls the rope so that it tightens around the cow's abdomen: this will force her to lie down. In this example the cow will go into lateral recumbency on her left side. Maintaining tension on the rope (2) will prevent her rising.

1.6 Pre-medication and sedation

Pre-medication and sedation (see Table 1.6) have six aims:

- to improve handling and restraint; improve safety
- to enhance the analgesic effect produced by other anaesthetic agents
- to reduce the induction and maintenance doses of general anaesthesia (GA) agents
- to reduce the possible disadvantageous side-effects of anaesthesia
- to promote smooth post-operative recovery
- to improve the well-being of the animal

Very few anaesthetic drugs are approved for use in farm animals. Those known to the authors include azaperone, procaine, lignocaine (lidocaine), methoxyflurane and thiamylal (USA). Xylazine is approved for use in cattle in Canada, the UK and Switzerland, and acepromazine (ACP) is also approved for

Table 1.6   Activity and dosage of selected analgesic, anti-inflammatory and sedative drugs in cattle.

Drug (example trade name)	Analgesic	NSAID	Sedative	Dosage (mg/kg)	
				i.m.	i.v.
Butylscopolamine bromide/metamizole (Buscopan® Boehringer)	+	+	−	5 ml/100 kg^a	
Meloxicam (e.g. Metacam® Boehringer)	+	+	−	0.5^b	0.5
Carprofen (Rimadyl® LA soln, Zoetis)	+	+	−	1.4^b	1.4
Xylazine (e.g. Sedaxylan® 2%, Dechra)	+	−	+	0.05–0.3	0.03–0.1
Diazepam (Valium®)*	+	−	+	0.5–1.0	0.2–0.5
Flunixin meglumine (e.g. Finadyne®, MSD)	+	+	−	−	2.2
Ketoprofen (e.g. Ketofen® 10%, Merial)	+	+	−	3	3
Acetylpromazine* (ACP®)	−	−	+	0.03–0.1	0.03–0.1

* Not authorised for use in cattle in UK and EU, may only be given 'off label' under cascade prescribing
^{a} not authorised in lactating cattle
^{b} by s.c. route, not i.v.

use in cattle in Canada. Lignocaine is not licensed in EU countries for food-producing animals.

Although possibly not approved for use in cattle in many countries (including the USA), several non-steroidal anti-inflammatory (NSAID) analgesics (e.g. flunixin meglumine, dipyrone 50% (metamizole), ketoprofen and meloxicam) are beneficial as adjunct therapy both pre- and post-operatively in cattle with obvious somatic pain and discomfort. Pre-operative use of analgesics reduces the degree of operative discomfort and post-operative pain.

Warning

For any medication for cattle in the USA, it is the veterinarian's responsibility to consult the Animal Medical Drug Use Clarification Act for guidelines for the extra-label use of drugs and the Food Animal Residue Avoidance Databank (FARAD) for withdrawal times. Under EU legislation, the prescribing cascade can be used to prescribe 'off licence' under certain conditions and following guidelines, but additional withdrawal periods are required. UK practitioners should consult Veterinary Medicines Directorate (VMD) guidelines for cascade regulations. Only medicines that have pharmacologically active substances listed in a Table of Allowed Substances (European Medicines Agency) may be used in animals intended for food production, regardless of the cascade.

Xylazine (e.g. Rompun 2%® [Bayer]; Sedaxylan [Dechra Veterinary products])

Advantages
Very useful analgesic and sedative. Licensed for use in cattle (EU). Xylazine also causes muscle relaxation.

Disadvantages
- Causes ruminal stasis, increases salivation, uterine tone and effects of higher dose rate are somewhat unpredictable as animal may or may not become recumbent.
- Xylazine is unsuitable as the sole agent for minor surgery when more than a single painful stimulus is anticipated (e.g. unsuitable as the method of analgesia in teat surgery; lancing and drainage of large flank abscess is a suitable indication).
- Xylazine is contra-indicated in the last trimester of pregnancy due to its stimulation of uterine smooth muscle (risk of abortion). It may be used if a uterine relaxant is given before xylazine.
- Xylazine is contra-indicated in extreme heat, as hyperthermia may result.

- Avoid accidental intra-carotid injection! Violent seizures and possibly temporary collapse are likely.
- Unsuitable for placing in dorsal recumbency (e.g. certain DA surgery techniques) due to the risk of ruminal regurgitation and subsequent aspiration pneumonia.

Dosage and antagonists
- For anaesthetic pre-medication: 0.1 mg/kg xylazine i.m.
- For minor procedures in combination with local analgesia: 0.2 mg/kg i.m.
- A faster and more predictable effect is seen following i.v. 0.1 mg/kg (not authorised for all preparations).
- Xylazine sedation, analgesia, cardiopulmonary depression and muscle relaxation are reversible. Also xylazine overdosage (e.g. by inadvertent use of the equine preparation) may be antagonised by different drugs including:
  - yohimbine alone (0.2 mg/kg i.v.)
  - tolazoline (4 mg/kg i.v.) – fast onset
  - atipamazole (Antisedan® [Zoetis]) 0.02–0.05 mg/kg i.v.
  - atropine (100 mg s.c.) to counteract bradycardia and hypotension
  - doxapram HCl or doxapram 4-aminopyridine respectively 1 mg/kg and 0.3 mg/kg i.v. significantly reduces recovery period
  - mixture of doxapram (1 mg/kg i.v.) and yohimbine (0.125 mg/kg i.v.)

Tip

Doxapram acts by direct action on aortic and carotid chemoreceptors and medullary respiratory centre, while yohimbine antagonises xylazine sedation by blocking central alpha 2-adrenergic receptors. Therefore an alpha 2 antagonist such as yohimbine, tolazoline or atipamazole would be preferable to reverse accidental overdosage, though there are no licensed preparations for cattle.

Atipamazole (Antisedan®) can be given 0.025 mg/kg i.v. and 0.025 mg/kg i.m. to avoid resedation. This roughly equates to using a similar volume of 2% xylazine used but splitting it 50:50 between i.v. and i.m. routes. Overdosage can cause hyperactivity and excitement.

Chloral hydrate

Advantages

- cheap
- given orally or i.v.
- dose-dependent narcosis

● patient generally maintains a swallow reflex at usual dose rates so less risk of regurgitation/aspiration pneumonia, particularly for placing the cow in dorsal recumbency (e.g. LDA surgery or teat repair)

Disadvantages
● very irritant: can cause severe necrosis if accidental perivascular injection
● narcosis deepens after i.v. infusion: risk of over-dosage
● hepatotoxic: avoid in neonates
● not licensed
● not analgesic: local anaesthesia required in addition when used prior to surgery

Dosage
● Orally: 50–100 mg/kg as 5% solution produces recumbency and light hypnosis in adult cow in 10–20 minutes. Equivalent to 35–70 g for adult Holstein cow.
● Adult bulls require much higher oral dose: 120–160 g. Oral solutions are unpalatable even at high dilution so drenching or stomach tube is required.
● I.V. infusion: 80–90 mg/kg in 10% solution has faster effect (2–3 minutes). Give slowly i.v. (over 5 minutes) as hepatic metabolism to the active trichloroethanal causes a delay in effect.
● 50–60 g made up with water in a 500 ml bottle and administered slowly i.v. via a flutter valve gives suitable sedation for recumbency and positioning in dorsal recumbency for most adult Holstein cows.

Warning

Chloral hydrate is very irritant perivascularly. It is safer to administer i.v. using a catheter. If extravascular injection occurs, the area should be infiltrated with up to 1 litre saline. Anaesthesia should then not be attempted for at least 24 hours unless the procedure is vital and life saving.

Acetylpromazine (ACP)

● i.m. or slow i.v. injection
● variable effect in cattle but may reduce stress response; **no analgesic effect**
● causes hypotension: avoid in depressed or hypovolaemic patients
● avoid prior to GA: increased risk of regurgitation
● causes penile prolapse in bulls (variable): may be advantageous for penile examination but risk of paraphimosis if left unattended

Diazepam

- produces sedation i.v.; expensive
- more predictable effect/useful in calves (economically more viable), particularly prior to GA
- good muscle relaxation but no analgesia

Pentobarbitone

- mainly used as sedative/anticonvulsant in cases of hypomagnesaemia
- 1.5–2 mg/kg i.v. can provide effective standing sedation in adult cattle for 60–90 minutes
- avoid in calves: hepatic recycling and re-sedation likely
- **do not use preparations intended for euthanasia:** the preservatives can cause massive haemolysis

Atropine sulphate

- reduces quantity and increases viscosity of saliva
- pre-medicant dose in adult cow is 60 mg s.c.

1.7 General anaesthesia

Indications

General anaesthesia (GA) is rarely indicated in cattle. It is practised if the usual techniques of regional and local analgesia either cannot be adopted or fail. Specific indications include extensive surgery of the head, neck, chest and abdomen, or body wall, as well as most long bone fractures when maximum relaxation is desired. GA has a relative surgical indication when complete asepsis is essential, such as in umbilical hernia repair in calves. For GA, food should be withheld for 6–12 hours in calves and for up to 36 hours in adult cattle. Restriction of water is not indicated in calves and should not exceed 12 hours in adults.

Disadvantages of GA

Risks of GA in cattle include regurgitation, ruminal tympany, poor oxygenation and skeletal injury.

(a) **Risk of regurgitation** and subsequent aspiration of ruminal contents and saliva into the trachea, bronchi and alveoli with potential lethal consequences (necrotic laryngotracheitis and necrotising broncho-pneumonia with pulmonary oedema). Endotracheal intubation is therefore *essential* to avoid this problem.

Factors affecting regurgitation include:
- depth of anaesthesia (see Table 1.7): light level provokes active regurgitation, deep level passive regurgitation
- degree of ruminal distension or tympany
- fluidity of ruminal contents
- body and head/neck position
- body movement: struggling and repositioning of animal
- volume of saliva
- duration of anaesthesia

Table 1.7 Main signs for assessing anaesthetic depth.

	Surgical anaesthesia	Excessive depth*
Cardiovascular system		
Heart rate and rhythm	within normal limit	bradycardia, impending arrest
Mucous membrane colour	pink	cyanotic
Capillary refill time	< 2 s	> 3 s
Respiratory system		
Respiratory rate	near normal	shallow, irregular, gasping, apnoea
Tidal volume	reduced	more reduced
Character	regular	irregular
Ocular signs		
Position and size of pupil	moderately constricted, possibly rotated down	very dilated, centrally fixed
Palpebral reflex	present	very slow or absent
Corneal reflex	present	slow
Musculoskeletal system		
Muscle tone		
(lower jaw, limbs)	moderate	poor or absent
Other signs		
Swallowing reflex	absent	absent
Salivary flow	present, profuse	absent
Lacrimal secretion	present	absent

* Actions to take in case of excessive depth:
- note time
- check patency of airway
- stop any volatile anaesthetic administration, give oxygen and artificial respiration
- check heart rate (for five seconds)
- check respiratory rate and character (for five seconds)
- check other vital signs (see above)

(b) **Risk of severe ruminal tympany**. During recumbency the cardia is submerged in ruminal fluid, preventing normal eructation. Meanwhile, fermentation continues and gas builds up. Less of a problem in calves, depending on the stage of rumen development.

(c) **Risk of severe compromise** of the effective expansion capacity of lungs as a result of:
- increased abdominal size following development of ruminal tympany causing pressure on diaphragm;
- relatively poor oxygenation of the dependent lower lung due to inadequate circulation and pressure (ventilation–perfusion mismatch). Poorly oxygenated blood from ventral lung mixes with better oxygenated blood from upper dorsal lung, giving lowered systemic oxygenation and hypercapnia.

(d) **Risk of skeletal injury** in induction and recovery, involving possible dislocation, myositis and nerve paralysis.

(e) Expense and size of gaseous anaesthetic equipment and appropriate expertise in its use.

Equipment

Apparatus for GA of cattle older than three to six months is similar to that available for horses. Endotracheal intubation is essential in bovine GA. Equipment for volatile and gaseous agents is of a circle and to-and-fro pattern, incorporating a soda-lime canister and re-breathing bag with calibrated vaporiser (0–5%) to volatilise isoflurane or halothane by means of oxygen delivered by a pre-set flowmeter. The minimum internal diameter of airways in such an apparatus should be 4 cm.

Equipment for GA of calves with gaseous agents is similar to that for larger breeds of dog. The airway diameter, although theoretically inadequate, is unlikely to produce disadvantageous side-effects. Endotracheal tubes for calves should have an internal diameter of 12–16 mm, while those for adult cattle should be about 24–30 mm. Tubes of siliconised PVC are approximately one quarter the price of rubber endotracheal tubes (adult cattle).

List of equipment for GA by gaseous or volatile agents:

- anaesthetic apparatus: circle or to-and-fro system
- endotracheal tubes (calf–adult: 12–25 mm)
- syringe for inflation and clamping-off of cuff
- mouth gag (e.g. Drinkwater model)
- laryngoscope (e.g. Rowson pattern): optional for adults
- nasogastric tube to act as a guide, over which the endotracheal tube is passed (alternative)
- halothane or isoflurane and oxygen supply
- ruminal trocar and cannula

Placing the endotracheal tube in adults is best done manually using a gag to hold open the mouth. For calves, a laryngoscope with a long blade is usually necessary.

> **Warning**
>
> Do not use local anaesthetic lubricants on endotracheal tubes in cattle: this will anaesthetise the larynx and abate the protective laryngeal and cough reflexes. A greater risk of inhalation of regurgitated material/saliva will occur during the recovery period.

Intravenous anaesthesia (induction) agents

Intravenous agents for GA of cattle include:

- **thiopentone sodium** (no longer available in North America). Give as 10% solution by rapid i.v. injection, dose 1 g/100 kg 10 minutes after xylazine pre-medication or 1.2 g/100 kg if unpre-medicated. Perivascular injection is irritant: infiltration of 500 ml saline with hyaluronidase is essential to prevent perivascular necrosis and skin slough. 2.5% (larger volume) is safer. Catheter is advisable. Induction within 45 seconds with usually a brief period of apnoea. Duration of GA 5–8 minutes. Recover to stand in 30–60 minutes. Unsuitable for young calves < 3 months (prolonged recovery). Unsuitable for incremental doses to prolong anaesthesia
- **ketamine and xylazine**. Xylazine is given i.v. (0.1 mg/kg) or i.m. (0.2 mg/kg), followed immediately by i.m. ketamine (2 mg/kg). GA lasts for 10–20 minutes. Recovery is fairly rapid (on feet within 25–45 minutes). The two drugs may be mixed in one syringe and given i.m. (for calves: GA approximately 30 minutes and recovery in a further 90 minutes). Incremental doses (quarter or half doses of each agent) may be used successfully, but do not use ketamine on its own
- **ketamine, xylazine and guaiphenesin**. A mixture of 500 mg of ketamine and 50 mg of xylazine is added to a 500 ml bag or bottle of a 5% guaiphenesin solution. This combination is infused at 0.55 ml/kg to induce anaesthesia followed by 2.2 ml/kg/hour (adults) or 1.65 ml/kg/hour (calves) for maintenance. This combination produces good muscle relaxation and smooth recovery

After any intravenous GA technique endotracheal intubation should be carried out as soon as possible after injection. The tube should only be removed following a demonstrable cough reflex or swallowing movement. Extubation is performed with the head lower than the trunk and with the cuff inflated until it reaches the pharynx, preventing material moving between the tube and tracheal mucosa, dribbling towards the bifurcation of the bronchi and causing a necrotic bronchotracheitis.

Immobilon™/Revivon™ is a large animal product that is a reversible neuroleptanalgesia (narcosis) with analgesia for restraint and surgical procedures with LA Immobilon, the active principle of which is etorphine, combined with acetylpromazine. It is not licensed for use in cattle, but is sometimes used in exceptional circumstances where other methods of restraint are considered too hazardous. The drug is extensively used in various species in tropical Africa, but rarely now in the UK except for restraint of dangerous animals, e.g. a bull or steer amok in public places.

Warning

Immobilon is highly toxic, causing dizziness, nausea, pinpoint pupils, rapidly followed by respiratory depression, hypotension, cyanosis, loss of consciousness and cardiac arrest.

Etorphine can be life-threatening to the operator if absorbed by any route, including through skin or mucous membranes. Extreme care should be taken. Before any use of Immobilon the appropriate dose of the antagonist Revivon (contained in the same pack) should be drawn up first into a second syringe connected to a second sterile needle, which should then be kept close at hand for immediate intravenous use in the event of an accident. A second competent person should always be instructed clearly beforehand what action should be taken with the reversing agent, which should then be injected before calling medical assistance.

Indications and dosage

- Use with a dart gun (i.e. intramuscular injection) for restraint of dangerous and uncontrollable cattle.
- 0.5–1 ml Immobilon per 50 kg bodyweight i.m. by dart syringe. Cattle become recumbent some minutes later and remain immobile for about 45 minutes. Generalised muscle tremors and poor muscle relaxation are usually apparent.
- To reverse the drug an equal volume of Revivon (diprenorphine HCl) should be injected i.v. Recovery generally occurs with minimal disturbance and noise. A second half dose of Revivon may be given s.c. after the initial i.v. dose if required.

The reader should consult specialised textbooks for further details of bovine GA.

1.8 Local analgesics

The four local analgesics of greatest value today are the hydrochloride salts of lignocaine, procaine, bupivacaine and cinchocaine (see Table 1.8). In the EU, only procaine is licensed for use in cattle.

Lignocaine

In North America, lignocaine has largely replaced procaine as it has the advantages of:

- extreme stability
- more rapid diffusion (rapid onset)

Table 1.8 Properties of four local analgesic drugs (all hydrochloride salts).

Generic name (example trade name)	Lignocaine (Lidocaine®)	Procaine (Ethocaine®)	Bupivacaine (Marcain®)	Cinchocaine (Dibucaine®)
Main indications:				
surface analgesia %	2–10	NS	NS	0.25
infiltration %	0.5–1	2–3	0.25	0.25–0.5
Nerve block %	2–3	3–5	0.5	0.5
Epidural block %	2–3	3–5	0.5–0.75	0.5
Rate of diffusion	fast	slow	fast	slow
Duration of action	60–90 mins	<60 min	≃8 hours	≃8 hours
Analgesic potency	+	+	+	+++
Toxicity	+	+	+	++
Tissue irritation	low	low	low	low
Stability at boiling point	?	good	?	?
Cost (low → high: + → +++)	++	+	+++	++
Other properties	good safety margin, non-vasodilator	vasodilator, used with adrenalin	—	decomposes if mixed with alkalis

NS = not suitable

- longer duration of action
- useful surface analgesic activity on mucous membranes and cornea

It is, however, no longer authorised for cattle in the UK and EU states, as it has no MRL. See the discussion box.

Preparations:

- injectable solutions are usually 2–3%, though 1% is adequate for most uses
- often contain adrenaline at 0.002% to prolong the activity and reduce the possibility of toxic side-effects
- 1% or 2% gel with chlorhexidine gluconate solution 0.25%, or hydro-benzoates in a sterile lubricant water-miscible base
- aerosol spray (lignocaine 10%) with cetylpyridinium chloride 0.1%
- 5% cream

Discussion

There is, in the UK at least, some confusion regarding the use of lignocaine in cattle. The only licensed local anaesthetics for cattle in the UK are two products containing procaine hydrochloride 5% and adrenaline 0.002%. These are licensed only for minor surgical procedures at doses between 2 and 5 ml and have specific contra-indications for epidural anaesthesia. It therefore follows that for any procedure requiring a higher dose than 5 ml, or for epidural anaesthesia, it will be in any case necessary to prescribe under the cascade ('off-label'). Whilst this might include the use of procaine, it can also include lignocaine, including lignocaine combined with adrenaline. The usual cascade considerations, including advising appropriate withdrawal periods, apply.

The European Medicines Agency's Committee for Medicinal Products for Veterinary Use has stated that the minimum cascade withdrawal period for meat (28 days) is suitable for lignocaine, but that an extended **15 day withdrawal period for milk** should be used.

It is therefore legal to use lignocaine-containing products, licensed in other species, in bovine caesareans, DAs and epidurals, etc., under cascade rules. However, it would not be legal to use these products for disbudding and castration where volumes of 5 ml or less are sufficient. The appropriate extended withdrawal periods must be used.

> **Warning**
>
> Use caution with preparations containing epinephrine (adrenaline) for teat and digit surgery, due to the risk of vasoconstriction and potential tissue hypoxia and necrosis. This can also be a risk for large volume infiltration of muscle tissue.
>
> Toxic effects from lignocaine are rarely encountered (e.g. accidental i.v. injection); they include drowsiness, muscle tremors and respiratory depression, convulsions and hypotension. In sufficient dosage, cardiac arrest will occur.
>
> Toxicity is more likely in calves. As a general guide, administer no more than 25 ml 1% lignocaine (15 ml 2%) to a 50 kg calf.

Procaine

- procaine (novocaine) largely replaced cocaine, and has in turn been displaced by lignocaine
- may have economic advantages over lignocaine
- duration of action is shorter than lignocaine
- combined with adrenaline hydrochloride, procaine absorption is slow (N.B. vasoconstriction)
- solutions may be sterilised by boiling
- minimal tissue irritation
- metabolite para-amino benzoic acid inhibits action of sulphonamides

Bupivacaine

- marketed as Marcain® with and without adrenaline (1:4 000 000) as a 0.25, 0.5 and 0.75% (plain) solution
- analgesic potency and speed of action of lignocaine
- considerably longer ($\times$ 4) duration of activity
- very well tolerated by tissues
- indicated where prolonged epidural or perineural analgesia is required
- no MRL in the EU
- costs considerably more than lignocaine
- can be toxic (cardiotoxicity) if given intravenously

Cinchocaine and Mepivicaine

- Cinchocaine (Nupercaine™, Dibucaine®) is more toxic than procaine, but concentrations for epidural block and surface analgesia are lower (0.5%)
- longer analgesia than with procaine
- drug readily decomposed by action of alkalis and therefore syringes and needles should, if not sterile, be boiled in bicarbonate-free water

- Mepivicaine 2% (Carbocaine®-V) solution is sometimes used for infiltration and epidural block: equivalent to lignocaine and has several hours duration of activity

1.9 Regional analgesia

> **Tip**
>
> Local or regional anaesthesia is most successful when combined with adequate sedation and/or restraint. See Sections 1.5 and 1.6.

Regional analgesia is the preferred method of anaesthesia for many surgical procedures in cattle. Advantages over general anaesthesia (GA) include:

- relatively simple technique
- general availability (and licensed products)
- minimal apparatus, e.g. syringe, needles and drug
- generally low risk of toxic side-effects
- safety

Analgesia of the head

Analgesia of the horn is the most common local analgesic procedure carried out in cattle and is relatively straightforward. However, innervation of the eye is more complex and requires careful analgesia.

Cornual nerve block

- sensitive horn corium is largely innervated by the cornual branch of the zygomatico-temporal division of the maxillary nerve (from cranial V)
- caudally a few twigs of the first cervical nerve make a variable contribution to innervation
- the cornual nerve leaves the lacrimal nerve within the orbit, passes through the temporal fossa and around the lateral edge of the frontal bone, covered by fascia and thin frontalis muscle. The nerve is blocked a little below the lateral ridge of the frontal crest, about halfway between the lateral canthus of the eye and the horn (bud) base (see Figure 1.4). The cornual artery and vein are close to the site of the block

Equipment:

- disposable syringe, 10 ml for adults, 5 ml for calves; 2.4 cm 20 gauge needle; 5% procaine solution (or 2% lignocaine without adrenaline, where licensed)

Technique:

- insert the needle, with syringe attached, midway along lateral edge of crest of frontal bone, directing the needle at a 30° angle through skin towards the horn base (see Figure 1.4)
- draw back plunger to ensure that the needle is not inadvertently intravascular

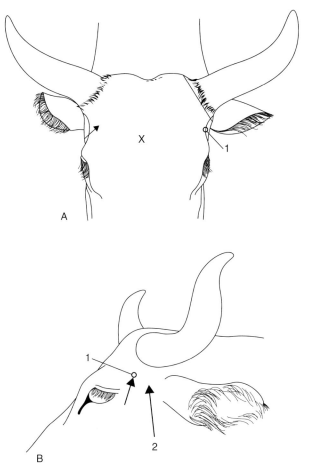

Figure 1.4   Site for cornual nerve block.
A. rostral view
B. lateral view
1 = cornual branch of zygomatico-temporal nerve. Note angle of insertion of the needle.
2 = site of auriculopalpebral block (subcutaneous)
X = site on skull for captive bolt euthanasia.

- inject solution in the arc just below the edge of frontal bone over a distance of 1 cm in adults and 0.5 cm in young calves; 2 ml per horn for small calves ($\leq$ 50 kg), up to 10 ml per horn for adults/large calves
- repeat procedure on the other side of the head
- time to analgesia 3–5 minutes, shown by skin analgesia and upper eyelid ptosis

Complications:

- failures are due to inadvertent i.v. injection or imprecise location of the site (e.g. subcutaneous injection)
- in adults and particularly bulls, significant innervation occurs from the caudal aspect to the horn base and subcutaneous infiltration is required here in addition to a cornual block

Infratrochlear block

- exotic breeds sometimes have an additional nerve supply from the infratrochlear nerve to the medial aspect of the horns (similar to that seen in goats)
- it is blocked by subcutaneous infiltration across the forehead, transversely and level with the site of the cornual block

---

Tip

Debudding is less stressful for both the calf and operator when the patient is sedated. Mild sedation to accompany local analgesia can be easily achieved by adding xylazine to a bottle of local anaesthetic (4 ml 2% xylazine per 100 ml bottle of 2% lignocaine or 5% procaine) and using this local anaesthetic mixture for the cornual block in normal quantities.

Onset and duration of sedation is similar to that of analgesia. At this dose rate, calves may lie down initially but usually stand up for the debudding to be done.

Supraorbital block
Indications:

- surgery of upper eyelid
- trephination of frontal sinus

Technique:

- see landmarks in Figure 1.5. The supraorbital foramen is dorsal to the medial canthus of the eye, approximately a third of the distance from the eye to the poll (3 cm from the medial canthus in an adult cow)

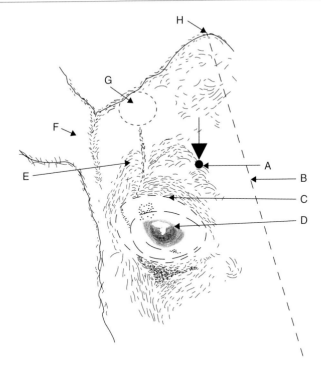

Figure 1.5 Supraorbital nerve block.
Oblique diagrammatic view of right side of head. Foramen is palpable about 3 cm dorsal to upper bony margin of orbit. Long dotted line is midline; dotted line is horn base. A. supraorbital foramen; B. median line; C. margin of bony orbit; D. orbit; E. frontal bone; F. right ear; G. horn base; H. poll.

- insert 1.1 metric (19G) 2.5 cm long needle into foramen to a depth of 1.5 cm
- inject 5 ml of 2% lignocaine or 5% procaine

Local infiltration may be used as an alternative.

Auriculopalpebral block
Indications:

- this block causes paralysis of the eyelids. Note that it produces akinesia but not analgesia
- very useful for removal of foreign bodies, eye examination or prior to subconjunctival injections

Technique:

- see Figure 1.4 for landmark. The auriculopalpebral nerve runs from the base of the ear along the facial crest. The nerve may be palpable in a notch at the end of the zygomatic ridge
- a 1.1 metric (19G) needle is inserted subcutaneously anterior to the base of the auricular muscles, just anterior to the base of the ear. The point of the needle should be at the dorsal border of the zygomatic ridge
- 5–10 ml of local anaesthetic are injected and then massaged into the surrounding area
- may be used in conjunction with topical analgesia of the eyeball (proparacaine hydrochloride, 0.5% ophthalmic solution)

Discussion

Nerve supply to ocular structures
Innervation of ocular structures is complex:

- eyelids: motor supply – auriculopalpebral branch of facial; sensory supply – ophthalmic and maxillary branches of trigeminal
- straight and oblique muscles of eyeball: motor supply – oculomotor, abducens and trochlear
- eyeball: sensory – ciliary branch of ophthalmic
- the oculomotor, trochlear, ophthalmic and maxillary branches of the trigeminal and abducens nerve emerge from the *orbitorotundum foramen* (see Figure 1.6)

Analgesia for enucleation (e.g. squamous cell carcinoma) is by one of two methods: the retrobulbar block or Peterson's block.

Retrobulbar block
Indications:

- intraocular neoplasia (e.g. SCC)
- severe trauma

Technique:

- produce topical analgesia of the cornea with proparacaine HCl 0.5% ophthalmic solution
- insert a forefinger into the lateral canthus between the eyeball and conjunctival sac
- alongside the finger pass a 1.25 metric (18G) 10 cm curved needle through the fornix of conjunctiva advancing along the floor of the orbit until the

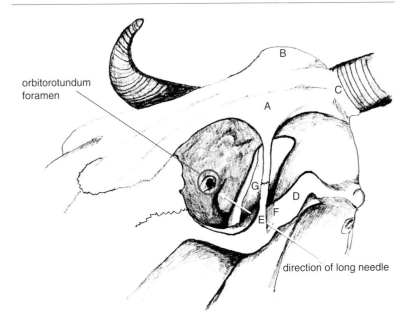

orbitorotundum
foramen

B

C

A

G

D

F

E

direction of long needle

A = frontal bone
B = nuchal crest (poll)
C = horn base
D = zygomatic arch

E = frontal process of zygomatic bone
F = temporal process of zygomatic bone
G = coronoid process of mandible

Figure 1.6   Bony landmarks for Peterson's nerve block.

point is retrobulbar (see Figure 1.7). The penetration of the tough periorbita should be obvious
- inject small increments of local analgesic solution as the needle is advanced
- ensure that the needle point does not enter the optic foramen (risk of intrathecal (CSF) injection) and attempt an aspiration check
- inject 20–30 ml l.a. solution beneath the periorbita, which blocks nerves to ocular muscles causing paralysis of the eyeball and analgesia
- do not attempt to anaesthetise the optic nerve, since this may stimulate the animal sufficiently to cause fatality (respiratory arrest)
- anaesthetise the upper and lower lids by local infiltration as required
- an alternative technique of retrobulbar injection is placement of 10 ml local anaesthetic at each of four sites (lateral, medial, dorsal and ventral canthi) through the conjunctiva, followed by infiltration of the eyelid margins (see Figure 1.7)

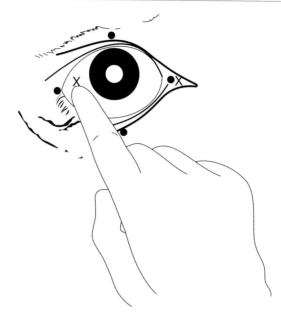

Figure 1.7   Retrobulbar block (two methods).
(a) needle insertion at four points (black circles) through eyelid and conjunctiva under careful digital guidance (4 × 8–10 ml) (b) needle insertion at lateral or medial (X) canthus, again perforating conjunctiva to deposit solution at orbital apex (20–30 ml). Use 18 gauge needle 15 cm long with marked curvature, advancing tip slowly.

Peterson's block
Technique:

- local analgesic solution is injected near the *orbitorotundum foramen*, some 8–10 cm deep, located behind the eyeball. The technique requires more skill than the retrobulbar block but is probably safer (less risk of intrathecal injection)
- two needles are required: a short (2.5 cm) wide bore (12 or 14G) needle acts as a cannula for the passage of a longer (12 cm) 18G needle to the injection site
- first, inject a small amount (5 ml) of local analgesic subcutaneously at the notch formed by the supraorbital process (frontal process of zygomatic bone) and zygomatic arch (see Figure 1.6). Place the short, wide needle through the skin, as far anterior and ventral as possible
- direct the 12 cm 18G needle through the wider needle horizontally and slightly caudally. The point of the needle will make contact with bone: the anterior edge of the coronoid process of the mandible. A slight redirection rostrally will allow the needle to advance medially, off the coronoid process towards the *orbitorotundum foramen*

- aspirate to check that the point of the needle is not in the large ventral maxillary artery
- inject 10–15 ml 2% lignocaine
- the technique does not block the eyelids: the needle can be withdrawn until it is just subcutaneous and redirected 5 cm caudally to block the auriculopalpebral nerve with a further 10 ml l.a. solution close to the zygomatic ridge

---

Tip

For Peterson's block, making a slight curve in the long narrow needle will facilitate advancement off the ventral edge of the coronoid process. Sometimes it is not possible to advance medially to the coronoid process and injection of l.a. solution at this point may still be effective.

It is useful to practise the technique on a cadaver before using for the first time.

Warning

Adverse effects of both the retrobulbar and Peterson's techniques may include haemorrhage from nearby blood vessels, direct pressure on the eyeball, penetration of the globe and optic nerve damage. These are of little consequence for enucleation but could be of considerable significance for other procedures.

Both blocks will prevent blinking for several hours so, except in the case of enucleation, it will be necessary to lubricate the cornea or suture the eyelids together for a period.

Analgesia of the flank

Mastering effective analgesia of the flank is invaluable to the bovine practitioner, for abdominal surgery including caesarean section. Most practitioners stick to the technique they first learn in early years of clinical practice. Lack of confidence often means this is the simple line block or inverse L block. We strongly recommend gaining confidence in mastering the paravertebral block as this gives distinct advantages:

- superior muscle relaxation: easier wound closure
- usually superior analgesia: better welfare
- better wound healing: no l.a. agent near to incision

Paravertebral block

Indications:

- laparotomy, omentopexy, rumenotomy, caesarean section (flank incision); midline incision: bilateral paravertebral

Equipment:

- disposable 30 ml syringe; disposable 18G 90 mm spinal needle with stilette (dairy breeds) or re-usable 150 mm 16G needle and stilette for beef cattle; 2% lignocaine or 5% procaine with adrenalin. Total volume of solution is 100 ml (four sites)

Technique:

- block dorsal and ventral branches of spinal nerves emerging from thoracic 13, lumbar 1, 2 and 3 (T13, L1, L2, L3) by 'walking' the needle off cranial edges of L1, L2, L3 and L4 transverse processes
- best practice is to clip and scrub skin from last rib to *tuber coxae* along a band 15 cm wide, to left or right of dorsal midline as appropriate; not essential
- locate all four injection sites (see below) and put a 5 ml bleb of l.a. subcutaneously and into the dorsal epaxial muscles at each
- block nerve L3 first: identify L4 transverse process by counting forwards from the last palpable process (L5), which is just cranial to the *tuber coxae* of the ilium
- work cranially to find all four injection sites (nerve L2 = cranial edge of transverse process L3; nerve L1 = cranial edge of L2; nerve T13 = cranial edge of L1)
- correct site for each injection (in adult Holstein/Friesian cow) is 5 cm from midline, near cranial lateral edge of each transverse process (see Figure 1.8)
- wait 5 minutes for s.c. analgesia to take effect
- push needle vigorously through the skin and *longissimus dorsi* musculature, directed almost perpendicularly but with shaft inclined 10° medially
- advance needle firmly to contact and pass over cranial border of each transverse process; you may feel the needle 'popping' through the inter-transverse ligament (more difficult with a sharp, single use spinal needle and stilette) and advance 1 cm further. The needle point should now lie close to where the dorsal and ventral branches of spinal nerves have just emerged and separated adjacent to the spinal foramen
- remove the needle stilette and attach the syringe with 25 ml solution and after applying negative pressure (check needle is not in blood vessel) inject 15–20 ml solution in an area about 1 cm below the ligament, moving the shaft and needle point around very slightly
- inject the remaining 5–10 ml solution during the first stage of withdrawal of the needle above the level of the ligament to block aberrant dorsal cutaneous fibres

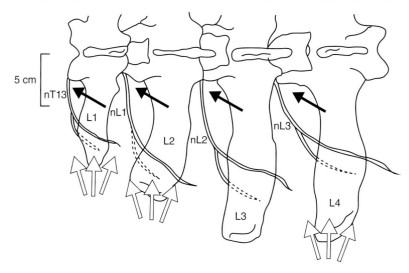

Figure 1.8   Paravertebral anaesthesia: diagrammatic view of left lumbar vertebrae 1–4 to show the course of nerves T13, L1, L2 and L3 and the position of the needle. Black arrows indicate the direction in which the vertical needle point is 'walked off' the transverse process (proximal technique). White arrows show the area of infiltration above and below tips of process in the distal technique.
Note: the lumbar transverse process tip, which can be palpated immediately cranially to the *tuber coxae*, is L5. It can be palpated in all but the fattest of cattle. Count forwards from this landmark. The short stumpy L1 transverse process can only be palpated in very thin cattle: its position must be estimated using the relative positions of L2, L3, L4, etc.

- the most cranial site (nerve T13) is the most difficult and least well tolerated by the patient; the distance travelled by needle shaft is usually slightly more than for preceding sites
- allow 20 minutes for analgesia to take effect; use this time to surgically prepare the operation site

Variations:

- some operators prefer to walk the needle off the caudal and cranial edges of the transverse processes. Thus, nerves T13 and L1 may be accessed from a single point above transverse process L1. However, the required needle angles would be too acute to access both nerves L2 and L3 from a single injection site over transverse process L3. It is easier to walk off the cranial edges --and easier to remember – though the nerve is actually closer to the caudal edge when injecting 5 cm from the midline

- some operators omit the initial s.c. bleb of local anaesthetic: this leads to greater discomfort of the patient and difficulty for the operator
- for more caudal incisions (e.g. caesarean) it may be possible to omit nerve T13; for cranial approaches to the abdomen, it may be possible to omit nerve L3
- the technique described above is the **proximal** paravertebral approach. The **distal** approach employs a horizontal needle insertion (see Figure 1.8). The local anaesthetic solution is deposited above and below the tips of transverse processes L1, L2 and L4 (not L3); 10–15 ml of l.a. is injected in a fan-shaped area ventral and dorsal to the transverse process tips, to a depth of approximately 3–4 cm

Field of analgesia:
Commencing analgesia is noted by a convex curvature of the spine on the injection side resulting from relaxation of *longissimus dorsi* and flank musculature. The field of analgesia runs slightly obliquely ventrally and caudally to the midline. Innervation of the individual dermatomes overlap so that a block of a single nerve produces a very narrow (1–4 cm wide) analgesic skin band over the flank. T13 innervates skin over the middle of the last 1–2 ribs (12–13), while an L3 block causes analgesia as far caudal as *os coxae*. The dorsal nerve ramus innervates the skin over the upper one third of flank skin, while the ventral ramus innervates the remainder of the flank (see Figure 1.9).

- T13: dorsocranial flank, ventrally to umbilicus
- L1 (*n. iliohypogastricus*): dorsal midflank abdominal wall
- L2 (*n. ilioinguinalis*): caudal flank skin over stifle and inguinal region, scrotum and prepuce, or udder
- L3 (*n. genitofemoralis*): caudal flank, especially ventrally, stifle, inguinal region, scrotum and prepuce, or udder

---

Tip

In the proximal paravertebral technique the needle may be inserted too far and enter the peritoneal cavity; there is usually a slight negative pressure, but aspiration can be used to check the needle placement (it should not be possible to aspirate).

In well conditioned cattle (particularly beef breeds), landmarks are more difficult to see and palpate. In such cases take particular care that the injection site remains close to the midline (5–8 cm) and that a long enough needle is being used to penetrate the intertransverse ligament.

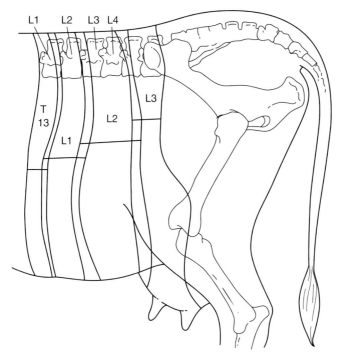

Figure 1.9   Diagram of innervation of the left flank: paravertebral anaesthesia. Horizontal bars indicate width of skin analgesia from the block of individual nerves. Note the degree of overlap of dermatomes and caudal displacement of the analgesic field relative to the particular nerve root. (Modified from Dyce and Wensing, 1971.)

Discussion

The paravertebral block is easier in cattle with a poor body condition because identifying the landmarks is easy and the required needle depth is less. The analgesic technique in exceptionally large-framed and fat cattle requires a longer needle (≥12 cm long). A successful block results in localised hyperthermia and moderate convexity of the spine, which, particularly with a block of L4, may cause mild ataxia.

Advantages of the paravertebral block over flank infiltration include:

- minimal volume of anaesthetic solution
- absence of anaesthetic solution in the surgical field
- large area of desensitisation
- rapid onset of action
- analgesia of peritoneum

Line block, T block or inverted L (7) pattern

Indication:

Anaesthetic infiltration at or around the incision site can produce adequate analgesia. It can also be used following an unsuccessful paravertebral block. Its advantage is simplicity. Its disadvantages include:

- large volume of solution, local oedema and haemorrhage
- distortion of tissue layers
- poor analgesia of peritoneum
- poor muscle relaxation
- increased post-operative swelling
- increased risk of wound infection

Technique:

- infiltrate subcutaneous tissues, muscularis and the sub-peritoneal layers in three distinct movements
- insert the needle at the point where horizontal and vertical bars of imaginary 'T' join (see Figure 1.10). This point forms the dorsal commissure of intended flank incision
- pass the needle (18G 10 cm) cranially to the full extent subcutaneously, and infiltrate with 2% lignocaine or 5% procaine (without adrenaline) during slow withdrawal
- detach the syringe and, without removing the needle from the skin, direct the point caudally and advance, and likewise infiltrate during withdrawal

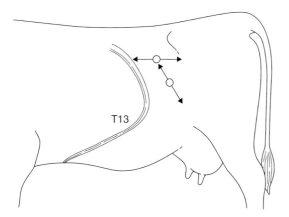

Figure 1.10   Method of infiltration of the body wall of flank in the 'T block'; the technique can also be used in 'reverse 7 block'. Note that the needle is only inserted through the skin twice in the whole analgesic procedure.

- repeat with infiltration of deeper tissues (total of about 80 ml in a horizontal line)
- insert the needle 10 cm ventral to the previous point and similarly infiltrate the proposed incision line (another 80 ml, i.e. total of about 160 ml in an adult cow

Note that in this technique the needle is only inserted through skin twice in the entire infiltration.

Inverted L block ('reverse 7' left flank; '7' right flank)

- A slight variation in the linear infiltration of the flank is the 'reverse 7 block' or 'inverted L block', which are self-explanatory (see Figure 1.10). The nerves are blocked a little further proximally in their paths, cranially and dorsally to the incision site. This avoids some of the tissue distortion that a line block produces.

Analgesia of the pelvic and mammary regions

Epidural block
Indications:
Caudal epidural

- reduce abdominal straining and discomfort, e.g. after calving
- intravaginal and intrauterine manipulations (e.g. embryotomy), dystocia (abolishes tenesmus)
- replacement of vaginal and uterine prolapse, rectal prolapse
- perineal and tail surgery

Cranial epidural

- same site, larger volume of analgesic solution
- flank laparotomy, surgery of hind limbs and digits, penis, inguinal surgery, udder and teat surgery

An analgesic solution is injected into the epidural space, which caudally contains branches of spinal nerves (*cauda equina*) invested with epineurium (*dura mater*), small dorsal and ventral venous plexuses, and a variable amount of fatty tissue.

Equipment:

- 5 ml (caudal epidural) or 30 ml syringe (cranial)
- short bevelled 5 cm 19G needle
- 2% lignocaine or 5% procaine without adrenaline
- ± 2% xylazine

> **Tip**
>
> Preparations containing preservatives, such as chlorocresol and sodium metabisulphite, and adrenaline are contra-indicated for epidural injection. In practice, many practitioners use the commercially available local anaesthetic preparations, which contain both preservative and adrenaline for caudal epidurals without adverse effects.

Technique:

- locate first intercoccygeal space (Co1–Co2), which undergoes significant movement when the tail is elevated (sacrococcygeal space is virtually immobile). It measures about 1.5 cm transversely and 2 cm craniocaudally (see Figure 1.11)
- this should be an aseptic procedure, so clip the site with scissors and disinfect. Entry of infection is a serious problem and could lead to permanent paralysis of the tail, resulting in persistent faecal contamination of the perineal skin and udder, and subsequent culling. This is a very rare complication
- insert the needle precisely in the midline, directed very slightly cranially, the shaft forming an angle of 15–20° with the vertical in a standing animal. Note that structures penetrated are skin, fat and interarcuate supraspinous and interspinous ligaments
- appreciate at a depth of about 2 cm that the point of the needle is freely movable
- inject 5 ml of lignocaine solution slowly; there should be no appreciable resistance

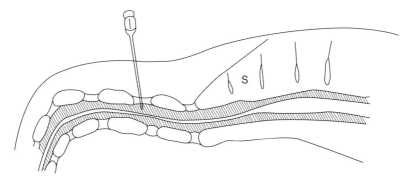

Figure 1.11 Caudal epidural block at the intercoccygeal (Co1–Co2) space. s = sacrum; shaded area is spinal canal with *cauda equina*.

- a palpable "popping" sensation may be noticed when the needle is advanced into the epidural space (less so with sharp needles)
- if resistance to injection is encountered, the needle has been inserted too deeply and has entered cartilaginous tissue of an intervertebral disc (point cannot be moved from side to side) or, though free in epidural space, needle lumen may be blocked by fibrous tissue. In either case remove the needle and repeat with a new needle
- the tail becomes flaccid within 5 minutes, which is an obvious method of ensuring a successful technique

Caudal (low) block

The dose is 5–7 ml of lignocaine or procaine in adult cows, 7–10 ml in bulls, 1–2 ml in calves (approximately 1 ml/100 kg). The field of analgesia with a caudal block extends from the tail base to ventral perineal skin and approximately 25–30 cm lateral to the midline. Increased dosage to 30 ml invariably causes severe ataxia, with recumbency in most individuals.

Cranial (high caudal) block

The dose is 40–80 ml in adult cattle, 5–25 ml in calves. The hind limb function is affected by desensitisation of L6 and sacral (S) 1 and 2 nerves (sciatic supply) L5 and L6 (obturator and femoral) and more cranial nerves. Dysfunction, depending on the degree of involvement, ranges from mild ataxia and slight spasmodic flexion and extension of stifle and hock joints to complete posterior paralysis.

Discussion

A major disadvantage of high volume epidural is the risk of injury during the onset (ataxia) or recovery phase (e.g. hip dislocation). Recovery to standing takes several hours, and the patient should not be permitted to attempt to stand until tail sensation has returned. Keep in sternal recumbency with the hind legs roped together above the hock or sedate with xylazine or acetylpromazine to prevent attempts to stand. A straw-bedded box or yard is advised.

Prior sedation may also reduce the patient's anxiety and struggling.

Factors affecting the extent of epidural block include volume, concentration of the drug, bodyweight, pregnancy and position of the cow.

Xylazine and xylazine-lignocaine/procaine combinations:

- analgesia after epidural administration of xylazine lasts more than twice as long (approximately four hours) as after an equivalent use of lignocaine or procaine alone

- a dose of 0.05–0.1 mg/kg body-weight of 2% xylazine (20 mg/ml) may be used. Dilute to total volume of 5–10 ml with sterile 0.9% saline solution or distilled water, e.g. 1.75 ml 2% xylazine in 3.25 ml saline solution for a 700 kg cow
- alternatively, use 0.02–0.03 mg/kg xylazine diluted with 2% lignocaine or 5% procaine to 5 ml total volume for an adult cow. This has the advantage of faster onset than xylazine alone and requires a lower dose, which reduces the sedation
- very useful in cows with chronic tenesmus (see Section 5.16). The extent of perineal analgesia is more variable than with lignocaine, but may include the entire perineal region, including the udder and flank
- side-effects may include marked transient sedation, hind limb ataxia, bradycardia and hypotension. These can potentially be reversed using a peripheral vasodilator without affecting analgesia. There are no such products licensed for food-producing animals in the EU

> **Tip**
>
> Add 0.75 ml of xylazine 2% to 5 ml of 2% lignocaine or 5% of procaine in the same syringe. This gives a suitable mixture sufficient for a long-acting caudal epidural in an adult Holstein cow. This is equivalent to approximately 0.025 mg/kg of xylazine.

Internal pudendal block
Indications:

- penile surgery distal to sigmoid flexure
- examination of prolapsed penis in standing animal
- reducing straining after vaginal trauma
- desensitises perineal region, anus, rectum, penis, scrotum, outer lamina of prepuce (male), vagina, cervix and distal urethra (female). Does not desensitise the testes

Equipment:

- 16G 10–15 cm needle, 30 ml syringe
- 2% lignocaine or 5% procaine

Technique:

- the Larsen method involves a block of the pudendal nerve (fibres of ventral branches of S3 and S4) and anastomotic branch of caudal rectal nerve (S3 and S4) via an ischiorectal fossa approach
- scrub the perineal region clean and inject a small bleb of anaesthetic either side of the rectum

- insert a gloved hand in the rectum to locate the nerve lying on the sacrosciatic ligament immediately dorsal and lateral to the obturator foramen, which is less than a hand's breadth cranial to the anal sphincter
- note pulsation of the internal pudendal artery just ventral to the nerve
- insert the needle forward at the deepest point of ischiorectal fossa, directed slightly downwards for a distance of 6 cm (see Figure 1.12)
- check the position of the needle point by rectal digital control and inject 20–25 ml solution (e.g. 2–3% lignocaine) around the nerve, spreading by massage
- withdraw the needle slightly and redirect slightly more caudally and dorsally to inject a further 10–15 ml (caudal rectal branch of the pudendal nerve)
- again, slightly withdraw before redirecting slightly cranially and ventrally to inject 10–15 ml at the cranial border of the foramen (communicating branch from the sciatic nerve)
- repeat the procedure on the other side of the pelvis, reversing the position of the hands
- allow 30–40 minutes for the block to take effect. Penile prolapse is followed by a loss of sensation

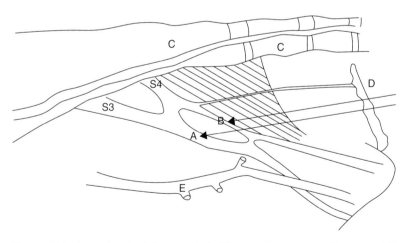

Figure 1.12 Internal pudendal nerve block. Diagram shows nerves (from sacral 3 and 4) and injection sites A and B on the medial surface of the right pelvic wall and floor of the cow (pelvic viscera removed).
A is just dorsal and lateral to obturator foramen; B is slightly more caudal and dorsal; C is the sacrum and coccygeal vertebrae 1–3; D is the anus through which the hand is inserted only to wrist level; E is the internal pudendal artery (pulsation) and lies just ventral to sites A and B.

Discussion

Manipulation of a long needle is easier if a short stout (14G 2–3 cm) needle is inserted through the skin (and analgesic skin wheal) serving as a cannula for the longer needle. Alternatively, a caudal epidural block (5 ml) rapidly desensitises the area of intended needle insertion.

The pudendal block persists for several hours. The main advantage is that the patient remains standing. The volume of l.a. necessary to block the nerve supply to the penis by an epidural technique almost invariably causes posterior paralysis. Cleanliness and experience of the pelvic landmarks are the main criteria for success with the pudendal block. Technical failures are common in inexperienced hands. A long delay (30–40 minutes) before the onset of analgesia is a further drawback.

Block of dorsal nerve of penis

The alternative technique to pudendal block for penile relaxation and analgesia involves analgesia of the dorsal nerve of the penis as it passes over the ischial arch.

Technique:

- infiltrate skin 2.5 cm from the midline adjacent to the penile body
- insert the needle, advancing to contact the pelvic floor and withdraw 1 cm (see Figure 1.13)
- check that needle is not intravascular (dorsal artery of penis)
- infiltrate 20–30 ml 2% lignocaine (plain) into region
- repeat procedure on opposite side of penis
- onset of analgesia in about 20 minutes; duration one to two hours

Intratesticular block
Technique:

- single injection of 3–5 ml l.a. into the body of each testicle prior to castration
- very fast onset (3 minutes) but short duration (10 minutes)
- achieves analgesia of the spermatic cord as well as the testicle, but the scrotal skin remains sensitive
- for open surgical castration, a small bleb of l.a. subcutaneously at the incision site may be beneficial
- aseptic technique is particularly important where bloodless castration is used

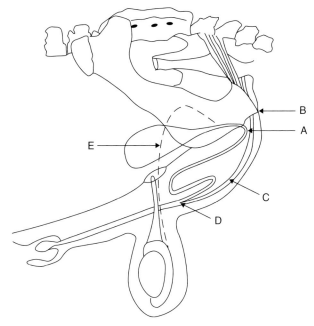

Figure 1.13   Block of dorsal nerve of the penis at the ischial arch.
A. insertion of needle horizontally 2.5 cm from midline where the penile body is palpable below the level of *tuber ischii*; B. *tuber ischii*; C. retractor penis muscles and penis; D. point of insertion of retractor penis muscles; E. *vas deferens*.

Teat block
Indications:

- teat analgesia is required for repair of teat lacerations (perforating fistula and severe lacerations), polyp removal, mucosal flaps of the rosette of Fürstenberg and supernumerary teats
- analgesia is also needed for teat endoscopy (not discussed further)

Equipment:

- 10 ml syringe, 21G 2.4 cm needle, catapult elastic and large curved artery forceps, or dog tourniquet
- 2% lignocaine or 5% procaine

Technique:

- sedate patient and lift one hind leg in the crush
- perform local infiltration of the teat base after removing any obtruding hairs from the udder

- insert the needle subcutaneously transverse to the direction of the teat and make an s.c. injection of 10–20 ml l.a. solution as a peripheral (ring) block (see Figure 1.14)
- accidental injection of anaesthetic into the teat cistern or circular veins at the teat base is not harmful but is ineffective in producing analgesia
- analgesia develops in 5–10 minutes
- place the tourniquet, teat clamp or intestinal clamp (with rubbers) on the teat base to reduce bleeding and dripping of blood and milk

---

Discussion

Partial analgesia can be achieved by infusion of the teat cistern with 2–5 ml l.a., but is not recommended. Even cases of polyps and stenosed teat orifices prove difficult to block in this way because only the mucous membrane becomes desensitised. The intermediate layer is also involved in the surgical trauma and will remain sensitive.

Using a ring block, the entire teat is anaesthetised distal to the site of injection. An alternative technique is by i.v. injection of any superficial teat vein distal to a tourniquet. This produces analgesia throughout the teat but is virtually only possible in a recumbent cow.

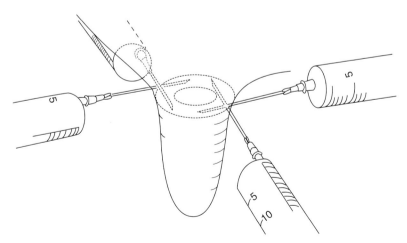

Figure 1.14 Teat ring block: 10–20 ml of 2% lignocaine or 5% procaine evenly distributed around the teat base.

Analgesia of the distal limbs

Intravenous regional analgesia (IVRA) of digit

This technique is simple and effective and supersedes the cumbersome local infiltration or nerve block procedures. It is indicated in any painful interference distal to the hock and carpus, and is ideal for digital surgery. No additional tourniquet is required for foot surgery on a cow in a Wopa-type crush (see Figure 1.15).

Equipment:

- If required, a tourniquet of stout rubber tubing, metal clamp to fix the tourniquet, two rolls of muslin bandages (or similar padding material)
- 30 ml syringe and 21G winged infusion set (butterfly catheter)

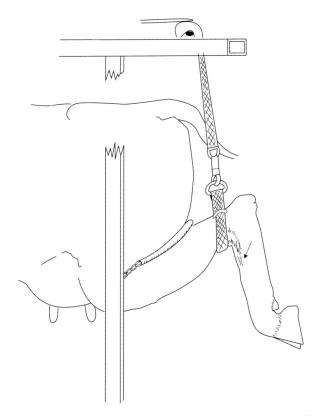

Figure 1.15　Intravenous regional anaesthesia (IVRA) in cow standing in a Wopa-type crush, using the lateral saphenous vein. The strap above the hock forms a sufficient tourniquet for this technique. Arrow shows injection site. A 19G butterfly catheter (winged infusion set) is recommended.

Technique:

Cow standing in Wopa crush (hind limb):

- elevate the limb using strap and buckle, fixed overhead (strap above hock is an efficient tourniquet)
- note lateral saphenous vein prominent in the proximal quarter of metatarsus (see Figure 1.15)
- push vein sideways to make it more prominent and relatively immobile
- place needle of a 21G winged infusion set (bung removed from the end) into the vein, aiming distally (against the blood flow); blood will quickly flow into infusion line and should be under pressure
- inject 25–30 ml of 2% lignocaine or 5% procaine quickly (adult cattle)
- analgesia develops in the entire limb distal to the tourniquet after about 5–10 minutes and is optimal after 20 minutes. Test the block with a needle-prick in the interdigital cleft
- anaesthesia persists for at least 90 minutes if the tourniquet is left in place

Cow in lateral recumbency:

- restrain animal in lateral recumbency, preferably after an i.v. or i.m. injection of xylazine for sedation, with the affected limb uppermost
- wrap the rubber tourniquet firmly around the limb proximal or distal to the hock or carpus (see Figure 1.16)
- in the hind limb place a rolled bandage in the depression on either side of the limb between the Achilles tendon and tibia to increase pressure on the underlying vessels
- clip the hair over any convenient and visible superficial limb vein distal to the tourniquet. The lateral saphenous or lateral plantar digital vein is a suitable site in the hind limb (see Figure 1.16)
- insert the needle of 21G winged infusion set, either in a proximal or distal direction, into the vein; observe for flow of blood and inject 20–30 ml 2% lignocaine or 5% procaine as rapidly as possible
- remove the needle from the vein and massage the site well for one minute to prevent development of subcutaneous haematoma

Forelimb:

- tourniquet is placed around the distal radius or proximal metacarpus
- make an injection into a superficial vein medially, e.g. large radial vein passing medially across the carpus (clipping site helps to visualise) or cephalic over the distal radius
- alternatively, use a low tourniquet (mid metacarpal region) and inject into a deep digital vein that is midline halfway between the accessory digits and the heel bulbs on the palmar aspect (see Figure 1.16). Use a 19 G 4 cm needle (observe blood before connecting a syringe and injecting).

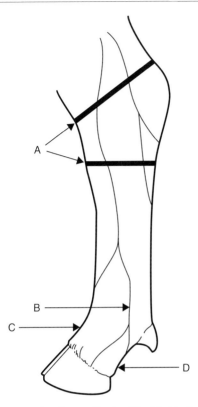

Figure 1.16 Intravenous regional anaesthesia of the hind foot–distal sites. Lateral aspect of the left hind limb of the cow showing two possible positions for a tourniquet (A) and sites for injection into the lateral digital vein (B) and dorsal common digital vein (C), lying deep, at the pastern between the proximal phalanges. A third site (D) is the deep digital vein accessed exactly midline halfway between the bulbs of the heel and the accessory digits.

Discussion

- The speed of onset is governed to some extent by the volume of the l.a. solution used, since higher intraluminal pressure causes more rapid diffusion of the solution (e.g. 30 ml versus 20 ml).
- The tourniquet may safely be left for two hours, although few surgical procedures ever require this length of time. Usually surgery is finished in 10–30 minutes, when the tourniquet may be safely released. Sensation returns within 5–10 minutes.
- Ideally the tourniquet remains in place for over 20 minutes: l.a. solution (and adrenaline) gaining access to the systemic circulation

could cause severe arrhythmias. Signs of toxicity might include drowsiness, minor convulsions and seizures, trembling and profuse salivation with hypotension. In reality, the risks appear relatively small and rarely reported, perhaps due to rapid detoxification in the liver.

● Lack of success is generally due to slackness of the tourniquet, which has failed to occlude the vascular drainage of some deeper vessels or perivascular injection. Analgesia occurs latest in the interdigital region.

● Lignocaine or procaine without adrenaline is preferred, but in practice, commercial preparations with adrenaline are usually used.

● The winged infusion set is not essential but makes the technique much easier because if the limb moves during injection of the l.a. solution, the needle is more likely to stay in place.

Warning

IVRA may be impossible to perform if there is severe swelling of the distal limb (e.g. cellulitis). In such cases, even if it is possible to locate a suitable vein, it is unlikely that sufficient intraluminal pressure of l.a. solution will be achieved. Regional nerve blocks should be used in preference.

Distal limb local anaesthesia (not IVRA)

Indications:

● distal limb surgery where IVRA fails or is not suitable (e.g. severe swelling)

Technique:

● inject 5–10 ml l.a. solution over peripheral nerves at four sites subcutaneously (depending on which digit requires anaesthesia):
  i. two sites 1 cm distal to both accessory digits (palmar or plantar axial nerves). Block both nerves regardless of digit requiring anaesthesia
  ii. midline dorsally just proximal to the metacarpal or metatarsal joint (dorsal common digital nerve, a branch of dorsal metatarsal/metacarpal nerve)
  iii. for lateral claw: 1 cm proximal to an accessory digit on the lateral aspect (lateral plantar/palmar nerve)
  iv. for medial claw: 1 cm proximal to an accessory digit on the medial aspect (medial plantar/palmar nerve)
● onset of anaesthesia in 10–15 minutes
● alternatively, a ring block (subcutaneous injection) may be used approximately 3 cm proximal to the digit to be anaesthetised

CHAPTER 2

Fluid and supportive therapy

2.1 General principles of fluid therapy

Considerations

- dehydration
- acid–base disturbance
- electrolyte disturbance
- fluid therapy in the field primarily depends on clinical acumen (lack of pen-side tests)
- bovine PCV (packed cell volume) normal range is very variable
- economical and practical constraints

2.2 Shock

Stems from inadequate perfusion of tissues. Shock lesions result from:

- failure of homeostatic mechanisms to maintain adequate perfusion
- homeostatic mechanisms themselves reduce perfusion by eliciting excessive production of various vasoactive hormones, amides, peptides and kinins

Shock may eventually become refractory to treatment. Inadequate perfusion is due to failure of blood flow, not of blood pressure. Changes are due to hypoxia and accumulated metabolites from defective perfusion. Basic

Bovine Surgery and Lameness, Third Edition. A. David Weaver, Owen Atkinson, Guy St. Jean and Adrian Steiner.
© 2018 John Wiley & Sons Ltd. Published 2018 by John Wiley & Sons Ltd.
Companion website: www.wiley.com/go/weaver/bovine-surgery

pathology: necrosis of cells and tissue, haemorrhages and fibrin thrombi in venous circulation (Shwartzman reaction). Almost every organ displays lesions.

Shock in cattle may be due to various reasons, for example:

- hypovolaemic shock as a result of massive haemorrhage: reduction of circulating blood volume to less than 80%; <65% is critical
- dehydration: 10–12% is severe; >15% is critical
- burns, e.g. third degree burns over more than 25% of the body surface
- infection: septic shock, especially gram-negative bacteria releasing endotoxins (e.g. toxic mastitis)
- peripheral vascular disease with gangrene (e.g. 'Fescue foot'; ergot poisoning)
- spinal anaesthesia (cranial or caudal epidural, see Section 1.9)
- acute haemolytic conditions

> **Discussion**
>
> A fall in blood pressure as a result of shock due to severe systemic blood loss triggers a sequence of events in which the animal attempts to maintain an adequate blood supply to the brain and coronary vessels, but which may compromise other tissues (see Figure 2.1). Prompt fluid therapy is often the most important corrective measure in such cattle.

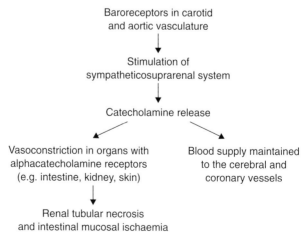

Figure 2.1   A summary of some reactions following severe blood loss and shock.

Table 2.1 A guide to hydration status (more reliable for calves than adults).

Dehydration (%)	0	2	4	6	8	10	12	14
Eyeball recession (mm)	0	1	2	3	4	6	7	8
Cervical skin tent duration (seconds)	2	3	4	5	6	7	8	9
Capillary refill time (seconds)	1	2	2	3	4	>4	>4	>4
Other signs		increased thirst			cold, dry nose		weak; depressed; cold; collapsed	

2.3 Hydration status

Dehydration is expressed as a percentage of total reduction of body fluids and is estimated using the indicators in Table 2.1:

● Volume of fluid required for replacement is calculated very simply: litres required = bodyweight in kg × % dehydration. For example, a 700 kg cow with 10% dehydration requires 70 litres of fluid to correct her deficit.
● Around 8–10% dehydration certainly indicates the need for fluid therapy. In calves, recumbency and suck reflex might be used to determine if i.v. fluids will be needed or if oral fluids will suffice.

In cows, although oral (intraruminal) rehydration has become easier and more practical with the ready availability of guarded stomach tubes, the general rule is that ≥8% dehydration warrants i.v. fluids. This is because the absorptive ability is reduced from the rumen mucosa due to reduced perfusion. Combination therapy (i.v. and oral) is often successful.

Avoid oral fluids in cattle with an impaired ability to swallow (e.g. milk fever).

Avoid oral fluids in calves when fluid pools in fore-stomachs (sloshing on ballotment); the calf is unable to stand or has no suck reflex. The latter two conditions increase the risk of aspiration pneumonia.

2.4 Acid–base status

Metabolic alkalosis

● most likely in dehydrated cows (exceptions: see the box below)
● corrected with Cl^- and K^+
● when the cow eats, she will have adequate K^+ intake, particularly from grass/grass silage

- fluid therapy usually provides Cl^-
- given adequate circulatory volume and electrolytes, the kidneys can usually correct the alkalosis. K^+ supplementation may be included in oral electrolytes

Metabolic acidosis

- likely with diarrhoeic calves
- also diarrhoeic cows; cereal engorgement; choke (bicarbonate loss in saliva)
- in practice, correction of acidosis is most commonly required for calves with a disturbed acid–base balance, which can be corrected with i.v. 8.4% (1 molar) sodium bicarbonate solution

---

Tip

Is my cow patient with intestinal obstruction likely to be acidotic or alkalotic?

A left displaced abomasum can result in either metabolic alkalosis or sometimes acidosis. Caecal torsions = alkalosis. Small intestine obstruction (e.g. strangulation/mesenteric torsion) = acidosis

---

Estimating acidosis in calves

- an out-of-fashion method of estimating whole blood CO_2 pressure in the field is with a Harleco apparatus (barometer). Not commonly used as it is fiddly and prone to experimental error
- hand-held electronic blood analysers may be available (e.g. i-STAT®) which can be used quickly in the field to aid decision making
- clinical examination is the usual method: physical weakness, depressed mental demeanour, ataxia, impaired palpebral reflex. Limited accuracy (see Table 2.2)

Table 2.2   Table of clinical signs associated with degrees of acidosis in calves.

Severity of acidosis	Signs	Base deficit (mEq/litre)
Clinically normal	scouring, clinically normal, strong sucking	5
Mild	weak sucking, standing but depressed	10
Moderate	recumbent, depressed, only stands with help, impaired palpebral reflex	15
Severe	unable to stand, no suck reflex, absent palpebral reflex	20

Tip

Clinical experience can help elucidate the likelihood of acidosis in calves:

- suckler calves that are 7–42 days old are more likely to be severely acidotic than dairy calves or young (<7 days old) calves
- diarrhoeic calves sick enough to warrant i.v. fluids may arguably benefit from bicarbonate
- if the calf is more depressed than the level of dehydration would suggest (or pooling fluid in its abomasum), it is probably acidotic (and would benefit from i.v. bicarbonate)
- faecal consistency is an unreliable sign: more watery does not mean more severe acidosis or dehydration

Calculating and correcting base deficits

- bicarbonate requirements for calves: base deficit (mEq/l) × weight (kg) × 0.6 (proportion of extracellular fluid in calves)
- base deficit in cows: base deficit (mEq/l) × weight (kg) × 0.3 (proportion of extracellular fluid in adults)
- e.g. a moderate acidosis in a 50 kg calf (15 mEq/l deficit) = 15 × 50 × 0.6 = 450 mEq HCO_3, so for $NaHCO_3$ = 450/12 = 37.5 g
- aim to correct half of a base deficit with bicarbonate and allow the kidney function to correct the rest
- **practical acidosis correction for calves**: when unable to estimate the base deficit, 'spiking' a 5 litre isotonic i.v. saline drip with 200 ml of a 8.4% solution of $NaHCO_3$ is practical and therapeutic in many dehydrated scouring calves. Deliver over 6–8 hours
- if very severe acidosis is likely, give up to 400 ml of 8.4% of solution over a prolonged period (e.g. 12 hours)
- **practical acidosis correction in adult cattle**: $NaHCO_3$ required for a moderately acidotic cow (600 kg) = (10 × 600 × 0.3)/12 = 150 g. Correct with 75 g (i.e. half) of $NaHCO_3$ dissolved in at least 1 litre of sterile water delivered i.v. over 2–3 hours

Tip

Production of a home-made 1 molar (8.4%) $NaHCO_3$ solution: dissolve 35 g in 400 ml of sterilised warm water (soft tap water is fine; purified demineralised water is better).

Acidotic neonates

- hypoxic acidosis is common after a difficult birth
- inject (slow i.v.) 50 ml of 8.4% $NaHCO_3$ to newborn calves that show poor responsiveness
- can be very useful after dystocia

Discussion

The administration of i.v. bicarbonate to correct acidosis is controversial. In most species, acidosis due to hypoperfusion (metabolic acidosis) resolves once the hypovolaemia is corrected. However, acidosis in diarrhoeic calves is, at least in part, due to absorption of lactic acid from the large intestine following fermentation of undigested solids. This D isomer of lactate cannot be metabolised and so whereas i.v. bicarbonate is rarely warranted in other species, there is a stronger argument for its use in diarrhoeic calves.

Warning

- Intravenous bicarbonate therapy can cause overshoot alkalosis and/or a paradoxical respiratory acidosis. Use with caution.
- Avoid administering i.v. bicarbonate alongside other fluids containing calcium (e.g. Hartmann's): it is likely to produce a precipitate.

2.5 Other electrolytes

- **Potassium:** in practice, NaCl is typically used for i.v. fluid replacement (hypertonic or isotonic) in calves and adult cattle; see Table 2.3 for the

Table 2.3   Composition of fluids that might be given as replacement therapy to cattle.

Fluid	\multicolumn{6}{c}{Electrolyte concentration (mmol/litre)}
	Na^+	K^+	Ca^{2+}	Cl^-	HCO_3^-	$Lactate^-$
Normal plasma	140	4	2.5	103	25	5
0.9% NaCl (isotonic)	154	0	0	154	0	0
7.2% NaCl (hypertonic)	1232	0	0	1232	0	0
Ringers solution	145	4	3	155	0	0
Hartmann's solution (lactated ringers)	131	5	2	111	0	29

composition of fluids. Cows and calves can become hypokalaemic either after correcting acidosis or with probable metabolic alkalosis, so following up i.v. fluids with an oral solution containing potassium is a good idea (as KCl or K_2CO_3); 60 g KCl = 800 mEq, which is sufficient for a cow with moderate hypokalaemia. Excess potassium will be excreted by the kidneys.

- **Calcium:** acidotic animals may develop hypocalcaemia once corrected, but take care with potential cardiotoxicity when administering Ca i.v. to dehydrated animals. Do not mix with i.v. bicarbonate. It is safe to give s.c. or orally.
- **Glucose:** may be indicated for ketosis or for calves to aid nutrition but be aware of limitations to supply actual energy requirements. A 50 kg calf would require approximately 800 g/day of glucose to provide maintenance energy requirements (impractical and likely to cause severe electrolyte imbalances). 500 ml of 50% dextrose provides 250 g of glucose, which is hypertonic, so administer concurrently with 0.9% saline or Hartmann's solution.

2.6 Oral fluid therapy

Indications

- diarrhoeic calf where not recumbent; dehydration in cattle <8%

Contra-indications

- animals with impaired ability to swallow
- rumen stasis or hypocalcaemia (risk of regurgitation/aspiration pneumonia)
- heavily sedated/anaesthetised patients

Equipment

- oesophageal tubing
- small volumes can be gravity fed (e.g. calf feeder bag) but larger volumes require a pump
- gag to prevent chewing of tube (or via nasogastric tube). In practice, Aggers™ or Selekt™ pumps are readily available (Europe), which have modified Frick specula, to guard the stomach tube in the mouth (see Figure 2.2)

Restraint

- adults: halter or crush
- calves: manual restraint

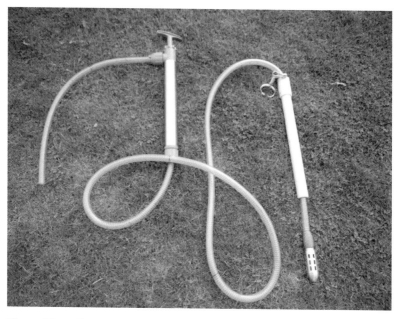

Figure 2.2   A Selekt pump connected up for collection of rumen fluid. The tube is passed into the rumen via the mouth guard held in place with the nose clip. The heavy metal end penetrates the fibre mat and the fenestrations reduce clogging of the tube. Negative pressure is applied via the reversible stirrup pump and rumen fluid can be collected into a bucket via the short tube from the pump.

Method

- gently apply a gag or insert a tube centrally into the animal's mouth
- maintain the head in a natural position, avoiding neck extension, and slowly introduce the oesophageal tube and allow the animal to swallow
- feed the tube down to its required position; some models remain oesophageal (calf feeders), sometimes intraruminal
- check the tube has not entered the trachea by either feeling the tube on the left side of the neck and/or by smelling rumen gas
- administer the desired fluids and any other oral medication slowly, as reflux and aspiration are possible
- remove the tube fully then the gag

Warning
● Many farmers will be adept at using their own calf stomach tubes or rumen pumps. However, without a little training first, mistakes will happen and either fluid can be administered directly into the lungs or aspiration of regurgitated fluid occurs. Both result in aspiration pneumonia and are invariably fatal. In worse cases, death is within minutes.   ● The Veterinary Defence Society (UK) has several claims a year against vets using rumen fluid pumps: always check the tube placement.   ● Be very careful in moribund or weak cattle; consider i.v. fluids instead.   ● Ensure the tube does not slowly slide out after the correct initial placement.

Discussion
Oral rehydration therapy (ORT) for diarrhoeic calves has undergone several developments over the last few decades, which has led to a system of categorisation: ● first generation ORT: an equimolar solution of glucose and sodium   ● second generation ORT: contains additional bicarbonate (to correct acidosis)   ● third generation ORT: increased energy (e.g. glucose) and osmolarity   ● fourth generation ORT: contains glutamine (amino acid, the predominant intestinal epithelial fuel)   Remember that the underlying principle function of ORT remains the transport of sodium-coupled glucose across the small intestinal epithelial membrane to stimulate absorption of water and electrolytes; this is achieved using first generation ORT products.

2.7 Intravenous fluid therapy

Indications

● cows or calves judged to be >8% dehydrated
● very useful in toxic mastitis, even if dehydration is less marked
● surgery where supportive fluid therapy is likely to help, particularly where endotoxic or hypovolaemic shock develops after surgical correction of volvulus

- severe: haemorrhage
- calves with intestinal hypomotility/abomasal dilation, where oral fluid is unlikely to be effective

Contra-indications

- none; i.v. fluids are very valuable in most circumstances of surgery or pathology, but using the correct fluid type and infusion rate are always important

Equipment

- razor/clippers, surgical scrub and spirit, scalpel blade
- narrow rope: to raise vein in collapsed calf
- 16G 2 cm needle; 5 or 6 metric nylon suture, pre-cut into 3–4 15 cm lengths
- catheter: 12 or 14G for calves; 10G for cows (certainly no smaller for gravity fed hypertonic saline)
- giving set: wide bore infusion set without drip chamber for adult cattle
- garden pump (modified) for hypertonic saline given under pressure (e.g. 12G catheter or needle)
- 5 litre bags isotonic (0.9%) saline or Hartmann's solution: for calves
- 3 or 5 litres hypertonic saline (7.2%): for adult cattle
- proprietary sterile fluid bags are readily available and economically justifiable. Home-made solutions can be used with tap water, but equipment is harder to maintain or keep acceptably clean

---

Tip

- A 10G 3 inch catheter is available from BD Supplies (BD Angiocath™) in the US, Canada, Australia, New Zealand and Europe.
- A wide bore (8 mm) 200 cm long infusion set with a single spike, no chamber and a rotating luer lock connector is available from Smiths Medical (SurgiVet®) in Europe, the US, and Australasia.

Restraint

- calves: lateral recumbency, manually restrained. Choose a clear, unrestricted flat site, or place the calf's head slightly downhill (for jugular vein)
- adult cattle: halter plus assistant. Sometimes possible in a crush, if not recumbent

Method

- set up a fluid bag and connect an infusion set. Large bore infusion sets without drip chambers can be re-used if necessary. Extended length (240 cm) disposable i.v. giving sets with a drip chamber (20 drops per ml) are very cheap (£2–3) and practical for calves. Run fluid through the giving set and clamp off
- adults: clip hair with scissors. No need to surgically prepare. Incise full depth skin with scalpel, over the jugular vein
- calves: raise the vein with a rope around the neck and an assistant. Clip and surgically prepare a 10 cm^2 site over the jugular, mid neck. Incise the skin full thickness with a scalpel for approximately 1 cm long incision
- raise the vein. Insert the needle and cannula through the skin incision and into the vein, in the direction of the blood flow. Once blood flows, run the cannula off the needle to the hilt, and immediately connect the giving set
- suture the cannula in place in skin using a 16G needle and nylon (more secure than tape or glue)
- speed of transfusion:

  hypertonic saline (cows): as fast as it can flow through the catheter. Typically, 5 litres takes 10–15 minutes through a 10G catheter

  isotonic saline (calves): quickly for first 1–2 litres (1 litre in 15 minutes is typically the fastest flow through a 12G catheter), then slowly give the remaining 3–4 litres over 6–8 hours

---

Tip

To calculate calf i.v. fluid requirements (50 kg) and drip speed:

Maintenance requirement = 120 ml/kg/day or 250 ml/hour
Plus fluid deficit : e.g. 8% = 4 litres

Administer 1–2 litres quickly. Deficit will now be around 3 litres. Aim to replace the remaining deficit over the next 8 hours (375 ml/hour). To provide maintenance plus deficit (250 ml/hour + 375 ml/hour = 625 ml/hour) requires 5 litres over 8 hours. Using a typical small animal giving set (20 drops/ml), set at 3–4 drips per second (200 drips per minute).

Hypertonic saline

- convenient and quick compared with isotonic saline due to a lower volume required
- allows sterile i.v. fluids to be administered to cows more practically in the field

- arguably not as physiologically effective as isotonic saline, but excellent for rapid reversal of hypovolaemic shock; transient increase in cardiac output and tissue perfusion occurs for about 30 minutes
- animal **must** receive a higher volume of oral fluids post-infusion, for lasting benefits. Cows usually drink 20–40 litres from buckets; otherwise give with stomach tube. Offer fresh water in buckets; can add electrolyte if delivered by tube
- avoid perivascular injection (slough/tissue necrosis: dilute with normal saline)
- may be repeated after 24 hours
- occasional sudden death after rapid administration to very moribund patients
- contra-indicated in obstructive disease (LDA/RDA)
- can be used as a bolus in calves, 4–5 ml/kg ≈ 200 ml, but isotonic recommended (just as easy).

Warning

Hypertonic saline (7.2%) draws water from interstitial spaces into the intravascular space. In the short term it can behave in a similar way to a colloid in that it boosts circulatory volume. However, in dehydrated patients such as diarrhoeic calves interstitial fluid is already depleted and hypertonic saline is contra-indicated.

Home-made i.v. solutions:
- may be useful if poor availability of proprietary solutions or for economy
- practical for an isotonic i.v. drip for a cow (e.g. using a 25 litre chemical drum)
- **hypertonic saline (7.2%):** 180 g NaCl in 2.5 litres water
- **isotonic saline (0.9%):** 45 g NaCl in 5 litres water (or 225 g in 25 litres)
- **isotonic electrolyte solution:** in 5 litres water, 35 g NaCl, 6.25 g KCl, 2.5 g $CaCl_2$
- **1 molar (8.4%) sodium bicarbonate:** 35 g $NaHCO_3$ in 400 ml water (difficult to dissolve); avoid 'hard' water containing high mineral content: use purified or demineralised water (e.g. for autoclaves). Warm the water to help dissolving but not too hot or CO_2 will evaporate. Can be sealed and kept in the vehicle or emergency kit for future use

Possible complications:
- thrombophlebitis: be clean; consider systemic antibiotics; use antibiotic spray after catheter removal

- difficulty finding a vein: more likely with calves. Ensure incision is through full skin thickness; prepare site well
- pulmonary oedema: too rapid or over-perfusion (more likely with calves)
- potential paradoxical CSF acidosis with bicarbonate therapy: fits/neurological signs, particularly if infused too fast
- overshoot alkalosis with bicarbonate therapy: therefore aim for half a base deficit correction

2.8 Blood transfusions

Indications

- blood loss and/or uncompensated anaemia, e.g. abomasal ulcers; postcalving haemorrhage; babesiosis
- PCV not valuable in cattle, but mucous membrane colour, heart rate and sound are useful indicators
- failure of passive immunoglobulin transfer (calves): valuable
- no need to cross-match as no antibodies to other blood group antigens unless previously exposed

Contra-indications

- previous transfusion: recipient must then be matched with donor

Equipment

- healthy donor (preferably of known disease status). If transfusing a calf, preferably use dam
- sodium citrate: 19 g/5 litres blood. Can be diluted in saline or water easily: e.g. 19 g in 500 ml (3.8% solution)
- 2 × 10G 3 inch catheter, or trocar needle for collection
- 5 litre collection bag, e.g. emptied 5 litre hypertonic or isotonic saline bag. Large animal giving set (without filter or drip chamber); proprietary blood collection bags can be used. A blood infusion set will reduce the risk of microclot administration
- scalpel; surgical scrub; clippers or razor; suture (for catheters)
- rope (tourniquet)

Restraint

- halter donor in crush for good head restraint. Sometimes xylazine is useful. Local anaesthetic before catheterisation
- for recipient: halter (as for i.v. fluid therapy)

Method

- prepare jugular site for donor, as per i.v. therapy, but include clipping and surgical scrub
- prepare the collection bag: empty saline/electrolyte from a 5 litre bag (administering some i.v. fluid to the recipient first may in any case be useful) or use a proprietary blood collection bag
- take some saline from the bag and dissolve sodium citrate in a 100 ml bottle (or in a sterile water bottle) or have 500 ml of a pre-mixed 3.8% solution ready. Inject via the injection port into the blood collection bag
- connect a large animal giving set to the collection bag and place on the floor by the donor. Allow anticoagulant to coat the inner surface of the whole bag and giving set. Keep the inlet port lowermost so blood flows into the anticoagulant first
- incise the skin and suture in place a 10G catheter in the donor. A tourniquet is rarely needed
- collect 4–5 litres from an adult, healthy cow (takes 10–15 minutes). Slowly agitate the blood in the bag during collection
- close off the giving set. Remove and discard the catheter. Suture/staple the incision if needed. This 'closed' method of collection is preferable to 'open' methods
- prepare the recipient as for i.v. fluids, including a surgical scrub
- suture in place a 10G catheter and infuse blood by gravity from the bag, over 30–40 minutes (slower than the maximum flow)
- calves: 500 ml as a bolus or 2–4 litres over several hours (use a 14G catheter)

Possible complications

- anaphylactic reaction: rare on the first transfusion. Stop the transfusion and treat with corticosteroids
- preferably transfuse slowly to see if symptoms develop (increased respiratory rate; hiccoughing; sweating; violent movements; tachycardia)
- inadvertent infection, e.g. BVD virus
- continued blood loss, e.g. uncontrolled uterine or vaginal artery haemorrhage: as blood pressure increases, bleeding may re-start.
- fatal stress: a severely anaemic animal is at risk and cardiac failure possible
- fatal thromboembolism: rare complication even without a microclot filter

Tip

To calculate whole blood requirement for calf with failure of passive transfer:

>Minimum IgG requirement = 10 g/litre blood
>Blood volume ≈ 9% body weight: $0.09 \times 45 = 4$ litres
>→ calf requires 40 g of IgG

Adult serum ≈ 18.9 g/litre IgG, so to receive the full amount of IgG from a blood transfusion would require at least 2 litres of blood. In practice ≈ 500 ml can be very easily administered, which provides around 25% of IgG requirements.

2.9 Transfaunation

Introduction

- introducing rumen contents from one animal into another
- easy with a specially designed stomach tube and pump
- abattoir-obtained rumen fluid contravenes Food Standard Agency regulations (UK)

Indications

- treatment of indigestion/grain overload
- supportive therapy for inappetent cattle, e.g. recovering from surgery

Equipment

- special collection fitting for an Aggers or Selekt pump, a weighted metal perforated end that sinks below the rumen fibre mat into the liquor layer (see Figure 2.2). The standard fitting may work but tends to float on the rumen fibre mat, limiting the volume collected
- fit, healthy donor, preferably on same diet and from the same group as the patient

Procedure

- pass the collection tube into the rumen as described in Section 2.6. Check the placement carefully
- reverse the pump and start to draw; rumen fluid should appear in the tube. At this stage, fluid can be collected by the siphon effect or repeated pumping
- collect 2–10 litres of fluid into a bucket, release the donor, and pump the fluid into the recipient as soon as possible using a standard rumen fluid pump (which may be the collection pump)

Possible complications

- aspiration pneumonia: care with the tube placement; avoid with animals with swallowing difficulties
- always kink off tubes or ensure they are fully pumped through with air before withdrawing them: even a small amount of aspirated rumen fluid can cause a severe pneumonia
- clogging of tubes is common, even with a perforated metal collection end
- retracting the tube through the cardiac sphincter can be difficult if a bolus of fibre is attached to the metal end of the collector: try reverse pumping to blow clear and patiently allow fibre to loosen
- potential disease spread, for example *Salmonella*
- improved demeanour is often seen within a few hours. If not, the primary problem may have been missed. Pumping 10 litres of fresh, healthy rumen liquor into a rumen that still contains a lot of cereal (cereal over-eating) might have very limited effect.

2.10 Antimicrobial therapy

Introduction

- antimicrobials are no substitute for a sound surgical technique in sterile aseptic procedures and neither will they control deep-seated necrotic and purulent foci
- antimicrobials should be considered as adjuncts to the natural host defence mechanisms
- primary aim should be proper preparation of the surgical field, surgeon and instruments
- appropriate debridement, excision of necrotic tissue, drainage and lavage will aid recovery better than antimicrobials alone (e.g. deep digital sepsis)
- antibiotic prophylaxis is not required during clean surgical procedures in cattle (e.g. LDA, entropion surgery)
- prophylactic antibiotic therapy is indicated in extensive abdominal surgery, open fracture repair and non-sterile invasive procedures, starting before the surgical intervention; therapeutic concentration should already be adequate at the start of surgery; intravenous route may be preferable
- dose rates of prophylactic and therapeutic antimicrobials are similar; continue therapy for at least three to five days after surgery.

Antimicrobial selection

- initial antimicrobial drug selection is often arbitrary (broad spectrum) and may be altered following results of sensitivity testing

Table 2.4   Some guidelines for the antimicrobial sensitivity of certain antimicrobials against common bovine pathogens (see footnote).

Organism	Antimicrobial drug	
	First choice	Alternative choice (s)
Trueperella pyogenes	Amoxicillin (c)	Penicillin G (c)
Staphylococcus aureus		
Non-penicillinase	Penicillin G (c)	amoxy/clav (c)
Penicillinase	Cephalosporins (c)	Amoxy/clavulanic acid (c)
Clostridium spp.	Penicillin G (c)	Tetracycline (Cl. tetani) (s)
Escherichia coli	Trimethoprim + sulpha (s and c)	Ampicillin (c)
Fusobacterium	Amoxycillin (c)	Amoxy/clavulanic acid (c)
		Tetracycline (s)
Enterobacteriaceae	Aminoglycosides (s)	Fluoroquinolones (c)
		3/4 gen Cephalosporins (c)
Klebsiella	Aminoglycosides (s)	Cephalosporins (c)
		Fluoroquinolones (c)
Pasteurella	Amoxicillin (c)	Florfenicol (s and c)
	Tetracycline[†] (s)	Macrolides (s)
Proteus mirabilis	Ampicillin (c)	Cephalosporins (c)
Other *Proteus*	Amoxy/clavulanic acid (c)	Aminoglycosides (s)
Salmonella	Trimethoprim + sulpha (s and c)	Fluoroquinolones (c)
Streptococcus	Penicillin (c)	Amoxy/clavulanic acid (c)

Notes:

- (c) = bactericidal; (s) = bacteriostatic
- enormous variations exist between different laboratories and countries
- antibiotic legislation is very variable, therefore obtain local specialist advice

[†] widespread resistance of *Pasteurella* spp. to tetracycline is recognised

- selection should be based on the organism's sensitivity, predicted drug tissue levels, confidence in drug safety and cost. The most common bovine pathogens and their sensitivity are shown in Table 2.4. Sensitivity may be variable depending on the area and country
- approval of use in each country is a key consideration, including extra-label use (e.g. following cascade principles in the UK)
- routine use of 'critically important' antimicrobials should be avoided, reserving their use only when indicated after resistance to other antimicrobials has been demonstrated by culture and sensitivity. (Critically

Table 2.5   Failure of response to antimicrobial therapy: list of possible factors.

Absence of concurrent surgical/mechanical measures, e.g. inadequate drainage

Inappropriate drug selection or dosage; impaired absorption, penetration or accelerated elimination

Sensitivity testing: organism resistant *in vitro*

Predisposing and management factors remaining uncorrected

Misdiagnosis, as condition not of bacterial origin

Impaired immune function; reduced phagocytosis

Fluid electrolyte, acid–base imbalance, nutritional defects

Inflammation, with release of mediators, cellular breakdown products, oedema, tissue destruction, coagulation, impaired perfusion and penetration

Poor management of mixed infections involving anaerobes

Toxin elaboration before antibacterial concentration is obtained at infection site

Compliance issues: course not completed; incorrect route of administration; incorrect dose

Underlying disease or concurrent medication; adverse drug interactions and/or drug antagonism

Adverse reactions: toxicity

important antimicrobials include the fluoroquinolones, 3rd and 4th generation cephalosporins and most macrolides)

A failure of response to antimicrobial therapy can be due to various reasons other than resistance to the prescribed antimicrobial. Table 2.5 lists possible reasons.

2.11 Peri-operative analgesia

Introduction

- pain management is a critical part of the surgeon's role
- non-steroidal anti-inflammatory drugs (NSAIDs) are widely available, licensed, inexpensive and usually the first choice
- peri-operative analgesia deserves careful consideration, not just from a welfare perspective but also to improve surgical success rates and reduce post-surgical production losses
- see Chapter 1 for local analgesia and general anaesthesia techniques

Pain assessment

- objective methods measure **physiological** parameters (e.g. heart rate, respiration rate, temperature, biochemical markers such as acute phase proteins, cortisol levels and activity levels) or **production** parameters (e.g. feed intake, weight gain and milk production)

- subjective methods are observations and categorisations of behaviour, e.g. mobility scoring for lameness (see Chapter 9). Evaluator differences often lead to poor repeatability (improved through training)

- despite its limitations, observation of behaviour is important in pain assessment

- **pain scales** widely used in human and companion animal pain assessments are not available in bovine medicine and surgery, but usually combine several evaluations: e.g. psychological/behavioural characteristics; nociceptive responses; body posture

- UK bovine practitioners identified the following as common pain signs in cattle: anorexia, vocalisation, grinding of teeth, dull and depressed attitude, abnormal movements, abnormal posture, increased heart rate, changes in respiration, flinching, recumbency, reduced rumination and reduced milk yield

- studies of calves have also included the following behavioural pain signals after routine management tasks (ear-tagging; dehorning; castration): tail wagging, head and ear movement, rearing, tripping, feet stomping, licking at the site and vocalisation

---

Discussion

Cattle are prey animals and have evolutionarily developed a strong ability to mask signs of pain. Use a combination of physiological, production and behavioural measures to assess likely pain and do not assume that absence of clear pain behaviours means the absence of pain.

Chemotherapeutic approaches to analgesia

- intercepts the pain pathways in order to prevent transduction or transmission of the nociceptive signal, thus stopping perception of pain

- in the UK, analgesic drugs available for use in cattle include: carprofen, flunixin meglumine, ketoprofen, meloxicam and tolfenamic acid (nonsteroidal anti-inflammatory drugs (NSAIDs)); xylazine and detomidine (alpha-2-agonists); procaine (local anaesthetic nerve blocks); ketamine (anaesthetic) and thiopental barbituate (see Chapter 1)

- opioids are not licensed for food-producing animals but act at the spinal and central nervous system level and can produce profound analgesia in cattle (e.g. butorphanol)

- steroids may have some local analgesic properties based on their anti-inflammatory action and their ability to inhibit prostaglandin synthesis – not as profound as NSAIDs. Some value for short-term pain relief only

- whilst the sedative properties of xylazine may last 1–2 hours, note that the analgesia effects last only 15–30 minutes
- procaine and lignocaine local analgesia lasts 30–90 minutes
- management of chronic pain requires repeated administration of NSAIDs as none of those available are long acting
- initial administration should be pre-operative

Alternative therapeutic approaches to analgesia

- make the animal as comfortable as possible post-surgery (e.g. deep, soft bedding; warmth; unrestricted feed access)
- amniotic fluid drunk by cows post-partum provides some analgesic effect from endogenous opiates
- grooming brush may have some analgesia benefits similar to massage therapy in humans

Practical benefits of routine use of post-operative analgesia

- NSAID analgesia post-castration or dehorning decreases signs of behavioural and physiological signs of pain in calves and increases growth rates
- NSAIDs improve mastitis treatment success rates (meloxicam)
- NSAIDs improve outcomes of treating claw horn lesions with therapeutic trims; quicker recovery and less risk of relapse (ketoprofen for 3 consecutive days)
- decreased milk production, lower dry matter intake and changes in lying behaviour are commonly seen after abdominal surgery. NSAIDs improve appetite and lying behaviour but do not completely alleviate surgical pain

CHAPTER 3

Diagnostic techniques and procedures

3.1 Abdominocentesis

Indications

- suspected peritonitis, e.g. traumatic reticulitis, abomasal ulceration, intussusception
- uroperitoneum, e.g. bladder or ureteral rupture
- gut contents in abdomen, e.g. intestinal rupture, abomasal perforation in calves
- haemorrhage, e.g. splenic or hepatic rupture, tumours, perforated abomasal ulcer
- ascites, e.g. right-sided heart failure

Restraint

- restrain the animal to safely access the midline ventral abdomen, e.g. open-sided crush
- usually not necessary but may sedate if wished, e.g. xylazine 0.1 mg/kg i.v.
- where possible lift one hind leg
- alternatively apply a kick bar and/or have an assistant elevate the tail

Bovine Surgery and Lameness, Third Edition. A. David Weaver, Owen Atkinson, Guy St. Jean and Adrian Steiner.
© 2018 John Wiley & Sons Ltd. Published 2018 by John Wiley & Sons Ltd.
Companion website: www.wiley.com/go/weaver/bovine-surgery

Equipment

- 18 or 19G 5 cm needle (20G 2.5 cm needle for calf)
- alternatively, a sterile steel teat cannula: skin incision necessary
- possibly preliminary ultrasound check for depth of abdominal fluid

Technique

- clip and surgical scrub (diluted povidone-iodine) right ventral abdominal wall
- two possible sites: **1: cranial** to umbilicus over the most pendulous part of the abdomen 5 cm to the right of midline or **2: caudal**, in the triangle between the fold of the stifle and the 'milk vein' (see Figure 3.1)
- insert the needle through the skin and slowly advance to 'pop' through the fascia and parietal peritoneum
- needle tip is palpably free in the abdominal cavity
- if no fluid drips out, first rotate the needle and slightly change the angle
- attach a 5 ml sterile syringe and slowly withdraw the plunger (negative pressure may hinder collection due to omentum blocking the needle)
- normal fluid is pale yellow (volume <5 ml, odourless)

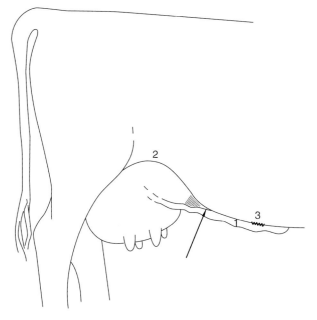

Figure 3.1 Possible caudal site for abdominocentesis on the right side of the abdominal wall in an angle between the right abdominal ('milk') vein (1) and stifle fold (2). Arrow shows the site of the needle puncture; (3) shows the level of the umbilicus.

- if abdominal viscus such as omental fat or bowel is entered, another site should be selected with a new needle

Limitations

- the cow normally has a very small volume of peritoneal fluid (except in late pregnancy)
- any peritonitis is usually localised ('walled off') very effectively in the cow
- the omentum easily blocks the needle
- iatrogenic blood contamination of the sample is not uncommon

> **Warning**
>
> Abdominocentesis alone is not a particularly sensitive test for peritonitis: in a study of 50 veal calves with abomasal perforated ulcers, abdominocentesis was only diagnostic for 30% of cases.

Fluid analysis and diagnostic tests

Fluid may be collected in EDTA tubes for a total white blood cell count, or sterile tubes for culture. Visual inspection alone should differentiate conditions such as diffuse peritonitis, haemoperitoneum and uroperitoneum from normal fluid. Table 3.1 summarises normal and abnormal peritoneal characteristics.

Table 3.1   Summary of different peritoneal fluid characteristics.

	Normal fluid	Gut contents	Transudate	Exudate (peritonitis)
Colour	straw/light yellow	brown/green; gritty	clear	turbid, darker yellow
Smell	mild metallic	characteristic abomasal or rumen fluid smell	none	putrid
Volume	up to 5 ml	>5 ml	>5 ml	variable
Specific gravity	<1.016	variable	<1.018	>1.018
Total protein (g/dl)	<25 g/l	variable	<25 g/l	>25 g/l (froths on shaking)
Cell count	$<10 \times 10^9$/l	n/a	$<0.5 \times 10^9$/l	$20–100 \times 10^9$/l
pH	6–8	<4 if abomasal contents	6–8	6–8

3.2 Rumenocentesis

Indications

- to investigate sub-acute rumen acidosis (SARA) problems in herds; a component of rumen health monitoring
- to determine rumen pH in individuals if acidosis/cereal over-eating is suspected

Restraint

- restrain animal for safe access to ventral left flank
- crush; insemination stalls; palpation rails or head yokes
- tail restraint by the assistant

Equipment

- local anaesthetic using a 2 cm 18G needle
- 16G 10 cm (4 inch) long needle (e.g. Air-Tite Products, USA) for sample collection. *Do not use shorter needles*
- 20 ml syringe
- scissors
- 20 ml sample pots

Technique

- mark the site with a small scissor clip: left side, 2–10 cm caudal to last rib and level with stifle (see Figure 3.2)
- pinch the skin and inject 3–5 ml of local anaesthetic s.c. and into superficial and deeper muscle layers, using 2 cm 18G needle. Wait 5 minutes
- clean flank (no need to surgically scrub)
- fully advance to hub 4 inch 16G needle through an anaesthetic bleb in a single stroke. Once the needle tip is embedded in rumen lumen, no risk of traumatic injury
- connect a 20 ml syringe and aspirate gently. Inject air through the needle if it blocks with food material (common). In theory, aspiration can lower CO_2 tension (and raise pH) in the sample: unlikely to be significant in practice
- collect 3–10 ml of fluid into a 20 ml container

Possible complications

- discomfort after needle insertion: select another cow and repeat (if herd test)
- similarly, select another animal if blood is present or the needle becomes grossly bent

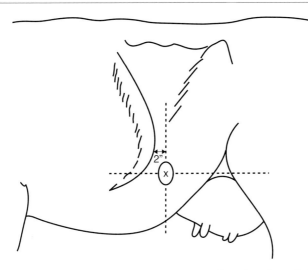

Figure 3.2   Site (x) for rumenocentesis, level with the stifle and two fingers' width behind the last rib.

- post-sampling skin swelling: possibly localised infection
- shorter needles may lacerate the rumen wall: localised peritonitis (rare)
- a gravid uterus might appose the flank site; therefore avoid cows in the last trimester
- a left displaced abomasum could rarely result in abomasocentesis

Animal selection (herd test)

- non-TMR (total mixed ration) fed herds: sample cows 2 hours after a main concentrate meal
- TMR fed herds: sample 4–6 hours after delivery of mix. Ensure cows do not miss a normal feed, e.g. due to shedding after milking
- sample 6 cows that are more than 3 weeks calved ('adapted' group) plus 6 cows that are 1–3 weeks calved. Include animals on the highest concentrate ration. Select cows from a herd management list, rather than a farmer selection

Fluid analysis and tests

- timing of fluid analysis: samples can be stored for several hours: redox test as soon as possible
- visual assessment: healthy is green, pleasant smell (not sour), viscous, small bubbles of fermentation, larger particles float to the top
- pH: use calibrated meter, not litmus paper

Table 3.2   Description of protozoal scores (score 2 or 3 is the target).

Description	Protozoal score
Highly motile and very crowded: a dense field of small and large protozoa darting randomly over the field of view. Large protozoa are uncountable as they transect a 1 cm line on the coverslip. Movement is visible to the naked eye.	+++ (3)
Motile and crowded, a mixture of small and large protozoa. Large protozoa are countable as they cross a 1 cm transect line on the coverslip.	++ (2)
Sluggish motility and low numbers, mainly small protozoa. Large protozoa in a 1 cm diameter field of view are countable.	+ (1)
No or sporadic live fauna: < 2 large protozoa detectable in a 1 cm diameter field of view.	0

Table 3.3   Factors affecting rumen protozoa activity and number.

Low pH: below 5.5; expect to see fewer numbers and activity. Larger protozoa species affected first

Temperature: colder temperatures depress movement considerably. Examine at 37 °C

Dilution, e.g. after a large fluid intake: expect numbers to be reduced

Mycotoxins: may depress protozoal numbers and activity

Oral antimicrobials: may depress numbers and activity, e.g. monensin (effect is short-lived)

- methylene blue reduction test: 0.5 ml 0.03% methylene blue decolourised in 125 ml fluid at 37 °C < 5 minutes. Assessment of redox potential of bacteria
- microscopy (× 10–40): protozoal activity estimated at 37 °C (±2 °C) on a pre-warmed slide
- score graded 0 (only sporadic live protozoa) to 3 (highly motile dense field). See Table 3.2
- factors affecting protozoa scores are listed in Table 3.3

Limitations

- uncertainty as to excessively low rumen pH: <5.5 is too acidic and 5.5–5.8 borderline
- timing of sampling is important: aim to sample at the time of lowest likely pH; problems with out-of-parlour feeders, inaccurate in-parlour feeders or variable feeding regimes

- SARA can only be diagnosed if rumen pH remains <5.5 for 3 or more hours (impossible with single time-point sampling). A practical convention of ≥5/ 12 cows ≤ pH 5.5 is diagnostic of the herd problem
- when cows stop eating, pH rises again, so a single time-point pH measurement is very limited in usefulness due to *low sensitivity*. Assessment of rumen health using protozoal interpretation is less problematical
- even if timing of sampling is correct, a low rumen pH at a single time point is not *specific* for SARA and diagnosis should not be based on the pH alone

Discussion

Diagnosis of SARA in a herd is not easy. If timing of sampling is correct and feeding of cows very uniform, it is quite possible to have ≥5/12 cows with a low pH, having selected them at the pH nadir, which can be *quite normal*. Many high producing cows with high dry matter intakes will normally have a pH that dips below 5.5 for at least part of the day without suffering any ill effects. Conversely, inappetent cows are likely to have a high rumen pH. A low rumen pH at a single time point is perhaps less useful, therefore, than poor protozoa scores for a SARA diagnosis.

Reticular telemetric pH boluses measure pH fluctuations over a long period of time and can provide very useful data to aid in the diagnosis of SARA. However, they are expensive and limited to a single use.

3.3 Liver biopsy

Indications

- to investigate the trace mineral status of cows, especially copper
- to diagnose 'fatty liver' disease
- investigate other hepatic pathology
- consider use of ultrasound (particularly for neoplasia or abscessation)

Restraint

- a good rumen fill keeps the liver firmly pushed up against the diaphragm: ensure selected animals are not starved beforehand
- access required to right flank: crush or shute
- sedation rarely required (xylazine)

Animal selection

- Cu **deficiency** (usually in grazing systems): sample 6 or more first lactation animals that are 5–6 months pregnant or second lactation cows that have calved in the last two months
- Cu **excess**, i.e. toxicity (usually concentrate-fed and supplemented cattle): sample 6 older mid-lactation cattle or representative cattle in the suspect group (e.g. replacement heifers)
- in groups with different feeding in a six month period before biopsy (e.g. bought-in cattle), test 6 as a separate group
- for fatty liver diagnosis: calved 1–3 weeks; usually with a history of ketosis and/or weight loss
- avoid animals < 350 kg or > 7 months pregnant

Equipment

- razor/clippers and surgical preparation equipment; local anaesthetic
- scalpel, tissue forceps
- gauze swabs
- 25 cm long 4 mm external diameter percutaneous liver biopsy trocar and cannula (Shoof International; UK agent: Agrihealth NI), or a 14G 6 inch Tru-cut™ biopsy needle
- antibiotic and antibiotic spray

Technique

- identify landmarks on the right-hand side and clip and disinfect a 10 × 10 cm window
- landmarks (see Figure 3.3)
- **site (1)**: find the 10th intercostal space. There are 13 ribs (normally) so the last space is the 12th; then count back. Draw an imaginary line level with the greater femoral trochanter (15–20 cm below transverse processes). Where this line crosses the 10th intercostal space is the point of needle insertion
- **site (2)**: alternative for larger cows is slightly more ventrally in the 11th intercostal space
- infuse 5–10 ml local anaesthetic s.c. and in intercostal muscle layers. Wait 10 minutes
- make a 1 cm stab incision through skin in the caudal part of the intercostal space to avoid blood vessels close to the caudal border of the rib. Pull the skin caudally when making a stab incision to offset the skin incision with a puncture site to reduce the risk of pneumothorax
- insert the trocar and cannula or biopsy needle through the stab incision

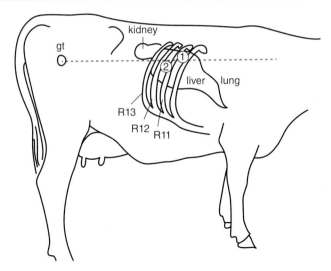

Figure 3.3 Diagram of the right side of the abdominal wall of a cow, showing sites for a liver biopsy. The cranial boundary of the liver is usually around rib 9. Auscultation may help to identify the area of hepatic dullness. The site for the biopsy is approximately one third of the distance down the rib cage, level with the greater trochanter (gt). 1 and 2 are possible sites for biopsy.

- needle penetrates the skin, intercostal muscles and diaphragm before entering the liver: 3–5 cm in most animals. A distinct popping sensation is often noticed as the instrument punctures the diaphragm and then a soft grainy sensation of liver tissue. If necessary, partly withdraw the cannula and repeat in a slightly different direction. Advance slightly ventrally and cranially (towards the left shoulder)
- **Tru-cut needle**: insert the needle with the stylet withdrawn into the needle. Once in the liver, advance the stylet, holding the needle stationary. Liver tissue fills the notch. Cut the tissue by advancing the needle, now holding the stylet stationary. Once the needle is fully advanced over the stylet, the instrument can be withdrawn with the biopsy in place. A single sample contains 10–15 mg of liver, so two samples are required for many assays (check with lab)
- **trocar and cannula**: insert the trocar and cannula into the liver and continue for a further 3–5 cm. Withdraw the trocar. Attach a 5 ml tight fitting syringe and with continuous negative pressure advance (punch) with a slight twist and then withdraw the cannula with tissue within it
- expel tissue (typically 4 cm × 3 mm diameter) on to a dry gauze swab by positive pressure or reinsertion of the trocar (see Figure 3.4). A 4 cm core is equivalent to circa 0.3 g of tissue, sufficient for most investigations

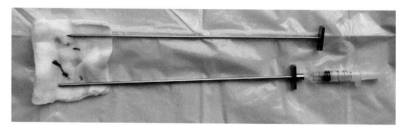

Figure 3.4   A liver biopsy trocar and cannula and a typical sample on a swab.

- often 2 or 3 biopsy samples can be obtained via a single stab incision
- place a single interrupted suture in the skin
- administer a systemic antibiotic to reduce the risk of clostridial infection

Tissue handling and tests

- minerals (Cu; S; Co/vit B12): place in a dry transport pot. Avoid a rubber plug if testing for zinc
- histopathology: transport in 10% buffered formal saline
- fatty liver diagnosis: oil RedO (lipid) stain is used to see fat; normal liver 5–15% surface area is fat; mild fatty liver 15–25%; fatty liver 25–33%; severe fatty liver ≥33%
- specific gravity test measures flotation in different strengths of $CuSo_4$ solutions (higher fat content is lower density); not commercially available. 0.1–0.2 g required for histopathology
- mineral assay: labs have different requirements for tissue (0.2 g for single mineral, e.g. Cu to ≥1 g). Consult lab for advice. Table 3.4 shows reference liver copper levels

Table 3.4   Reference liver copper levels (AHVLA 2015).

	Liver copper mg/kg wet matter	Liver copper μmol/kg dry matter
Below normal	<25	<1405
'Safe' normal range (adequate)	25–100	1406–5615
Upper normal range (high; toxicity unlikely)	100–145	5616–8000
'High" but not necessarily toxic (copper loading)	200–550	11 238–30 903
Toxicity range	250–800	14 047–44 950
Level above which liver is considered toxic for food safety	>500	>28 094

Tip

Consider samples for mineral assay from cull cows (abattoir) or dead stock (farm) to avoid live cow biopsy. Mineral status estimation does not require fresh tissue.

Discussion

- Over-supplementation of copper for dairy cows is very common.
- There is considerable overlap between liver copper ranges considered normal or toxic (see Table 3.4) due to different animals' abilities to store excess copper in the liver (copper loading).
- Clinical copper toxicity occurs where the ability of the liver to store excess copper is exceeded, leading to a rapid efflux of liver copper and widespread (usually fatal) haemolysis.
- Cattle with liver copper in excess of 14 047 µmol/kg dry matter are at risk of clinical copper toxicity.
- There is some controversy over whether copper loading *per se* causes harm.
- Diagnosis of *clinical* copper toxicity requires demonstration of hepatic pathology or haemolysis as well as high kidney or liver copper levels.

Possible complications

- serious complications are unusual
- some cows develop transient hiccups (1–2 hours)
- accidental entry into hepatic vessel: immediate bleeding from cannula. Avoid by stopping the advance of the cannula if any firm structure (perivascular fibrous tissue) is encountered; change direction
- accidental entry into hepatic abscess with gross peritonitis: usually fatal
- localised peritonitis: dirty technique
- wound infection: dirty technique
- clostridial necrotic hepatitis: systemic prophylactic antibiotic advised
- pneumothorax: unilateral, partial and temporary. Limited by skin suture

3.4 Bronchoalveolar lavage (BAL)

Indications

- collecting a cell sample for virus fluorescent antibody testing (FAT), particularly bovine respiratory syncytial virus (BRSV)

- differential cell counts: can be diagnostic for lungworm
- virology: preferably in early disease stage (pyrexia but limited lung pathology)
- mycoplasma isolation: diagnosis and for farm-specific vaccine production

Restraint

- firm restraint: crush and halter; assistant required to extend the neck

Equipment

- either a dedicated BAL tube, available from the USA (Bivona; Smiths Medical), or use Portex silicone tubing: outer tube: 1 m long, 8 mm internal diameter, 11.5 mm external diameter; inner tube: 2 m long, 3.5 mm internal diameter, 6.5 mm external diameter
- 50 ml phosphate buffered saline
- 50 ml luer-fitting syringes
- three-way tap

Technique

- clean external nares thoroughly. Lightly lubricate tubes with aqueous lubricant gel
- if using the Portex tubing method, take the outer tube and mark the length from the nose to the larynx with a pen
- guide the outer tube into the ventral nasal meatus
- extend the neck of the calf/cow and push the tube to the opening of the trachea; feel it contact the larynx; wait for an intake of breath and advance the tube; a cough follows and expiration through the tube is evident
- if the patient swallows, withdraw the tube to the larynx, extend the neck further and try again. If this happens repeatedly, use a new, clean tube
- insert the outer tube until resistance is felt as it encounters smaller bronchi
- feed the smaller tube through the outer tube until it meets resistance, i.e. lodges in a bronchus
- inject 60 ml of phosphate-buffered saline down the inner tube, wait 20 seconds and then aspirate it back; should yield a 10–30 ml frothy sample
- BAL tube (Bivona) is an all-in-one double tube with an inflatable cuff

Sample handling

- transfer the aspirate into sterile containers
- transport within a day (ideally ≤1 hour) to the lab for virus detection

Limitations

- viruses (particularly BRSV) are labile, so rapid lab work is required
- BAL tube normally lodges in the right diaphragmatic lobe, whereas primary sites of viral disease are normally the anterior lobes. The diaphragmatic lobe is an advantage for lungworm diagnosis
- not as useful for bacterial culture: often no growth; limited advantage over nasopharyngeal swabs

3.5 Trans-tracheal aspiration

Indications

- preferable to BAL for bacteriology but less useful for cytology: less fluid and cells collected
- IBR FAT: no advantage over nasopharyngeal or ocular swabs

Restraint

- firm restraint required with neck extended and restricted lateral head movement: two halters
- sedation (xylazine) advisable

Technique

- clip and disinfect 5 × 5 cm midline over the midcervical trachea
- inject 2–3 ml local anaesthetic s.c.
- stab full thickness through the skin with a scalpel blade
- insert a 10 or 12G needle perpendicular to the trachea between two tracheal rings; the patient will react when the needle enters the tracheal lumen
- aim ventrally (down trachea) and push the needle to the hub
- insert a narrow bladder catheter through the needle. Inject 60 ml of saline. Withdraw the fluid repeatedly: anticipate 5–10 ml of sample collection
- carefully remove the catheter and then the needle. If the catheter snags on bevel of the needle, remove the needle first

Complications and limitations

- limitations as for BAL; less aspirate can be expected
- less well tolerated than BAL
- risk of losing a severed catheter in the trachea

3.6 Pleurocentesis

Indications

- confirming pleurisy diagnosis
- injecting intrapleural antibiotic in cases of pneumothorax or pleurisy
- might be possible to drain excessive pleural fluid

Technique

- auscultate to ascertain the fluid level
- use a 12–16G 8–10 cm long needle
- 6th or 7th intercostal space below the suspected fluid line
- ultrasonography may help guide the procedure
- clip and disinfect a 5 × 5 cm site; inject local anaesthetic s.c.; stab an incision through the skin and advance the needle until air is drawn in to the pleural cavity or the fluid drains

3.7 Pericardiocentesis

Indications

- confirm the diagnosis of pericarditis or other cardiac tamponade (e.g. bleeding into the pericardium; pericardial effusion associated with congestive heart failure)
- consider ultrasound first

Technique

- 5th intercostal space on the left-hand side
- clip and disinfect a 5 × 15 cm site; inject local anaesthetic s.c.; stab incision through the skin
- 15 cm 14–16G needle or catheter; advance towards the heart slowly, with the syringe attached; ultrasonography may assist needle guidance
- confirm in the pericardial sac (not pleural cavity); inject 20 ml air and auscultate on the right side to hear a sloshing sound
- aspirate fluid; if not sanguineous, measuring total protein/specific gravity with a refractometer may help distinguish transudate or exudate

3.8 Bladder catheterisation

Indications

- urinalysis: pH, normally 7.5–8 (monitoring dietary cation/anion balance)
- urinalysis: ketone testing

- to diagnose cystitis/confirm haematuria
- to empty bladder for animals with bladder paralysis/post-calving trauma
- to irrigate bladder in chronic cystitis

Technique

- epidural anaesthetic optional
- clean vulva with dry towel
- flexible catheter is best, e.g. a two-way foley catheter or a foal stomach tube
- locate the urethral opening on the midline of vaginal floor
- insert the first finger into the blind-ending suburethral diverticulum; lift the finger to its dorsal wall and slide it back slowly; urethral opening flips past the finger nail and insert the finger forwards again into the urethra
- either use the finger as a guide for the catheter or use the catheter itself to locate the true opening
- may need to insert the catheter >20 cm before the urine flows

Possible complications

- cystitis: dirty technique; trauma to the urethra due to a large finger/too wide a tube
- bladder rupture: avoid rigid catheter

Tip

For urinalysis, catheterisation is rarely required: without touching the tail, lightly stroke the perineal region and the cow will shortly urinate.

3.9 Coccygeal venepuncture

Indications

- collection of venous samples (volume up to 10 ml) with minimal restraint and little or no assistance
- advantages over collection from the jugular or abdominal (milk) vein (latter not recommended)

Technique

- collect into evacuated blood collection tubes (e.g. vacutainer®) with or without anticoagulant using a 19G 4 cm needle that is screwed into a plastic holder into which the collection tube is inserted

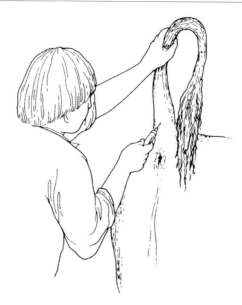

Figure 3.5   Restraint for obtaining blood samples from a coccygeal vein.

- alternatively, collect via an 18G 2 cm needle into a syringe (5–10 ml) with negative pressure
- restrain the head in a crush, chute or head yoke; manual restraint is rarely required
- grasp the tail in the mid third and slowly elevate it to almost a vertical position (see Figure 3.5)
- remove gross faecal contamination with a paper towel or cotton wool
- locate the palpable vein in the midline, just caudal to insertion of skin folds of the tail at the level of the coccygeal (Co) vertebrae 6–7
- insert the needle just cranial to the bony protuberance in midline to a depth of 8–12 mm (in the vacutainer system, insert the needle into the tube); withdraw slightly until blood flow starts
- if initially unsuccessful, reduce tension of the tail slightly and continue at the same site; otherwise attempt at Co 5–6
- do not massage the puncture site after venepuncture

Tip

Sites of Co 3–5 are sometimes used but anatomical studies show the vein lies to the right of midline in the ventral sulcus of the vertebral body at the more cranial site; the more distal Co 6-7 site is usually easier.

Possible complications

- minimal risk of infection
- sporadic haematoma formation insignificant: disappears in a few days
- does not cause thrombophlebitis or total occlusion of a vein: repeat samples are easily obtained days or weeks later
- tail paralysis: virtually unknown

CHAPTER 4

Head and neck surgery

4.1 Disbudding and dehorning

Indications

- improve stock management
- reduce aggressive behaviour towards other members of the herd and stock personnel
- reduce traumatic damage/injury

Anaesthesia, analgesia and selection of techniques

- in the UK all calves over one week old may only be disbudded or dehorned using anaesthesia or analgesia (Animal Anaesthetics Act 1964)
- in some countries (e.g. Switzerland), general anaesthesia is mandatory
- disbud at an early age: easier; less risk of infection; no haemorrhage; better animal welfare
- cornual nerve block is described in Section 1.9
- post-operative analgesia (NSAIDs) strongly recommended

Bovine Surgery and Lameness, Third Edition. A. David Weaver, Owen Atkinson, Guy St. Jean and Adrian Steiner.
© 2018 John Wiley & Sons Ltd. Published 2018 by John Wiley & Sons Ltd.
Companion website: www.wiley.com/go/weaver/bovine-surgery

Chemical cautery
- may be suitable for very young calves (<1 week old)
- local caustic compound (NaOH, KOH, collodion) applied to horn buds
- wear protective gloves
- clip hair from the horn buds, protect the surrounding skin with petroleum gel and apply a thin film of paste
- confine calves afterwards for 30 minutes
- use of caustic preparations is hazardous and forbidden in some countries

Surgical and heat cautery
- ideal age for surgical disbudding is one to two weeks old, when the horn buds project 5–10 mm, are easily palpable and a disbudding iron can be used alone (see Figure 4.1)
- hot irons suitable for larger horns may be free standing with large copper heads (heated in a naked flame gas burner) or connected via a regulator and gas pipe to a portable butane/propane gas supply
- disbudding of young calves (<6 weeks old) has become much easier since the advance of portable hot gas or electric irons, butane gas-powered

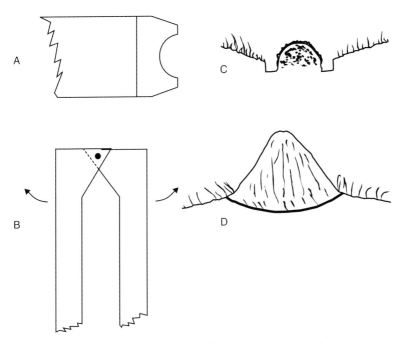

Figure 4.1   Two disbudding and dehorning instruments (not to scale).
A. Head of electrical or gas-powered calf disbudding iron; B. head of Barnes dehorner; C and D are cross-sections of the effect in C of burning a circular trough around the bud and in D the blades cut away the horn and rim of the adjacent skin.

dehorners (e.g. Portasol™ gas dehorner mark 3; Gas Buddex™) and rechargeable electric irons (e.g. Dairymac Steribud™; Horn'up™)

- from 1 to 4 months old (horn length 3–5 cm) a Barnes dehorning gouge (see Figure 4.1), Roberts dehorning trephine, or double-action hoof shears may be applied, followed by a disbudding iron for haemostasis
- older animals (older calves, yearlings, adults) are dehorned either by embryotomy (Gigli) wire, Barnes gouge, dehorning (butcher's) saw or dehorning shears

Restraint

- a purpose-built calf disbudding crate is best for both operator and patient: holds the calf and head securely; superior models include a belly support
- manual restraint of calf: hindquarters in a corner and head held with fingers placed below the jaw; assistant leaning against the shoulder region; halter advised for larger calves
- calves may be adequately handled in pens, a group of 10–20 being blocked and marked in sequence before carrying out the dehorning
- xylazine may be used in addition to local anaesthetic (see Section 1.9)
- stock over six months (>200 kg) will require a crush/chute and a halter

Technique of disbudding

- place the hot disbudding iron on the bud and rotate several times, angling the instrument so that the edge burns the skin around the periphery of the bud to include adequate germinal epithelium (see Figure 4.1)
- press down on the instrument, scoop and flick off the horn bud, leaving a crater, in the middle of which is a residual small cartilaginous protrusion, which may be left since it is not germinal epithelium
- operate on older calves by placing the Barnes dehorner blades precisely around the base of the horn bud and removing a small (3–5 mm) strip of skin at the same time as the bud is guillotined off. Achieve haemostasis with the hot disbudding iron
- alternatively, remove horns as short as 5 cm rapidly with embryotomy wire (more physical effort but minimal haemorrhage due to the heat)

Tip

Removing the skin at the centre of the horn bud is not strictly necessary as long as the full thickness of skin is cauterised around the periphery. However, removing the central skin is a practical method of ensuring adequate cautery: too little and the horn will grow; too much time/ pressure applied and bone necrosis may occur ± brain damage

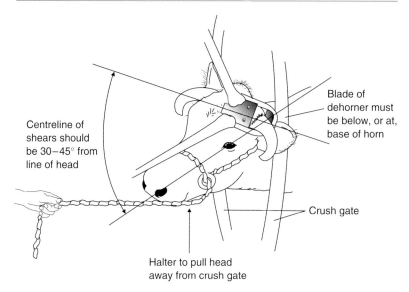

Centreline of
shears should
be 30–45° from
line of head

Blade of
dehorner must
be below, or at,
base of horn

Crush gate

Halter to pull head
away from crush gate

Figure 4.2 Position of the cow's head and of the dehorning shears (Keystone) or saw. Note that the haltered head is pulled forwards and to the side away from the crush gate, the cutting angle should be 30–45° and the blade or wire is placed on to the skin of the horn–skin junction.

Technique of dehorning

- sedation recommended
- cornual nerve block (see Section 1.9)
- for mature cattle (>18 months), inject additional 5–10 ml l.a. s.c. at the caudal base of the horn to block significant innervation from the first cervical nerve
- wait 10 minutes; then check with a needle that skin adjacent to the horn is painless
- ensure adequate restraint of the head in the gate of the crush and position the head (halter) so that considerable traction can be exerted on an embryotomy wire during sawing (see Figure 4.2)
- if using a saw, ensure the head is restrained so the operator is safe yet access to the medial aspect of the horn is possible
- wire: the first cut is made with wire on the caudolateral aspect; ensure the direction is caudolateral to the craniomedial; change of direction is difficult midcut
- saw: a cut can be made medial to lateral
- place the wire and saw so that the instrument passes through skin about 1 cm from the skin–horn junction

- blade or wire should emerge dorsally through the skin lateral to midline of the poll. In Friesian/Holstein cows residual width of midline skin should be 5–8 cm
- avoid interrupting the sawing movement in the middle of the dehorning process
- relatively narrow diameter horns (<5 cm) may be removed by a long-handled dehorning gouge (Barnes pattern). This instrument may also be useful in trimming off additional protruding lips of horn where the initial procedure has been too conservative

---

Discussion

- In yearling and adult cattle the preferred method is embryotomy (obstetrical, Gigli) wire, disadvantages being the physical effort and relatively slow speed. Advantages include neat appearance and less haemorrhage.
- The saw method is more unsightly and control of haemorrhage takes longer.
- Dehorning shears (e.g. Keystone dehorner) is the most rapid method but causes considerable haemorrhage. A major disadvantage is that a sudden violent head movement during closure of the guillotine blades can cause a shear fracture of the frontal bone and secondary wound problems including frontal sinusitis.

Haemostasis

- preferred method: torsion or torsion/traction on the 2–3 major vessels in the medial aspect (ventral crescent) of the peripheral skin; easily identified and picked up by haemostatic forceps; six to eight turns
- rubber tourniquet or string around the horn base applied in a pattern to exert pressure also on dorsal horn border
- if the horn is removed too high up: wooden toothpicks can be pushed into the bone canal, from which considerable blood can spurt (remove the toothpick the next day)
- cautery, e.g. hot iron: often ineffective by itself, particularly with large horns
- liberal use of bacteriostatic (e.g. sulfanilamide; not licensed in the EU) or haemostatic wound powder (Fe salts, tannic acid, alum)
- check dehorned cattle 2, 12 and 24 hours after surgery for any recurrence of bleeding, which may result from local irritation and pain leading to rubbing the cut surface against a wall

---

> **Warning**
>
> Do not expect heat from embryotomy wire to be sufficient alone to achieve adequate haemostasis; the effect will be temporary only.

Technique of cosmetic dehorning

- used in show cattle in North America
- gives an improved appearance following surgery, as the wound is closed by apposition of skin edges over the horn base
- carried out aseptically with the aim of primary healing; a sterile paper drape is optional
- should decrease the risk of post-operative sinusitis
- clip a skin band 8 cm wide over the poll and around each horn base; surgical skin preparation
- cornual nerve block (Section 1.9) and local analgesic infiltration caudal to the horn base and in midline
- make a transverse incision over the poll and laterally in a curved fashion, passing 0.5 cm from the horn–skin junction, the two wounds joining lateral to the horn base and continuing towards the mandibular joint for 5 cm (see Figure 4.3)
- undermine the skin peripherally from the incision far enough to avoid skin damage when the horn is removed by a saw or Barnes gouge
- avoid auricular muscle laterally
- remove more horn if necessary (sterile bone chisel and hammer, Barnes gouge) until the cut is exactly flush with the frontal bone
- clean the surface with sterile swabs and effect haemostasis
- undermine the skin further to enable edges to be apposed across the bone surface without excessive tension, and check cosmetic appearance; relief incisions are often required
- appose edges with interrupted sutures of monofilament polypropylene
- clean surface of all blood and debris; apply topical antibiotic
- remove sutures in 14 days

Possible complications of disbudding or dehorning

- side-effects (excessive salivation, mild ataxia, temporary collapse) caused by an inadvertent i.v. injection of analgesic solution in young calves
- failure to remove the horn bud completely in calves (inadequate depth of cautery) results in regrowth or 'scurs'

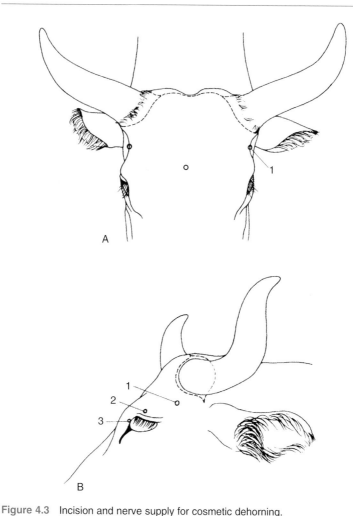

Figure 4.3 Incision and nerve supply for cosmetic dehorning.
(A) Rostral view: 'o' is the position for the captive bolt gun in euthanasia.
(B) Lateral view: 1. zygomaticotemporal nerve; 2. frontal nerve; 3. infratrochlear nerve; ---
skin incision.

- in older cattle frontal sinusitis (pneumatisation of the horn starts at eight to nine months) and empyema caused by entry of infection and fly strike in summer and autumn (see Section 4.2)
- poor surgical technique results in prolonged local irritation and an increased tendency for the cut surface to be rubbed against dirty surfaces (e.g. soil, bedding, walls)

Tip
• Avoid dehorning in the major fly season (e.g. in the UK from May to late September). • Avoid feeding hay or straw from overhead racks to reduce the risk of frontal sinusitis.

4.2 Trephination of frontal sinus (for empyema)

Indication

- frontal sinusitis with pus occupying this multiloculated structure and with chronic discharge through the horn base
- post-dehorning infection

Anatomy (Figures 4.4 and 4.5)

- the frontal sinus has several compartments: the large caudal frontal sinus is completely divided by an oblique partition into rostromedial and caudolateral sections
- the rostromedial compartment has a narrow nasofrontal opening and a post-orbital diverticulum
- the caudolateral compartment has the cornual diverticulum and nuchal diverticulum, which ends by also excavating the parietal, occipital and temporal bones
- two or three small chambers lie level with the rostral part of the orbit
- the borders of the frontal sinus are from the rostral part of the orbit to a transverse line drawn through the midline of the orbit, laterally to the frontal crest and caudally to the nuchal crest (poll). A midline septum separates the two frontal sinuses
- the normal small communication of the frontal sinus with the ethmoid sinus and the nasal cavity is usually occluded due to mucosal thickening and purulent discharge

Clinical signs of frontal sinus empyema

- chronic discharge of pus (e.g. from the dehorning wound)
- may pass into the maxillary region, sometimes with systemic illness (pyrexia, anorexia, loss of condition, head tilt, localised swelling and pain)
- some cases result from horn fracture, usually a direct result of uncontrolled movement of the head during dehorning (poor anaesthesia)
- sinusitis often confined initially to the caudal part of the sinus

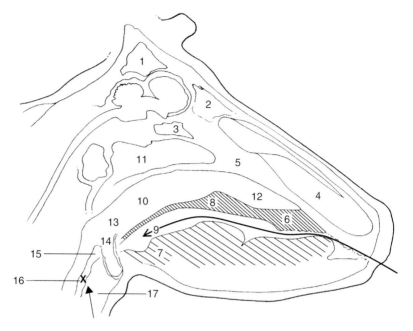

Figure 4.4   Median section through the head, left half. (From Pavaux, 1983.)
1. caudal frontal sinus; 2. medial rostral frontal sinus; 3. sphenoidal sinus; 4. nasal cavity; 5. nasal septum; 6. hard palate; 7. root of tongue; 8. soft palate; 9. isthmus faucium (oral part of pharynx, oropharynx); 10. nasal part of pharynx (nasopharynx); 11. pharyngeal septum; 12. nasopharyngeal meatus; 13. laryngeal part of pharynx (laryngopharynx); 14. entrance to larynx (laryngeal aditus); 15. vestibule of oesophagus; 16. oesophagus (cervical part); 17. cavity of larynx.
X shows the common site of the oesophageal obstruction; the long arrow shows the hand passed into the pharynx and the short arrow the retrograde pressure on oesophageal foreign body.

Restraint, anaesthesia and trephination landmarks

- restrain the animal adequately in a crush/chute and give a sedative
- clip the hair around the horn base and over the entire frontal region, cleanse and disinfect
- produce local analgesia by a supraorbital block (see Section 1.9) or infiltration over the site of the proposed trephine opening, located 5 cm dorsal to the line joining the two supraorbital processes and about 5 cm from the midline
- further landmark: 2–3 cm abaxial at the level of a horizontal line joining the axial parts of both orbits
- sometimes a soft area of bone indicates a suitable site

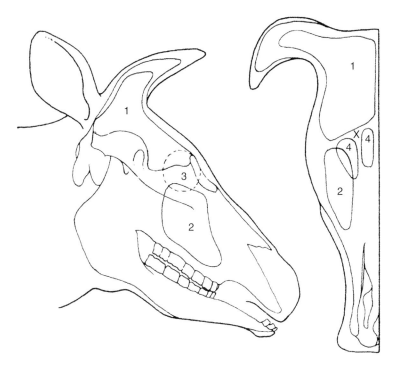

Figure 4.5 Diagram of longitudinal and rostral sections through the skull to show the extent of sinuses.
1. frontal sinus; 2. maxillary sinus; 3. position of orbit; 4. rostral compartments of frontal sinus; X trephine sites for empyema of frontal sinus. (Modified from Dyce and Wensing, 1971.)

- a ventral site is preferable if the horn sinus is still patent, permitting flushing from one opening to the other
- avoid the supraorbital foramen and vein (see Figure 1.5)

Technique

- remove a circular area of skin, subcutaneous tissue and cutaneous muscle 3 cm in diameter using a scalpel and forceps
- elevate the periosteum with a periosteal elevator and remove it with the scalpel
- trephine the bone over the sinus using a 2.5 cm diameter Galt or Horsley pattern trephine, and remove this bone disc
- flush the sinus initially with warm water using an enema pump
- insert the enema pump (Higginson's syringe) to direct an irrigation mixture into the various compartments

- continue irrigation through the horn sinus orifice
- irrigate finally with isotonic saline, flushing from top to bottom
- pick up any major bleeding points with artery forceps and keep the trephine opening patent for daily flushing by a stock person

Post-op care and possible complications

- avoid feeding hay/straw from an overhead rack
- in chronic cases, repeated lavage or a permanent through-and-through lavage system may be indicated
- the wound usually heals in three to four weeks
- parenteral medication (five to ten days with broad spectrum antibiotics) is indicated in animals with systemic signs and in all long-standing and severe cases
- as the trephine opening closes over, continue irrigation with a flexible polypropylene or PVC catheter attached to the syringe; it is helpful to suture the catheter in place
- prognosis is favourable (acute cases) to guarded (chronic cases)
- infection rarely (but sometimes!) extends to the opposite side of the skull or to the brain

4.3 Entropion

Introduction and signs

- low incidence, more common in over-conditioned beef breeds
- involves the lower lid more frequently than the upper lid
- often bilateral to a varying extent
- occasionally congenital, usually acquired (facial skin folds – particularly over-conditioned bulls)
- often exacerbated by halters (e.g. show animals)
- signs include mild blepharospasm, conjunctivitis, keratitis, and corneal ulceration if not corrected early
- rarely resolve spontaneously, progressing to blepharospasm and keratitis

Anaesthesia

- linear sub-conjunctival infiltration of anaesthetic solution parallel and 2 mm distant to the lid margin

Techniques

(a) careful insertion of 3 or 4 stainless steel staples into a horizontal fold of the lower lid is a simple and effective method of achieving eversion

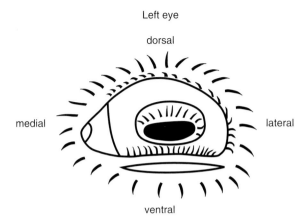

Left eye

dorsal

medial

lateral

ventral

Figure 4.6 Entropion correction involving the lower lid of the left eye with a skin incision 2 mm below the lid margin.

(b) alternatively the Holz–Celsus procedure is possible:
- estimate length and width of skin to be resected by pinching to produce an approximate skin fold to correct inversion of the lid margin
- scalpel incision to remove a ridge of skin previously measured (see Figure 4.6)
- close the wound margin with a single continuous or mattress absorbable suture e.g. PDS (avoiding the need for later removal)

(c) injection of a small volume (e.g. 1 ml) of long-acting antibiotic. The line in the lower lid may effect correction. This technique may allow temporary resolution during a weight-loss diet
- complications are unlikely, though under-correction may necessitate second surgery

4.4 Third eyelid flap

A suture placed in the third eyelid (nictitating membrane) is passed through the dorsal lateral conjunctival fornix to emerge through the skin. When tightened the third eyelid is drawn across the corneal surface.

Indications

- Cases of extensive but superficial corneal ulceration and of traumatic damage, often when antibiotic medication has failed to achieve early resolution of the lesion.

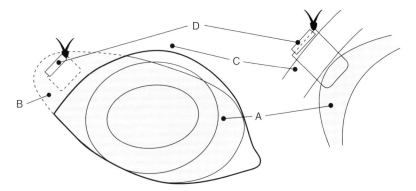

Figure 4.7 Third eyelid flap in the right eye. The shaded area is the third eyelid (A) sutured into the dorsolateral fornix, (B) by a suture through the skin and (C) supported by a 1.5 cm long plastic stent (D).
Note that the suture does not penetrate the full depth of the third eyelid and therefore does not contact the corneal surface.

Techniques (Figure 4.7)

- inject 2 ml of local anaesthetic into the third eyelid, which is grasped by fine Allis tissue forceps, and then 5 ml into the area of skin sutures
- thread PGA (Dexon®) or PDS 0 gauge suture material into a half-curved cutting needle
- grasp the edge of the third eyelid with Allis forceps again and place the suture through the palpebral surface of the lid about 5 mm from the edge. The suture should not penetrate the bulbar surface of the third eyelid (as this could cause subsequent corneal abrasion)
- now insert each end of the suture in turn through the lateral dorsal conjunctival fornix to emerge through the skin about 2–3 cm above the lateral commissure of the eyelids
- insert 1 cm of polypropylene stent on to the suture over the skin, and tie in a 'quick release' fashion with sufficient tension so that the third eyelid covers the entire visible surface of the cornea, including the lesion
- inspect the eyelid suture daily (stockperson), apply any local medication and possibly slacken off the suture to inspect the cornea in order to assess the healing process
- leave the suture for two to three weeks, then remove with scissors

Possible complications

- early tearing out of the suture from the third eyelid (insufficient tissue 'bite')
- failure to pull the flap sufficiently laterally (incorrect placement)
- tearing out of sutures through the skin due to the absence of a stent

- mechanical irritation of the corneal surface from the suture material (suture perforating the entire depth of the third eyelid, or is too slack, failing to pull the third eyelid completely across the cornea)

Discussion
No comparative studies are available on the success of this simple technique. Results are generally good as the bovine cornea heals well.

4.5 Eyelid lacerations

Introduction

- The upper or lower lid is sometimes torn following injury from a projecting nail, piece of metal or gate hinge
- sometimes a strip of the lower eyelid hangs down and the extent of the loss of the lid margin is very variable
- repair is urgently needed but initially the cornea should be carefully examined for damage

Restraint and clinical signs

- firm restraint in the crush with a halter applied
- topical anaesthesia and regional s.c. local anaesthesia
- consider xylazine for sedation
- examine the extent of the injury and check for any foreign bodies on the cornea and beneath the lids
- many lacerations are contaminated with vegetable matter and bleed profusely if seen shortly after an accident
- insert two drops of fluorescin dye to help identify a corneal laceration

Technique of repair

- do not trim off the strips of damaged eyelid, unless obviously non-viable; rub gently with a dry gauze swab to identify viable tissue
- do not clip the surrounding hair, since it is impossible to avoid hairs going on to the corneal surface, which leads to further trauma
- appose skin edges using figure of eight interrupted sutures (simple interrupted cruciate pattern) with fine (5-0) vicryl
- sutures should never contact the corneal surface
- maintenance of an intact eyelid margin is vital, so the first suture should precisely appose the eyelid margin, incorporating the firm tarsal plate and the *orbicularis oculi* muscle, which aids good wound apposition

- regular spraying with normal saline maintains clean field for sutures
- if the corneal surface is damaged, topical broad-spectrum antibiotics should be applied every few hours on the first day, and a least twice a day for a further week

Possible complications

- primary complications: dehiscence; suture rubbing on the cornea; ulcer not healing (if damaged cornea)
- secondary complications: trichiasis from irritation caused by eyelid hairs; exposure keratitis (poor tear film over the cornea) and chronic keratoconjunctivitis
- severe lacerations may require to be stented with the sutured lid being sutured to the opposing eyelid, and a trans-palpebral ocular lavage system built in for easy application of medication

4.6 Ocular foreign body

Indications and signs

- foreign bodies such as particles of chaff, burrs and thorns may lodge on the corneal surface, particularly in the lateral or medial canthus, and provoke a keratoconjunctivitis
- signs are obvious in recent cases with epiphora, ptosis, blepharospasm and discomfort
- chronic cases show corneal scarring and pigmented keratitis
- material may often be removed without local analgesia
- differential diagnosis includes conjunctivitis, iritis and uveitis

Techniques of removal

- place the animal in a chute with a halter attached; consider sedation
- suitable topical analgesics include amethocaine, xylocaine or proparacaine
- hold the head firmly and tilted in good light so that material is in midfield of the orbital fissure
- spray sterile saline through a 22 gauge needle hub tangentially at the foreign body in an attempt to dislodge it
- if unsuccessful then attempt removal with fine dissecting forceps or with a fine flat surface such as the blunt surface of a large scalpel blade
- assess superficial corneal damage subsequent to foreign body removal, following installation of one to two drops of fluorescein stain
- insert a topical broad spectrum antibiotic (e.g. cloxacillin) four times daily for three days after removal, or inject a subconjunctival antibiotic depot

- topical 1% atropine b.i.d. or to effect will maintain pupil dilatation; cortico-steroids are contraindicated as they hamper repair of any residual ulcer

Prognosis

- good, unless secondary infection is present, or secondary endophthalmitis has resulted from deep corneal perforation

4.7 Neoplasia of eyelids

Introduction

- most common neoplasm of the upper or lower lids and nictitating membrane (third eyelid) is squamous cell carcinoma (SCC) ('cancer eye')
- rarely, other tumours, such as papillomata, and fibrosarcoma
- SCC is most important in terms not only of incidence but also of economic importance and prognosis, especially in South West USA; the most common malignancy in cattle
- SCC is very invasive locally and may metastasise to the local lymph nodes (parotid, atlantal or retropharyngeal and the anterior cervical chain)

Warning

It is illegal in some countries to transport cattle with large (> 2 cm diameter) ocular tumours. In EU countries, generalised neoplasia renders the whole carcass unfit for human consumption. Quick action is advised with ocular neoplasia.

Clinical signs

- SCC is particularly common in Hereford and Simmental breeds and their crosses; approximately 85% of cattle with SCC lack pigment in the affected area
- the non-pigmented area is liable to develop neoplastic lesions under the influence of ultraviolet radiation from sunlight; there is often a precursor lesion
- affected cattle are usually four to nine years old
- lesion is often a proliferative irregular mass that may ulcerate through the skin and cause distress and blepharospasm
- early lesions appear either as rice-grain-like plaques on the sclera or corneal surface (which may regress), or as small firm nodules in the periocular dermis; this precursor of a greyish-white plaque at the nasal and temporal limbus develops into a papilloma and carcinoma in situ

- lid lesions often start as pale brown, horn-like teratomata
- differential diagnoses include ocular foreign body, traumatic injury and iritis

Treatment

- treatment is indicated in early lesions with no evidence of secondary spread either to adjacent structures (e.g. bone) or metastases to the drainage lymph nodes
- Several techniques are available and include:
  a. excisional surgery
  b. cryotherapy
  c. hyperthermia
  d. radiotherapy (rare)
  e. immunotherapy (rare)

(a) *Excisional surgery of third eyelid*

- sedation advised
- in a standing or recumbent animal induce analgesia by local anaesthetic infiltration of the base of the eyelid after instilling a topical anaesthetic solution (e.g. 0.5% proparacaine) into the conjunctival sac
- draw the third eyelid out by traction with forceps
- excise the eyelid as deep as possible to cartilage with curved scissors
- control haemorrhage with an adrenaline-soaked swab, or cryotherapy

(b) *Cryotherapy*

- cryotherapy is particularly advantageous since it avoids haemorrhage and is simple and relatively fast
- a small liquid nitrogen flask (e.g. Nitrospray®) is adequate for lesions up to 5 cm in diameter and 1 cm deep
- protect the globe from inadvertent freezing by inserting 'Styrofoam' strips or acrylic between the lid and corneal surface; apply water-soluble lubricants or vaseline to surrounding healthy skin
- clip and wash the affected area; wear latex gloves
- freeze the area twice (liquid nitrogen) or three times (nitrous oxide, carbon dioxide) initially using a spray tip
- freeze at least a 5 mm width border of clinically healthy tissue
- evert tissue lying close to the cornea by grasping with towel clips or Allis tissue forceps, before applying a probe head to deal with lesions of the third eyelid
- use thermocouples if available, inserting points 5 mm from the margin of lesion and stopping freezing when they indicate a temperature drop below $-20\,°C$

- disadvantages of cryotherapy are: lesions > 2.5 cm diameter require relatively prolonged application of a probe head for complete ice-ball formation; lesions exceeding 5 cm must be treated in two stages, or involve an initial surgical debulking procedure

(c) *Other techniques*
- radiofrequency hyperthermia: involves application of heat (50 °C for 30 seconds) to various surface points of the tumour and surrounding skin using a probe head; penetration is limited to 0.5–1 cm only
- radiotherapy: radon and gold seed implants have both been successfully used in valuable cattle; penetration again only to 0.5–1 cm
- immunotherapy: local infiltration of the mycobacterial cell wall fraction (Regressin-V®, no longer commercially available)

Possible complications

- recurrence possible: failure or inability to remove all the neoplastic tissue (SCC)
- wound breakdown

4.8 Enucleation (ocular exenteration)

Indications

- ocular neoplasia
- gross damage to the bulb, usually with severe primary or secondary infection
- trauma or rupture of the globe, resulting in anterior staphyloma or panophthalmitis, and a risk of ascending infection up the optic stalk
- enucleation (removal only of the globe) is rarely indicated in cattle; as a cosmetically satisfactory appearance it is not as important as in equines and small animals; exenteration (removal of the globe and orbital contents) is more common

Restraint and anaesthesia

- anaesthesia: GA if possible
- alternatively standing or recumbent under xylazine sedation and Peterson or retrobulbar block (see Section 1.9)
- or ophthalmic nerve analgesia and local infiltration of the lower lid and medial canthus

Technique of ocular exenteration

- clip, cleanse and disinfect peri-orbital area
- place continuous suture through the upper and lower lids

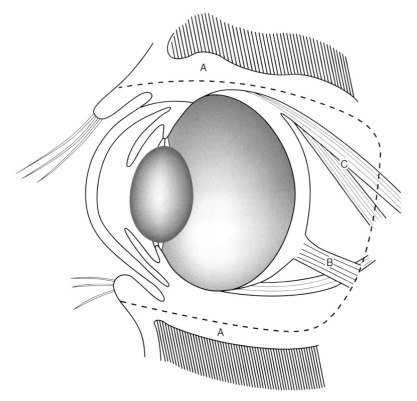

Figure 4.8 Exenteration of the eye (longitudinal diagrammatic section). Dotted line (A) starts in the lids, passes through the peri-orbital structures and results in removal of the globe, all orbital contents, eyelid margin and conjunctiva. B. optic nerve and vessels; C. muscles. Shaded areas above and below are frontal and zygomatic bones.

- perform lateral canthotomy (2 cm) to aid exposure of peri-orbital tissues
- using traction with towel clips or Allis tissue forceps, make a circumferential incision 1 cm from the skin–conjunctival junction, or as appropriate depending on the distribution of non-viable or neoplastic skin (see Figure 4.8)
- continue towards the orbital ridge down to, but not through, the conjunctiva
- exerting some digital traction on eye muscles, dissect the extraocular muscles bluntly with Mayo scissors from the lateral and medial canthus
- avoid excessive traction on the optic nerve (risk of vagal nerve stimulation and damage to optic chiasma)
- grasp the eyeball and use further gentle traction to dissect it free from surrounding retrobulbar tissue (excluding the conjunctival sac) and optic nerve

- if SCC, remove as much retrobulbar tissue as possible
- clamp the ophthalmic vessels, optic nerve and retractor bulbi muscle with slightly curved, long-handled artery forceps (Roberts 23 cm or Kelly 25 cm); ligate vessels with 7 metric chromic catgut (difficult: not essential)
- the third eyelid and Harderian gland will also be removed
- check the site for complete removal of all neoplastic or infected tissue
- meticulous haemostasis during enucleation is time-consuming and in most cases not necessary
- pressure pack the orbital space for a few minutes with sterile gauze swabs; remove and irrigate with aqueous antibiotic solution (20 ml)
- re-pack with a scrunched-up gauze bandage soaked in antibiotic, leaving a free end to protrude from the wound
- alternatively, insert absorbable gelatine sponges
- appose skin edges of lids using a simple continuous suture pattern (mono-filament nylon)
- leave the free end of the bandage packing (pressure haemostasis) protruding from one end of the wound
- administer systemic antibiotics for five to seven days, NSAIDs for three days, and tetanus prophylaxis as required
- insertion of a drain is rarely indicated
- remove the gauze bandage packing by pulling the free end gently after 2 days; this may be done in stages (i.e. half removed after 2 days and the remainder after 2 further days)
- remove the sutures two to three weeks later
- the resulting ankyloblepharon is cosmetically acceptable. Some cows become more nervous due to a restricted field of vision

Possible complications

- failure or inability to remove all neoplastic tissue (SCC)
- massive intraorbital haemorrhage
- abscess formation
- excessive dead space, and failure to appose the skin margin without excessive tension on sutures: relieving sutures may help

4.9 Insertion of a nose ring in a bull

Introduction

- a ring is used to aid restraint and control of a bull when being moved or in the show ring
- it is inserted into the soft tissue of the nasal septum immediately cranial to the cartilaginous septum
- a stock bull should have his ring inserted from 10 to 12 months old

Restraint

- confine the bull to a crush; sedation advised
- always apply a halter and firmly restrain to a fixed object (not a person)
- local anaesthetic injection is not helpful; some local anaesthesia via mucosal absorption is possible: hold cotton-wool soaked in procaine against the nasal septum. Wait 5 minutes

---

Warning

Take particular care working around adult stock bulls; each year several injuries and deaths are reported in the UK alone due to stock bulls. Common injuries include crushing and head trauma (e.g. fractured skull) resulting from being knocked over by the swipe of a bull's powerful head. This is far more likely than being charged.

Technique of insertion

- the septum must be punctured prior to inserting the sharp end of the open ring
- use a made-for-purpose bull ring hole punch (strongly advised)
- make a hole for the ring approximately 2–3 cm in, through the cartilaginous part of the septum
- a metal trocar and cannula can be used as an alternative: forced in one movement through the septum and the trocar is removed; the pointed end of the ring is placed into the cannula which is then slowly withdrawn so that the ring emerges through the wound
- once in place, the ring is quickly closed, and the screw inserted and turned rapidly
- smooth off the surface of the screw and the hinge section with sandpaper if necessary; most rings now incorporate a screw where the head can be snapped off so it is flush with the ring
- systemic antibiotics are usually not required but there is a small risk of tetanus

---

Tip

The small nose-ring screw is easily lost on the ground. Either attach a length of fine, coloured cotton on to the screw to ease detection if dropped or carry a spare.

Possible complications

- a nose ring is designed to last a lifetime
- if pulled out accidentally, as when caught on a sharp pointed object (e.g. fencing) then a nasal septum can potentially be repaired by careful surgery and heals after 4–6 weeks
- repair should be done as soon as possible, as granulation tissue development will hinder surgery
- it is unlikely that a repair will be strong enough for a new ring; possibly a larger ring, inserted more caudally in the septum, may be used

4.10 Tracheotomy

Introduction

- necrotic and purulent laryngitis is caused by *Fusobacterium necrophorum* infection and *Trueperella pyogenes* abscessation respectively, or may be secondary to intra- or retrolaryngeal foreign bodies or other mechanical irritants (dust, repeated coughing due to other pathogens)
- indications for tracheotomy rarely involve pharyngolaryngeal neoplasia, retropharyngeal abscessation, foreign bodies in the upper respiratory tract, or persistent laryngospasm
- surgical conditions of head involving haemorrhage and potential aspiration of blood and infected tissue should be managed with an endotracheal tube in position
- the tube should only be removed after the return of a cough and swallow reflexes

Clinical signs

- signs indicative of the need for tracheotomy, often an emergency procedure, include progressive dyspnoea, stridor, and mild cyanosis
- some animals have fetid breath (*F. necrophorum*) and pharyngeal lesions, which can be both seen and palpated
- a mouth gag should be inserted and a long-bladed laryngoscope or endoscope used to aid examination

Anatomy

- tracheal rings are readily appreciated on deep palpation of the upper part of the neck
- diameter is narrow compared with equine trachea
- depth is slightly greater than width

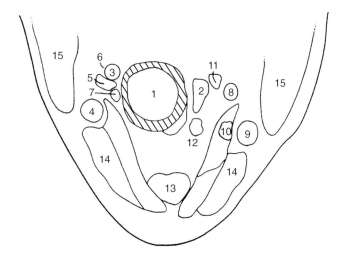

Figure 4.9   Cross-section of the neck at the level of the fifth cervical vertebra, ventral part, looking caudally.
1. trachea; 2. oesophagus; 3. right common carotid artery; 4. right external jugular vein; 5. right internal jugular vein; 6. right vagosympathetic trunk; 7. right recurrent laryngeal nerve; 8. left common carotid artery; 9. left external jugular vein; 10. left internal jugular vein; 11. left vagosympathetic trunk; 12. left recurrent laryngeal nerve; 13. sternohyoid and sternothyroid muscles; 14. sternocephalic muscle; 15. brachiocephalic muscle. (From Pavaux, 1983.)

- trachea is related at the junction of the upper and middle thirds of the neck to the oesophagus on the left side, and to the carotid sheath, enclosing the common carotid artery, vagosympathetic trunk and internal jugular vein on the right and to a lesser extent on the left. It is deep to the distinct and bulky sternomandibular and the finer sternothyrohyoid muscles, which are fine muscular bands on the ventral tracheal surface (see Figure 4.9, which is a cross-section somewhat distal to the preferred tracheostomy site)

Restraint and anaesthesia

- perform surgery preferably on a haltered animal in a crush with the head and neck extended
- sedate with xylazine only if necessary: not animals with signs of severe cardiovascular and respiratory dysfunction
- local s.c. infiltration of the surgical site with local anaesthetic

Technique

- keep the head and neck extended
- identify the midline in the upper third of the neck at the level of tracheal rings 4–6
- clip and disinfect the skin over this area and make a 6 cm longitudinal incision through the skin and subcutis directly over the tensed trachea
- separate the paired sternomandibular muscles in the midline by blunt dissection, followed by sternothyrohyoid muscles
- insert a self-retaining wound retractor (West or Gossett model): not essential
- **temporary tracheotomy tube**: incise the tracheal annular ligament; **do not incise tracheal rings**
- insert the tracheal tube; various models are available. In a calf the maximum diameter may be 13 mm; these are commercially available. Some tubes are up to 14 mm in diameter (Portex Blue Line®) and have external tapes for fixation
- anchor the tube to the skin at two points to prevent rotation. Tie loosely to allow removal for cleaning
- **permanent tracheotomy tube**: resect two half-moon shaped segments of adjacent tracheal rings corresponding to the size of the tracheal tube (see Figure 4.10). This form of tracheal incision maintains the tracheal lumen, which can otherwise collapse when incision involves an entire cranio-caudal section of ring
- use an equine steel tracheotomy tube (see Figure 4.11) with an internal diameter of 22 mm (Kruuse veterinary products)

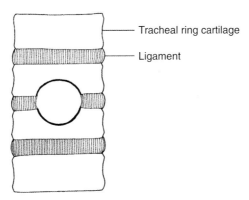

Tracheal ring cartilage

Ligament

Figure 4.10 Diagram of a tracheostomy incision to show a portion of two adjacent rings resected to permit insertion of a tracheotomy tube.

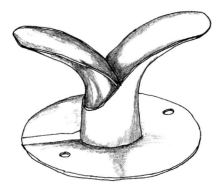

Figure 4.11 Stainless steel or nickel-plated brass tracheotomy tube (internal diameter 22 mm; external diameter 28 mm).

- insert one half and then thread the second part through the first; the fitting is usually tight and brings the trachea close to the skin
- suture in place (nylon), though a tight fit usually secures it in place

---

Warning: Risk of Tracheal Collapse

The C-shaped cartilage rings are completed dorsally by a flexible ligament; hasty section of the rings ventrally will result in a collapsing trachea under negative pressure during inspiration unless held open by a tracheotomy tube. Although often acute in onset and requiring rapid treatment, it may be preferable to treat laryngeal obstruction medically initially (e.g. corticosteroids) unless a permanent tracheotomy tube is immediately available (Figure 4.11).

Post-operative care

- silicone temporary tracheotomy tubes require frequent (minimal twice daily) cleaning of both the tracheal lumen and external surface
- the relative quantity of debris and inflammatory discharge is greater than in horses
- skin scalding by exudate is reduced by petrolatum jelly (petroleum jelly or Vaseline™)
- remove the tube after alleviation of the primary condition, which may require systemic antibiotics alone, or combined surgery (drainage of the laryngeal abscess in calves) and antibiotic therapy and NSAIDs
- do not suture the tracheal or skin wounds
- avoid hay dust in the immediate environment to reduce possible iatrogenic bronchopneumonia

Possible complications

- a major complication is the extension of granulation tissue from the wound margin to partially occlude the tracheal lumen. Resect proliferative tissue by electrocautery
- the prognosis for cattle requiring tracheotomy should always remain guarded

---

Discussion

Temporary tracheotomy tubes are *very* difficult to manage successfully, and swelling/chondroma formation after removal can cause tracheal stenosis and severe dyspnoea. Complete relapse and death is not uncommon. A temporary tracheotomy tube will necessarily have a restricted diameter because the cartilage must not be cut prior to insertion. They are more suitable for smaller (<200 kg) animals.

A permanent tracheotomy using a metal equine tube is more likely to be successful in a heavy beef animal until it can be slaughtered for human consumption. Tubes may stay in place with little maintenance for approximately six months.

4.11 Oesophageal obstruction ('choke')

Aetiology and signs

- usually due to round or irregular pieces of food material, e.g. potato, turnip or sugar beet, rarely to sugar beet pulp (cf. horse)
- copious salivation and rumen bloat are the most obvious signs
- bovine rabies or tetanus sometimes present with similar signs
- often can be relieved by medical means (e.g. tranquilizers such as phenothiazine derivatives, relaxants) and manual retrograde manipulation
- site of obstruction is usually the proximal cervical oesophagus, often in the first 20 cm (see Figure 4.4); rarely the distal cervical or thoracic oesophagus
- distal thoracic oesophageal obstruction is sometimes seen in calves due to swallowing of stomach feeders following oral rehydration therapy
- oesophageal obstruction causing recurrent bloat (but not usually salivation) can result from external compression (thymic lymphosarcoma, mediastinal lymphadenopathy, e.g. calves with pneumonia) and neurogenic dysfunction (rabies, tetany)
- rarely life-threatening as long as care is taken to control development of rumenal tympany: insert a temporary rumenal canula

---

Tip

Most cases of choke (obstruction) from feedstuffs will resolve spontaneously within 24 hours due to softening from saliva. Insert a rumen trocar and cannula to create a temporary rumen fistula, which will avoid life-threatening rumen tympany.

   This conservative approach is recommended over passing a probang or other tubing, which may cause oesophageal tear or rupture.

Warning

Oesophageal surgery in the field should be an absolute last resort: the oesophagus is not a forgiving tissue for surgery and the prognosis is always very guarded. Oesophagotomy is in any case only practical in proximal two-thirds of the cervical part, where the organ is relatively accessible.

Surgical techniques of oesophagotomy

- identify the site of obstruction and, if not palpable, ascertain by gently passing a stomach tube
- delay radical surgery a minimum of 24 hours, pending medical relief (e.g. xylazine)
- perform surgery under GA or with a sedated animal in right lateral recumbency with good head restraint
- infiltrate a local anaesthetic solution after routine skin preparation
- perform surgery with strict aseptic precautions
- the oesophagus lies in deep fascia to the left of the trachea and overlaid by the left jugular vein and the carotid sheath enclosing the carotid and vagosympathetic trunk
- keep tissues tense and the surgical field convex, elevated by an underlying pad or manually by a sterile assistant, and attempt again to move a foreign body retrograde into the pharynx
- incise the skin to an adequate length (twice the length of the foreign body) and bluntly dissect down to the oesophageal wall
- carefully identify and reflect the jugular and carotid trunk dorsally
- incise the thin oesophageal wall longitudinally, preferably in an undamaged section, and carefully remove the obstruction, using gauze swabs to avoid surgical field contamination by saliva and food debris
- close the oesophageal wall (unless necrotic) with simple interrupted absorbable sutures
- place sutures 5 mm apart through the mucosa and muscularis

- over-sew the muscularis in the second layer of simple continuous PGA sutures, including fascia for increased strength
- irrigate the area well with sterile saline before routine skin closure
- insert a Penrose drain along the external oesophageal wall to emerge at the ventral (caudal) commissure of the skin wound in cases where contamination is thought likely to result in infection and secondary healing
- systemic antibiotics for 5 days, tetanus prophylaxis
- remove the drain after 48 hours
- do not suture the oesophagus in cases of full depth mural necrosis, but leave as an open fistula with a supplementary drain
- though lying adjacent to the oesophagus, it should be easy to avoid damage to the common carotid artery (dorsolateral) and jugular vein (ventrolateral)
- a distal oesophageal obstruction (broken stomach feeders, see above) is treated by removal via rumenotomy

Possible complications

- always a guarded prognosis
- it is difficult to ensure the primary healing of an oesophageal incision, but chances are improved by keeping the animal on fluids for two days, followed by three days of mash and short-cut fodder
- post-operative oesophageal stricture may occur

CHAPTER 5

Abdominal surgery

5.1 Topography

Topography of the forestomachs and abomasum (see Figure 5.1) is incorporated in descriptions of approach (e.g. left flank laparotomy, traumatic reticulitis). The complex topography of the intestinal tract is considered in this introduction.

The intestinal tract

- the small intestine includes the duodenum (cranial including the S-shaped flexure, descending and ascending parts), jejunum and ileum
- the large intestine is comprised of the caecum, ascending colon (proximal loop, spiral loop (centripetal and centrifugal coils), distal loop), transverse colon, descending colon and rectum

Bovine Surgery and Lameness, Third Edition. A. David Weaver, Owen Atkinson, Guy St. Jean and Adrian Steiner.
© 2018 John Wiley & Sons Ltd. Published 2018 by John Wiley & Sons Ltd.
Companion website: www.wiley.com/go/weaver/bovine-surgery

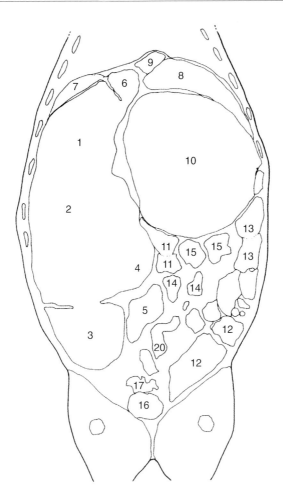

Figure 5.1 Horizontal section of the trunk at mid-height of the thorax and thighs, looking ventrally.
1–5. rumen: 1. atrium (cranial sac); 2. dorsal sac; 3. caudodorsal blind sac; 4. ventral sac; 5. caudoventral blind sac; 6. reticulum; 7. spleen; 8. liver; 9. caudal vena cava; 10. omasum; 11. jejunum; 12. caecum; 13–15. ascending colon: 13. proximal loop; 14. spiral loop; 15. distal loop; 16. urinary bladder; 17. uterine horns. (From Pavaux, 1983.)

Position and course

- The muscular pylorus is very movable but positioned between the lesser omentum dorsally and the greater omentum ventrally, and situated level with the costochondral junction of ribs 9 and 10 on the right side (see Figures 5.2 and 5.3). The cranial duodenal loop passes craniodorsally, initially freely mobile, but with the next portion firmly adherent to the visceral hepatic surface. It curves in an S-shaped manner near the bile and pancreatic duct openings, and becomes the descending loop, which is suspended dorsally by the mesoduodenum, and the loop passes caudally in the dorsal and right lateral part of the abdominal cavity (see Figure 5.2). Superficial and deep layers of the greater omentum attach to the ventral surface of the descending loop of the duodenum.

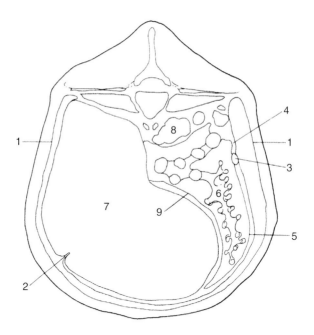

Figure 5.2 Distribution of the greater omentum, viewed diagrammatically through a vertical section of the abdomen, about lumbar vertebra 3.
1. parietal peritoneum; 2. insertion into left longitudinal groove of the rumen of the superficial layer of the greater omentum; 3. duodenum; 4. mesoduodenum (cranially the lesser omentum); 5. deep and superficial layers of greater omentum; 6. intestinal mass in supraepiploic recess; 7. rumen; 8. left kidney; 9. deep layer of greater omentum inserting on to right longitudinal groove of rumen. (Modified from Dyce and Wensing, 1971.)

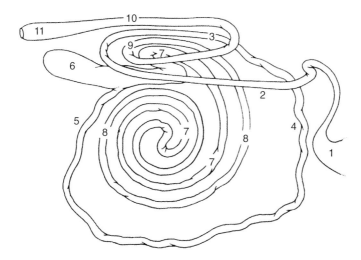

Figure 5.3 Diagrammatic representation of the small and large intestine, viewed from the right side.
1. pylorus; 2. descending limb of duodenum; 3. ascending limb of duodenum; 4. proximal jejunum; 5. distal jejunum and ileum; 6. caecum; 7. proximal loop and centripetal gyri of colon; 8. centrifugal gyri of colon; 9. ascending terminal colon; 10. descending colon; 11. rectum. Length (in adult) of small intestine is 35–50 m, that of the large intestine is 10 m.

- The duodenum turns cranially at the caudal flexure, where it is attached to the descending colon by the duodenocolic ligament, and becomes the ascending loop to pass cranially to the left side of the mesenteric root. It turns to the right side of the root to become the jejunum.
- The jejunum, 35–50 m long, comprises a mass of tight coils at the edge of the mesentery. The greatest intestinal mass is formed by these heaped coils of jejunum. The mesentery of the proximal and middle sections is short, that of the distal part and that attached to the ileum are longer, forming a mobile section that lies in the caudal aspect of the supraomental recess or caudally thereof. The ileum comprises a convoluted proximal segment and a distal straight part. The junction of the jejunum and ileum is the point where the cranial mesenteric artery ends and the cranial limit of the ileocaecal fold. The ileum is attached to the caecum ventrally, the orifice lying obliquely on the ventral surface of the caecum, and readily identified in adulthood due to the fat pad overlying it.
- The caecum is a mobile sac, with the blind end directed caudally. Cranially the caecum is continuous with the proximal loop of the ascending colon. The short caecocolic fold attaches the caecum to the colon dorsally.

The caecum often extends caudally to the limits of the supraomental recess.

- The proximal loop of the ascending colon passes cranially to the level of T12 and then turns caudally to pass dorsally to the first segment. It again turns cranially, but now to the left of the mesentery, and then ventrally to become the spiral loop of the ascending colon. The arrangement comprises two centripetal, followed by two centrifugal coils (see Figure 5.3). The central flexure is the midpoint and the change in direction of the spiral colon. The distal portion of the spiral colon is normally adjacent to the ileum. The distal loop of the ascending colon passes caudally along the left side of the mesentery, around which it turns to run cranially again, adjacent to the proximal colon. It then becomes the transverse colon, which passes from the right to the left side, around the cranial edge of the cranial mesenteric artery.
- The descending colon proceeds caudally along the dorsal surface of the abdomen, attached by the mesocolon. The mesocolon is rather elongated at the level of the duodenocolic ligament, affording it some mobility. The descending colon terminates in the rectum, which lies entirely within the pelvis.
- The relative shortness of the mesentery means that exteriorisation of the intestine is difficult in many areas. Vessels and lymph nodes within the mesentery are hard to identify due to the fat deposition. The ascending duodenum, proximal and distal loops of ascending colon and the cranial portion of the descending colon lie close to one another due to the near-fusion of their mesenteries. The cranial mesenteric vessels supply the small and large intestines, except for parts of the duodenum and colon.
- The greater omentum passes from its origin on the duodenum, pylorus and greater curvature of the abomasum, encircles the intestinal mass and inserts on the left longitudinal groove of the rumen (superficial part), while the deep part passes similarly ventral and to the left, to attach to the right longitudinal groove of the rumen. These two parts are fused caudally, forming the caudal fold. The lesser omentum extends from the oesophagus along the reticular groove and omasal base to attach to the lesser curvature of the abomasum and covers most of the parietal surface of the omasum.

Abdominal viscera (see also Figure 5.7 later)

Viscera that contact the left abdominal wall (see Figures 5.1, 5.2, 5.4 and 5.5):

- cranially and ventrally: reticulum
- laterally ribs 10–12 dorsally, ribs 7–8 ventrally: spleen
- laterally: rumen covered ventrally by the greater omentum from the left longitudinal groove
- laterally and (sublumbar) dorsally: perirenal fat
- ventrally and caudally: sometimes coils of jejunum and ileum

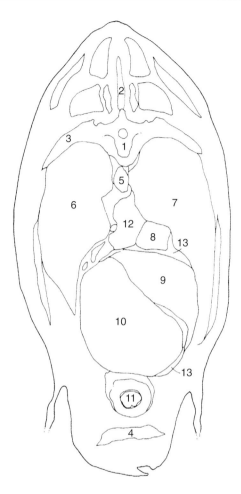

Figure 5.4   Cross-section of the thorax through the body of the seventh thoracic vertebra, looking cranially.
1. body of seventh thoracic vertebra; 2. spinous process of sixth thoracic vertebra; 3. seventh rib; 4. sternum; 5. thoracic duct and aorta; 6. left lung; 7. right lung; 8. caudal vena cava; 9. liver; 10. reticulum; 11. apex of heart; 12. accessory lobe of right lung; 13. central tendon and sternal part of diaphragm. (From Pavaux, 1983.)

Viscera that contact the right abdominal wall:

- cranially and ventrally: reticulum and abomasum
- laterally and cranially (ribs 7–12): liver
- laterally (rib 7 ventrally, rib 12 dorsally): descending loop of duodenum and greater omentum

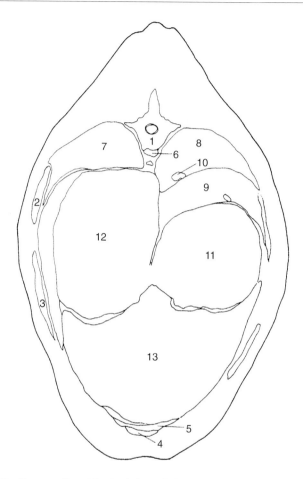

Figure 5.5 Cross-section of the trunk through the body of the ninth thoracic vertebra, looking cranially.
1. body of ninth thoracic vertebra and head of ninth rib; 2. eighth rib; 3. seventh rib; 4. xiphoid process of sternum; 5. sternal part; 6. thoracic aorta (thoracic duct, to right, and left azygos vein, to left, coursing along it dorsolaterally); 7. left lung (caudal lobe); 8. right lung (caudal lobe); 9. liver; 10. caudal vena cava; 11. omasum; 12. atrium (cranial sac) of rumen; 13. reticulum. (From Pavaux, 1983.)

Viscera that do not normally contact the body wall:

- omasum at the level of ribs 8–11, lying ventrally to the right of midline
- jejunum
- caecum and ascending colon (caudal midabdomen), transverse and descending colon

- left kidney (level with vertebrae 2–4) and right kidney (thoracic vertebra 13–lumbar 2)
- uterus and ovaries: uterus in advanced pregnancy (gestation month seven) may contact lower left and/or right flank

5.2 Exploratory laparotomy (celiotomy), left flank

Indications

- specific indications may include suspected left displaced abomasum (LDA) (see Section 5.6), rumenotomy, traumatic reticuloperitonitis (see Section 5.4) or caesarean section (see Section 6.1)
- LDA is evident on opening into the peritoneal cavity
- traumatic reticuloperitonitis may be suspected on exploration of the area between the cranial aspect of ruminoreticulum and the diaphragm-body wall area. In positive cases specific surgical correction is performed; indication is often not clear cut. Some cattle show persistent abdominal pain apparently localised to the ruminal area
- left flank exploratory laparotomy is rarely as useful or as practical as the right flank approach and is not recommended if a small or large intestinal surgical disorder is suspected

Technique

- paravertebral analgesia (nerves T13, L1 and L2) or local infiltration (see Section 1.9)
- clip, scrub and surgically prepare a wide area of the left flank including at least 30 cm around the proposed incision site (see Figure 5.6)
- drape with sterile cloths or plastic drape with an appropriate window
- make a paracostal incision 20 cm long about 5–8 cm behind the last rib, starting 10 cm below lumbar transverse processes (incision 2, Figure 5.6)
- incise the skin in a single movement and continue the scalpel incision through subcutaneous fat and fascia to expose the abdominal wall musculature
- insert the blade of straight scissors at an angle of 45° to the surface and into the external oblique abdominal muscle, which is separated by a blunt dissection
- make a 20 cm long scalpel incision through the internal oblique muscle to expose the underlying transverse fascia and transverse muscle
- make an 18 cm long incision with scissors through this fascia and muscle to reveal the parietal peritoneum beneath a variable amount of loose fat
- pick up the parietal peritoneum with rat-tooth forceps and make an incision with scissors; air rushes audibly into the abdominal cavity when opening the peritoneum, creating pneumoperitoneum, and the contact surface of the

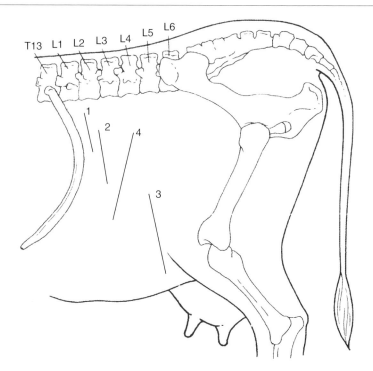

Figure 5.6   Position of various left flank incisions.
1. paracostal (15–25 cm), cranial in sublumbar fossa: rumenotomy (essential to be as far cranial as possible in large-framed cow and short surgeon); 2. left flank abomasopexy (Utrecht technique) or exploratory laparotomy (20 cm); 3. low flank incision in recumbent cow or heifer for caesarean section, where it is anticipated that it will be difficult to bring uterine wall to flank (35 cm); 4. oblique flank incision (35–40 cm) for caesarean section in standing animal.

ruminal wall (unless adhesed) drops away as the abdominal wall moves laterally
- occasionally some pneumoperitoneum is present before surgery, e.g. in traumatic reticulitis)
- left side of the abdominal cavity and part of the right side may now be explored (see Figure 5.7)

Visible and palpable features

- check the colour and volume of the peritoneal fluid; the normal colour is pale yellow and the normal volume is scant; a slight pink tinge may be due to contamination of some blood from the incision site

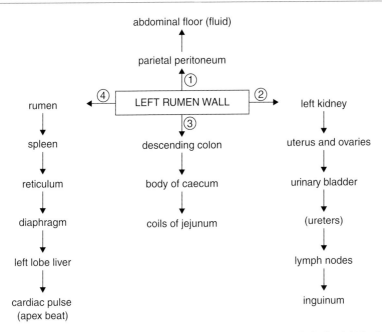

Figure 5.7 Flow diagram of the left flank exploratory examination. As in the right flank approach (see Figure 5.8) the entire accessible part of the abdominal cavity should be rapidly checked in any abdominal disease. Start from the left ruminal wall with palpation of the parietal peritoneum (1), then caudal abdomen (2) and the right side structures (3), before concentrating on the left flank and the left cranial and ventral regions (4).

- presence of any floccules, usually purulent, is abnormal and indicates an infective focus in the visceral or parietal peritoneum; possibly also an associated objectionable odour
- run fingers over the surface of both parietal and ruminal (visceral) peritoneum adjacent to the incision: the surface should be smooth. Irregularities may be in the form of discrete adhesions or generalised lesion ('sandpaper-like') consistent with chronic peritonitis
- LDA, if present, will be obvious as the abomasum will be between the rumen and body wall on the left-hand side, possibly quite high up in the flank
- structures palpated in the caudal abdominal area and pelvic area should include: left kidney through peri-renal fat, path of ureters (normally non-palpable unless thickened), bladder including the bladder neck, uterus, left and right ovaries, and descending colon
- pass the right hand and arm to the right abdominal wall by directing it caudally to the attachment of the ruminal wall to the abdominal roof, and ventrally to the left kidney and descending colon. Structures now accessible

include: spiral colon, duodenum, jejunum and ileum, caecum and caudal border of the greater omentum (see Figures 5.1 to 5.3)

- pass the hand cranially to check for adhesions between the body wall and spleen, reticulum and diaphragm or liver, or (rarely) between the rumen and abdominal wall, suggestive of traumatic reticuloperitonitis; adhesions may be of a recent origin and significant or long-standing and an incidental finding. Avoid breaking adhesions down unnecessarily as it is likely to be counterproductive
- it is usually not possible to palpate: abomasum (unless displaced), much of the visceral surface of the liver and the gall bladder, the omasum, right kidney, some of the small intestine and pylorus

5.3 Exploratory laparotomy, right flank

The right laparotomy site may be variable depending on purpose. Typically it is in the middle of the paralumbar fossa, the vertical incision starting 15–30 cm ventral to the transverse processes of the lumbar vertebrae and is 10–25 cm in length.

Tip

Take special care in the peritoneal incision on the right flank as the descending duodenum is immediately below.

A more dorsal incision is preferable to reduce the spontaneous prolapse of viscera through incision, but a more ventral incision (25–35 cm below the transverse process in Holstein) is easier for replacement of LDA and will allow a more anatomically correct fixation: use as small an incision as possible (small hands and arms are distinctly advantageous!). For LDA correction, it is also easier to make the incision close to the last rib (cranial) in order to reach beneath the rumen for the abomasum.

Visible and palpable features (see Figure 5.8)

- note the greater omentum below the incision, with the descending duodunum lying horizontally in the omentum
- pass a hand and arm cranioventrally to palpate abomasum (if not displaced); note some mobility is possible and the pyloric part of the abomasum may be grasped and pulled upwards towards the incision
- appreciate the cranially visceral surface of the liver (note any rounded edges, abscesses or surface irregularity) with the dependent gall bladder (normal size up to $10 \, cm \times 6 \, cm \times 4 \, cm$), and insert a hand between the

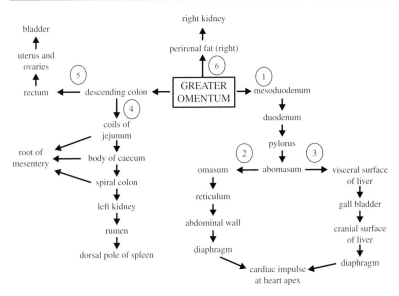

Figure 5.8   Flow diagram of the right flank exploratory laparotomy. The entire accessible abdominal cavity should be checked in any case of suspected abdominal disease. In a case of LDA the abomasum is not found on the right side (step 1), but against the left abdominal wall. Nevertheless, steps 2 and 3 should be followed to rule out co-existing traumatic reticulitis or liver abscessation. In suspect cases of small or large intestinal disease or displacement, step 4 should be followed, but exploration of the remainder of the abdominal cavity should be carried out at a later stage.

liver and diaphragm to palpate the cranial hepatic surface, e.g. discrete abscessation
- pass a hand along the lateral body wall ventrally to locate the omasum and reticulum (note any adhesions or foreign bodies)
- check the contact area of the reticulum with the diaphragm (possible adhesions)
- pass a hand dorsally to the incision and note that the mesoduodenum is dorsal to the duodenum and deep to this area is the perirenal fat and the right kidney
- pass a hand caudally to caudal edge of the greater omentum, which runs approximately midway between the last rib and the *tuber coxae*
- palpate the structures in this space, which include numerous coils of the jejunum and ileum, as well as the spiral colon, caecum, which is very variable in size, and the dorsally ascending colon and descending colon (see Figure 5.3)
- some intestine, which may be exteriorised for examination, includes much of the jejunum (except cranially), apex and body of the caecum, and more ventral loops of the ascending spiral colon

- note, suspended from the midline (palpable but cannot be exteriorised), the descending colon and part of the ascending colon, passing into the pelvic cavity together with the bladder, uterus and ovaries
- pass a hand dorsally within the supraomental recess to palpate the left kidney, which is to the right of the midline. To the left of the kidney, palpate the rumen with the dorsal and ventral blind sacs
- passing your hand over the dorsal blind sac of the rumen to the left side of the abdomen and passing further cranially, you reach the dorsal pole of the spleen, which is attached to the rumen; a left displaced abomasum can be palpated between the rumen and the left body wall

Closure of flank laparotomy incision

- there are many options for closing a flank incision
- **three layer technique** (see Figure 5.9a): appose the peritoneum and transverse fascia with a continuous suture of 4 metric PDS on a 3/8 circle round-bodied needle; commence the suture at the ventral commissure and tie off dorsally
- close the external and internal oblique abdominal muscles together with a similar single layer
- appose the skin with a Ford interlocking suture of monofilament nylon or Supramid® inserted with a cutting-edged semi-curved needle
- close the ventral 5 cm with interrupted sutures, which may be removed later for drainage of any wound infection
- note that in all three layers, sutures should be just tight enough to appose the wound edges. In the muscle layers the suture should be spaced about one every 2 cm, while in the skin slightly more are advised

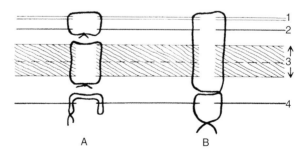

Figure 5.9 Transverse section through the flank (diagrammatic) showing two methods of closing laparotomy wounds. (A) a three layer closure; (B) a single layer figure-of-eight closure.
1. peritoneum; 2. transverse fascia/muscle, 3. internal and external oblique muscles; 4. skin.

- **four layer technique**: it is possible to suture internal and external oblique abdominal muscles separately, if the incision is caudal in the flank
- **two layer technique**: quick and efficient; all muscle layers and peritoneum (not essential) are closed with simple interrupted or simple interrupted cruciate sutures (figure of eight). The skin is closed with Ford interlocking or simple interrupted cruciate sutures
- **single layer technique** (see Figure 5.9b): is fast but less cosmetically pleasing and any wound infection is liable to be more severe
- avoid leaving any dead space

Intra-abdominal and systemic antimicrobial therapy

- routine intra-abdominal medication is unnecessary
- peritonitis is controlled by systemic medication if the animal is not culled
- drainage of purulent exudate is unlikely to help control if an active process
- intra-abdominal medication should be considered only if infection has been introduced into the peritoneal cavity; suitable drugs include antibiotic aqueous solutions or oleaginous suspensions as carriers. Intramammary preparations should not be inserted into the abdominal cavity or body wall
- most effective prophylactic medication is systemic injection of penicillin, amoxypenicillin or oxytetracycline hydrochloride

Possible complications

- collapse of patient: occasionally a weak patient undergoing a 'last-ditch' exploratory laparotomy collapses during intra-abdominal exploration, causing gross peritoneal contamination. Such cattle, usually thin cows, are unsuitable subjects for surgery and should be excluded on pre-operative clinical examination
- wound dehiscence: results from non-sterile, excessively fine material, material traumatised by forceps before or during insertion, massive wound swelling causing tearing out of sutures and development of a subcutaneous or subperitoneal abscess, or emphysema
- treatment of wound dehiscence: in such cases any remaining (nonfunctional) suture material should be removed and the wound cleansed, débrided and resutured. If healthy granulation tissue developed, infection is only superficial and this tissue can be resected (third intention healing), leaving a 3–10 cm opening in the ventral commissure for drainage purposes
- cases with copious purulent discharge involving a still relatively intact wound may be opened slightly, both dorsally and ventrally, to permit irrigation with clean tap water or isotonic saline (preferable). Note that infection may spread between tissue layers

5.4 Rumenotomy

Indications

- removal of perforating foreign body in traumatic reticulitis or reticuloperitonitis
- gross severe rumen overload ('grain overload') involving acidosis following sudden ingestion of a large volume of concentrates (barley, etc.), and, rarely, recent ingestion of toxic plant material (e.g. yew). The latter is usually fatal
- exploratory surgery, e.g. in chronic intermittent rumen tympany, for example for removal of a soft foreign body (rope), responsible for reticulo-omasal outflow obstruction

Traumatic reticulitis/reticuloperitonits

Incidence

- usually encountered sporadically in cattle over two years old
- occasionally farmers may experience a series of cases in a few weeks or months, associated with ingestion of a particular batch of feed or forage
- cases are more common when feeding conserved forage

Aetiology

- most foreign bodies ingested by cattle fail to penetrate the ruminoreticular wall and remain in the rumen (small stones, etc.) or are eventually voided in faeces
- long metallic foreign bodies such as pieces of wire, needles or nails (typically chopped wire strands from decomposing lorry or car tyres, or rusting fencing) and rarely broom bristles, etc., are thrown forwards by ruminal-reticular contractions into the honeycombed reticulum, which contracts and the foreign body may penetrate the mucosa
- common site is the cranial and ventral reticular wall
- penetration to depth of 5–7 mm results in perforation of the visceral peritoneum, and a point then traumatises opposing parietal peritoneum, usually the diaphragm and occasionally the abdominal wall, spleen or liver (see Figure 5.10)
- pain arises from irritation to the peritoneum and may be temporary, the foreign body dropping back loose into the reticular wall or lumen, either to repenetrate at another point or to pass further down the alimentary tract where further trouble is less likely

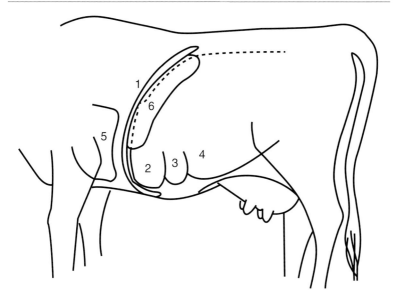

Figure 5.10 Sagittal section at the diaphragmatic area, seen from the left.
1. diaphragm; 2. reticulum; 3. cranial part of ventral sac of rumen; 4. rumen; 5. heart; 6. spleen.

- at the site of penetration an acute localised inflammatory reaction with exudate becomes slowly organised as an adhesion, or abscess
- in other cases, the foreign body slowly advances further, persistent pain is apparent for several days, and the foreign body may eventually enter the thorax and heart, liver, spleen or abdominal wall
- sequelae of reticular foreign body penetration and their signs are multiple and potentially fatal.

Clinical signs

Acute stage
- sudden onset anorexia, dullness and slightly apprehensive appearance
- severe drop in milk yield
- stiff gait, slightly hunched back
- ruminal tympany, possibly some pneumoperitoneum
- slight expiratory grunt
- animal may prefer to stand with forequarters relatively elevated. On lying down there may be an obvious grunt
- when forced to move the animal may show a stiff gait, abducted elbows and tucked up abdomen
- faeces hard and reduced in volume

- rectal temperature initially elevated to 39.7–41.1 °C and then falling to 39.2–39.4 °C with little or no or uncoordinated ruminoreticular activity
- urination may be initially suspended due to pain in adoption of the appropriate stance, followed later by passage of a large volume of urine
- ballottement or percussion of a cranioventral abdomen may be markedly resented, and pinching of withers may elicit a grunt and reluctance to depress the spine

Chronic stage

- starts five to seven days after the acute stage and is not striking or characteristic
- appetite is improved but not normal, often preferring concentrates to roughage
- slight ruminal tympany sometimes evident
- stance is almost normal although a slight stiffness is possible, while ruminal movements are present but of reduced intensity

Diagnosis

- usually easy in the early stages of an acute case and is based on the sudden onset of pyrexia, localised pain and ruminal stasis
- chronic cases diagnosis is often difficult: sporadic episodic flare-ups occur with persistent moderate pyrexia, abdominal pain, anorexia and lowered milk yield. Such recurrent attacks justify exploratory laparotomy and rumenotomy
- 60% of reticular punctures recover spontaneously, 30% remain as localised areas of chronic peritonitis and 10% develop serious sequelae
- radiography, ultrasonography, laparoscopy, abdominocentesis, haematology (leucocytosis with a left shift) and metal detector are ancillary aids to diagnose traumatic reticulitis/reticuloperitonitis. Such specialised diagnostic methods have obvious limitations even in the difficult chronic case:
  - ultrasonography permits visualisation of fibrin, exudate or abscess formation in the abdominal cavity and reduction of the rate and intensity of ruminal contractions
  - laparoscopy – expensive equipment is required and may require the cow to be in dorsal recumbency
  - radiography – powerful equipment is required and interpretation may be difficult
  - abdominocentesis – non-specific as any elevated protein and WBC count may be due to other causes of peritonitis; peritonitis is often localised
  - metal detector – non-specific for penetration and is only positive with ferrous material, and false positives with cobalt and magnesium boluses, slow release anthelmintics
  - haematology – raised white cell count possibly due to other causes

Conservative treatment

- often, as signs are assessed over a few days, conservative medical treatment is instituted
- traditionally, forequarters elevated 45 cm with boarding or earth
- systemic antibiotic therapy given for three days
- oral administration of permanent rumen/reticulum magnet
- many cases respond completely, some temporarily, to conservative treatment

Signs resulting from sequelae of traumatic reticuloperitonitis

- **intrathoracic penetration**: quite common, usually causing traumatic pericarditis (see Figure 5.10). Obvious illness about one week or more after an episode of vague indigestion. Signs of congestive cardiac failure (CCF) include ventral oedema, fast pulse, distended jugular veins and localised pain. Such cases usually die within one to two weeks. Less commonly, an intrathoracic foreign body causes localised abscessation in one lung lobe with chronic suppurative pneumonia and localised thoracic pain. Occasional entry into pleural space leads to fibrinopurulent pleuritis. Rarely reaction occurs in the mediastinum, and if extensive can cause pressure on the heart sufficient to cause CCF (i.e. pericarditis may not be the cause of CCF)
- **intra-abdominal penetration**: results in hepatic, reticular, omasal or abomasal wall adhesions and a more or less localised peritonitis. Signs are vague with dullness, pyrexia and anterior abdominal pain. Splenic abscession may cause septicaemia and pyaemic spread to other organs. In rare cases an abscess develops over the lower body wall and penetrates the skin, discharging foreign body as well as pus
- **chronic reticular adhesions and abscesses**: may be very extensive and involve the vagal nerve supply to the rumen. Some animals return to near-normal health, but some cases develop a syndrome of chronic ruminal distension or Hoflund syndrome

Technique of rumenotomy

- preferred treatment for acute traumatic reticuloperitonitis; also indicated in suspicious cases of chronic disease that are non-responsive to conservative treatment
- site is left flank as described in exploratory laparotomy (see Section 5.2)
- length of incision should be 25 cm, but varies somewhat with the particular technique selected to control possible contamination by ruminal contents:
  - Weingart frame: incision as above
  - McLintock cuff: incision length 16 cm
  - suture of ruminal wall to parietal peritoneum: no critical length

- ensure in all cases that dorsal commissure of incision is about 8–10 cm ventral to lateral extremity of lumbar transverse processes
- having entered the abdominal cavity (see Section 5.2) and before making rumenotomy incision check several points:
  - appearance of visible parietal and visceral (ruminal) peritoneum, e.g. roughening indicative of acute or chronic peritonitis
  - explore caudal and right side of abdominal cavity first
  - presence of excessive abdominal fluid: pass hand ventrally, and excessive abdominal fluid is easily obtained in handfuls, i.e. repeated volumes of 20–50 ml. A greyish-yellow colour with floccules of pus is evidence of acute or chronic peritonitis
  - presence of adhesions between reticulum, and diaphragm and adjacent viscera: indicative of past or present foreign body penetration
- to avoid potential contamination of the abdominal cavity by ruminal contents, the ruminal lumen is either exteriorised (Weingart frame or McLintock cuff) or the abdominal cavity is sealed off from the rumen by temporary insertion of a continuous suture

Weingart frame method (Figure 5.11)

- The stainless steel frame (size 27 cm × 18 cm) is used with two vulsellum forceps (23 cm) fixed with single hooks near the junction of the blade and handle, and with six small (7 cm) tenaculum hooks. Having entered abdominal cavity:
  - screw the Weingart frame into the skin at the dorsal commissure of the skin incision
  - push the ruminal contents inwards at the intended rumenotomy incision
  - grasp the rumen wall dorsally and about 25 cm ventrally with the two pairs of forceps, exteriorise and fix to two rings at top and bottom of the frame. This brings out the rumen but does not yet prevent contamination
  - place a sterile cloth or rubber drape or shroud completely around the exteriorised rumen between the frame and the abdominal wall
  - incise the rumen 3 cm below the dorsal forceps
  - insert one of the small ruminal hooks into the ruminal mucosa near the edge, pull back and clip the rumen on to the edge of the frame at an eleven o'clock position, followed by another at one o'clock
  - extend the ruminal incision ventrally to an appropriate length for entry of the arm and attach the rumen to the frame with four further hooks at nine, three, then seven and five o'clock positions.
- the ruminal lumen is now effectively isolated from the abdominal cavity

McLintock cuff method

- equally efficient but presents greater problems with sterilisation of equipment and rubber components eventually perish

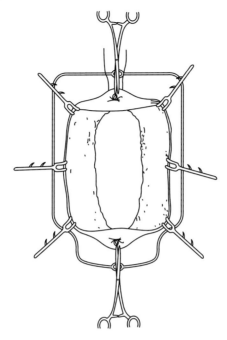

Figure 5.11 Weingart frame placed to exteriorise and fix the ruminal wall with six hooks and two vulsellum forceps.

- a special rubber cloth with an everted stiff cuff surrounding the abdominal incision is placed over the flank
- exteriorise the rumen and make a 2.5 cm incision in the upper position
- insert a rubber-covered hook, which is held temporarily by a non-sterile assistant
- extend the incision ventrally to 10–11 cm length
- insert the rim of a stiff rubber cuff through the incision, whereupon the lips of the ruminal incision will grip it tightly, and pull of the rumen draws the rim against the skin of the flank
- place a thin rubber sheet with a 15 cm elliptical hole between the rumen and skin
- place another, similar sheet over the rim and double back the edge of the ruminal cuff to form a seal

Suture method
- suture the ruminal wall to the skin by a simple continuous suture of non-absorbable material (6–8 metric) on a cutting needle; wide sutures are less likely to tear through the rumen wall
- after suturing, check the site for a good seal between the rumen and skin

- incise the rumen starting with a 2.5 cm ventral to dorsal commissure and ending with a 3 cm dorsal to ventral commissure
- evert the rumen wall with further sutures to the skin; this will also ensure a more secure fixation if the rumen is very full/taut
- for easy handling when working alone, dorsal and ventral parts of the exteriorised rumen may be temporarily fixed to the skin by towel clips (13 cm) for suturing purposes

Regardless of method, the next steps are similar:

- siphon off any excessive fluid with wide bore (≥ 3 cm internal diameter) plastic tubing filled with water, and remove any obstructing solid material
- pass an arm cranially and ventrally over the U-shaped ruminoreticular pillar and explore the reticulum methodically. Evidence of adhesions already palpated during intra-abdominal exploration may lead the hand to a particular area; otherwise make meticulous examination of the reticular floor and then of the cranial wall
- identify and examine the cardia, oesophageal groove and the reticulo-omasal opening as well as the medial wall: touching the reticulo-omasal orifice should provoke a contraction
- remove loose reticular foreign bodies, but search specifically for a pointed longitudinal foreign body lodged in secondary reticular cells between the secondary crests, which characterise this organ
- search with fingertips as only 1 cm or less length of foreign body may protrude into the lumen; in other cases it can subsequently be confirmed that the foreign body has passed right through the reticular wall
- it may be helpful to elevate the reticular wall with fingers to assess the presence of adhesions out of reach on the parietal surface, e.g. the right side
- palpate the reticular wall also for discrete abscesses
- if a penetrating foreign body is found, and before its removal, note the depth and direction of penetration to consider the likely structures damaged at this time. This aids prognosis. The wisdom of puncturing and draining reticular or ruminal wall abscesses from the ruminoreticular lumen should be carefully assessed
- use a magnet to retrieve loose ferrous material more easily
- place a permanent magnet into the reticulum

Tip

Difficulty in reaching the furthest points for exploration due to physical size of the animal or surgeon may be partially overcome by elevation of the forequarters, causing the reticulum to drop back slightly, elevation of the surgeon by standing on a pedestal or indirect pressure on the reticular area by upward pressure on the xiphoid region by an assistant (or two, using a wooden plank).

Warning
Do not attempt to break down adhesions: ● chronic adhesions: there is usually little or no benefit from breaking down chronic adhesions as they tend to reform very rapidly ● recent adhesions: they may mask and surround an abscess cavity so it is better to leave alone rather than risk a more widespread peritonitis

Closure of ruminal incision

● method varies slightly with the method of fixation, but in all instances two layers of inversion sutures should be placed. These should be:
  - continuous Cushing inversion suture of 4 metric PDS
  - continuous Lembert inversion suture of similar material
● **Weingart frame method**: remove the small ruminal clips and clean the peritoneal surface before and after placing the two suture layers, and clean again before releasing large forceps, permitting rumen to drop back into the abdominal cavity
● **McLintock cuff method**: remove the two rubber sheets, avoiding contamination, pull out the rumen and internal cuff further from the body wall and apply a foam-rubber edged special rumen clamp under the rim of the tube, which is then removed; the clamp then rests on the flank with the ruminal edges safely fixed; the contaminated surfaces may be easily cleaned and the two layer suture (Cushing or Lembert type) placed in position
● **Suture method**: after initial cleansing of the exposed ruminal surface, insert two layers of sutures and then carry out a thorough cleansing of the surfaces; débride any contaminated tissue from the body wall musculature
● intra-abdominal medication is not specifically indicated
● close the abdominal wall as described in Section 5.3
● all cases should receive systemic antibiotic therapy for three to ten days depending on the extent of peritonitis

Prevention of traumatic reticulitis/reticuloperitonitis

● prevention may be difficult to achieve
● whilst the advent of plastic bale twine in place of wire twine has removed a major source of potential foreign bodies, the widespread use of tyres on silage covering is now a very common source of small wire fragments (from perishing tyre walls)

- encourage farms to refrain from using tyres on silage clamps and remove ferrous and other potentially hazardous materials from the field and lane edges (e.g. during hedge-trimming)
- consider the use of permanent magnets (e.g. Bovivet® ruminal magnet, Kruuse) given orally, from one year old onwards; the best type is a cage model in which a plastic case surrounds the magnet so that most ferrous material lies within the grooves, avoiding any contact with the reticular epithelium (Hannover model cage magnet)
- magnets appear to be an effective prophylactic measure, but may lose effectiveness with age; a previously administered magnet should not preclude a diagnosis of traumatic reticulitis, not least because it will have no preventive effect with non-ferrous foreign bodies

Vagal indigestion (Hoflund syndrome)

Introduction

- vagal (vagus) indigestion is a chronic ruminoreticular condition of increasing abdominal distension and ruminoreticular dysmotility, thought to be associated with dysfunction of vagal nerve branches supplying the fore stomachs
- dysfunction involves hyper- or hypomotility, and may result in a secondary abomasal tympany

Anatomy

- the left and right vagal nerves (see Figure 5.12) form dorsal and ventral oesophageal trunks and supply direct branches to the ruminoreticular wall, including the sulcus and reticulo-omasal orifice, omasum and abomasum
- a section of both trunks completely abolishes coordinated motor activity of the fore stomachs
- a section of the dorsal branch alone results in almost complete, but not inevitably permanent, paralysis of the rumen, with lesser effects on the reticulum
- a section of the ventral branch alone results in less predictable effects, ranging from little to almost complete forestomach paralysis

Clinical signs

Signs develop following injury to the vagal nerves either in the thoracic mediastinum or in the cranial abdominal cavity, commonly due to extensive peritonitis secondary to traumatic reticulitis.

- movement of ingesta from the rumenoreticulum into the omasum and abomasum is grossly disturbed due to a functional stenosis and hypomotility of the omasum

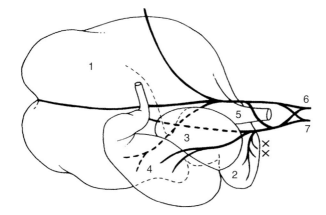

Figure 5.12 Vagal trunk innervation of bovine stomachs, viewed from the right side.
1. dorsal sac or rumen; 2. reticulum; 3. omasum; 4. abomasum; 5. cardia; 6 and 7. dorsal
and ventral trunks of vagus lying alongside oesophagus at cardia.
Note that abscessation in the reticular wall (x) is liable to interfere with innervation,
particularly of the omentum and abomasum. The dorsal vagal trunk (6) primarily
innervates the rumen. (Modified from Dyce and Wensing, 1971.)

- bradycardia is often present (<60/min)
- usually found in adult cows with a history of weight loss and increasing
  abdominal distension, often around parturition
- often a history of an episode of acute traumatic reticulitis
- viewed caudally, the animal has a 'ten-to-four' or 'papple' (pear right, apple
  left) distension, i.e. upper left flank and lower right flank
- ruminal distension possibly associated with hypomotility or atony, reduced
  feed intake, and scanty faeces. Other cattle show hypermotility but
  abnormal rumen contents
- careful deep palpation through the left flank reveals the ruminal contents to
  be completely mixed and not triple-layered (gas/firm solid material/fluid)

Treatment

- exploratory laparotomy and rumenotomy are indicated to check the
  abdominal cavity between the cranial surface of the reticulum and
  diaphragm
- rumenotomy may rarely reveal lesions of actinobacillosis: amenable to
  antibiotic treatment
- cases with massive adhesion formation involving vagal nerves: any treatment is purely palliative but fluids may be given for some days; lancing of a
  perireticular abscess may temporarily or completely resolve the problem
- prognosis in most adult chronic cases is poor.

5.5 Temporary rumen fistulation

Indications

Chronic recurrent rumen tympany in calves

- usually in calves three to nine months old, particularly barley-fed beef
- causes unthriftiness resulting from reduced feed intake
- **aetiology**: obstruction of the thoracic oesophagus and/or cardia by external pressure by mediastinal lymphadenopathy; usually a sequel to chronic pneumonia
- stomach tube can often be passed without any difficulty, excluding the possibility of mechanical stricture or stenosis
- fistula affords symptomatic relief and is rapidly produced

Signs

- slight but progressive loss of condition associated with more or less permanent overdistension of the rumen
- some calves eventually recover spontaneously (remove from barley feed)
- rumination is often unaffected
- collapse and death may occur with severe tympany (reduced venous return)

Technique

- pass a stomach tube to relieve any tympany
- paravertebral analgesia (T13, L1, see Section 1.9) or local infiltration
- site is the upper left paralumbar fossa, one third of the distance from the last rib to the tuber coxae, approximately a hand's width below the transverse processes
- clip the skin and disinfect
- remove a circular section of skin 4 cm in diameter, and split the muscularis by a blunt dissection (scissors)
- pick up the peritoneum with Allis forceps, incise, and grasp
- exteriorise the underlying ruminal wall with Allis forceps
- place sutures (nylon 6–7 metric) between the skin and rumen using an interrupted horizontal mattress pattern for the initial fixation (see Figure 5.13a)
- incise the rumen, removing a 3 cm diameter piece and place four or eight simple sutures to overlap the rumen and skin margin (see Figure 5.13b) using 6–7 metric nylon
- apply a topical antibiotic spray; a systemic antibiotic is only required to treat underlying lymphadenopathy/pneumonia complex

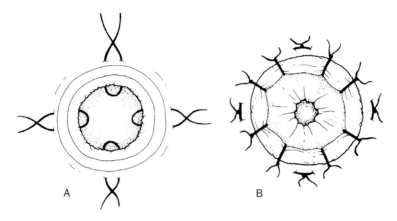

Figure 5.13   One technique of suturing the rumen to the body wall to create a ruminal fistula. A. four mattress sutures from the ruminal wall to the skin; B. eight simple sutures to overlap the rumen over skin edges; a fistula of an appropriate size may then be made.

- **alternative method**: a screw-in trocar and cannula (e.g. plastic 'red devil') may be inserted through the flank for several weeks as needed. Do not deflate the rumen before placing the screw trocar. Incise only the skin with a scalpel blade before firmly pushing and twisting in place, continuing to screw until the rumen wall is held tightly above the uppermost plastic thread. Remove the trocar and suture the outer ring of cannula to skin to hold it in place. This is an inferior method due to a greater risk of blockage (clean with the trocar), localised peritonitis and a tendency for the rumen wall to work loose from the screw.

> **Tip**
>
> There is no need for aftercare following the surgical creation of a temporary rumen fistula: the degree of continued tympany somewhat governs the speed of closure and keeps the fistula patent for as long as is necessary. In most cases, stricture and complete healing by secondary intention is complete in three to twelve weeks. The nylon sutures eventually slough.
>
> A permanent fistula requires a ruminal incision at least 6 cm long.

Chronic ruminal tympany in adult cattle

Causes include:

- chronic reticulitis commonly with adhesion formation: poor ruminal contractility subsequent to vagal nerve injury

- tetanus
- cancer of the oesophagus, oesophageal groove or cardia (alimentary lymphosarcoma): rare
- mediastinal lymph node enlargement: nodes resting dorsal to the oesophagus and effectively preventing eructation, due to chronic systemic lymphadenopathy, e.g. pneumonia or actinobacillosis
- visceral actinobacillosis of oesophageal groove, reticulum or cardia; usually cattle 1.5–3 years old
- thymic lymphosarcoma: cattle aged 6–18 months

Diagnosis

- easy to diagnose tympany but usually difficult to diagnose the cause
- oesophagoscopy may be helpful
- non-response to antibiotics may eliminate actinobacillosis
- some cases recover spontaneously; many persist and exploratory laparotomy and rumenotomy may sometimes be justified

Treatment and prognosis

- apart from actinobacillosis (antibiotics, e.g. penicillin/streptomycin) treatment of chronic ruminal tympany in adult cattle is usually unsuccessful
- creation of a semi-permanent ruminal fistula generally fails to alleviate the primary condition
- poor prognosis

5.6 Left displacement of abomasum (LDA)

Anatomy

- abomasum normally lies on the abdominal floor and its relations depend on the degree of distension of the rumen, reticulum and omasum
- has the fundic and pyloric regions; the distinction between the fundus and corpus (body) is imprecise and of no clinical importance
- narrower pyloric part passes transversely and possibly slightly cranially along the right body wall, to pass into the pylorus, which lies caudal and lateral to the ventral part of the omasum beneath ribs 11–12 (see Figure 5.14)

Aetiology

- left displacement of the abomasum (LDA), right dilatation and displacement (RDA), and abomasal volvulus probably have similar aetiologies despite differing symptoms

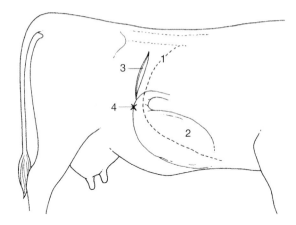

Figure 5.14 Diagram of the right flank of the cow to show the site of a laparotomy incision for right flank abomasopexy.
1. rib 13; 2. abomasal fundus and body; 3. flank incision; 4. pyloropexy or omentopexy site (x) sutured to body wall.

- LDA involves abomasal fundus hypomotility and hypotonicity resulting in delayed emptying. Predisposing factors include:
  - over-conditioned (fat) at parturition
  - high concentrate dietary intake and relatively low percentage of fibre
  - low dietary intakes or sudden change of feed (e.g. absence of roughage); stress factors (e.g. dystocia) or limited feed space reducing intakes
  - inherited factors?
  - rearrangement of viscera associated with parturition
  - concurrent disease, e.g. fatty liver, ketosis, metritis, mastitis and hypocalcaemia, are all associated with a higher risk of abomasal displacement

Signs

- dairy cattle, a winter-housed period and usually within six weeks of parturition; increased incidence in calved heifers on some farms
- drop in yield and selective anorexia, refusing most concentrates; often ketotic
- reduced or absent ruminal movements and reduced rumination
- usually low rumen fill; hollow left flank; occasionally distended by gaseous LDA
- animal fairly bright and without obvious abdominal pain except in rare cases (peptic ulceration, perforation and acute localised peritonitis)
- mild constipation initially
- afebrile (except with secondary peritonitis or concurrent disease)

- possible recent history of dystocia, milk fever, metritis or mastitis
- progressive and accelerating loss of condition

Diagnosis

- auscultation of left flank pathognomonic: high-pitched metallic tinkling sounds from the left flank over the middle area bounded by ribs 10–13
- corresponding area of resonance detected by applying a stethoscope and by flicking a forefinger against the rib cage: best heard when flicking the rib hard; echo-like 'steel band effect' or 'ping' sound is quite different from dullness appreciated with the rumen when closely applied to the left body wall
- in a doubtful case, ballotte the left abdominal cavity with a right fist while auscultating the left flank over ribs 10–12: splashing sounds are audible
- occasionally a slight distention of the dorsocranial part of the left paralumbar fossa just behind rib 13 results from severe abomasal tympani
- rarely can LDA be detected on rectal examination as a tympanitic viscus between the left dorsal sac of the rumen and the left abdominal wall

Differential diagnosis

- differential diagnosis of left flank resonance: hypotonic form of vagus indigestion may reveal peritoneal fluid and gas
- if necessary, a 'liptac test' can be used to confirm the diagnosis: 10 cm 16G needle pushed through the body wall into the centre of the area defined by a 'ping' to collect some fluid by centesis; pH <3.5 indicates LDA; pH >5.5 suggests rumen
- orogastric tube can be passed into the rumen to help differentiate a rumen 'ping' from that due to LDA
- ultrasonography: LDA can be visualised as a fluid- and gas-filled viscus covering the rumen

Conservative technique

Where economic factors (cost of surgery) dictate, treatment is primarily replacement by rolling.

- cast the cow on the right side (Reuff's method, see Figure 1.3)
- turn over on to the left side and while turning ballotte the ventral abdominal wall firmly in an attempt to move the abomasum into a midline position, using a knee to push anticlockwise
- alternatively, cast the cow on its back in dorsal recumbency and move from a 45° right lateral to a 45° left lateral position, 'shaking' the abomasum back into a normal position

- finally, in either rolling method, turn the cow into left lateral recumbency and maintain in this position for five to ten minutes to permit the organ to evacuate excessive gas
- check the absence of abomasum from the left side on auscultation and finger percussion
- reintroduce concentrates slowly over a one week period

Warning

Some cases of LDA corrected by rolling may at once or soon become cases of RDA. Many others have a recurrence of LDA within 48 hours and require rolling again or surgery. The long-term success rate of rolling is less than 20%.

Surgical techniques (LDA)

Numerous methods of surgical correction have been described since the first reports of LDA, around 1948, in Scotland.

Some options of sites and fixation techniques include:

- standing or recumbent surgery
- left or right flank or paramedian incision
- fixation of abomasum to the ventral body wall by an intra-abdominal approach or of greater omentum or pylorus to the right body wall
- one step or two step laparoscopy-guided fixations
- percutaneous fixation from the abdominal cavity (Utrecht technique)
- right paramedian blind percutaneous toggle-pin fixation

Advantages and disadvantages of various surgical sites are listed in Table 5.1. Personal preference varies enormously.

Right flank approach (Dirksen modified omentopexy or pyloropexy; Hanover method)

- paravertebral analgesia T13, L1 and L2; see Section 1.9
- skin preparation for aseptic surgery and drape
- paracostal skin incision 10–20 cm long starting 15–30 cm below the tip of the L2 transverse process and 4 cm behind the last rib (see Figure 5.14). A lower incision aids the reach for repositioning but increases the risk of omentum and the intestine prolapsing from the incision site, making closure more difficult
- entry into the abdomen as previously described (see Section 5.2)
- make a manual exploration of the abdominal cavity (see Figure 5.8): insert the left hand, passing it behind the caudal edge of the greater omentum and over the dorsal blind sac of the rumen to the left side of the abdominal

Table 5.1 Surgical correction of the left displaced abomasum: different methods.

Incision site	Right flank	Left flank (Utrecht)	Two step laparoscopic toggle fixation	Paramedian	One step laparoscopic toggle fixation	Percutaneous fixation (toggle)
Anaesthesia	paravertebral or local infiltration	paravertebral or local infiltration	local infiltration	sedation (xylazine or chloral hydrate) + local infiltration	local infiltration	sedation (e.g. xylazine) + local infiltration
Ease of decompression	+	++	++	++	++	N/A
Ease of reposition	+	+	++	++	+	(+)
Area of abomasal fixation	greater omentum caudal to pylorus or pylorus	fundus	fundus	fundus	fundus	fundus
Remarks	same approach as for correction of RDA	technical problems in inexperienced hands; rumenotomy also possible	use of tilting table advisable; need laparoscopy equipment	fast; possible restraint problems; good wound closure essential; risk of regurgitation and aspiration of rumen contents	fast, assistant necessary; need laparoscopy equipment	good, assistant needed, fast cheap, but risk of misdirected fixation (e.g. rumen) and risk of rumen regurgitation and aspiration
Personal preferences of authors						
(ADW)	1	2	3	5	6	4
(GSJ)	1	3	5	2	6	4
(AS)	1	2[a], 3[b]	1	3[b]	1	4[c]
(OA)	1	3	n/a	1	n/a	4

[a] = antepartum LDA.
[b] = long standing LDA.
[c] = low value cow.

cavity; appreciate the displaced abomasum between a relatively small rumen and the left body wall (abomasum may extend two thirds or often further up the left flank)

- check the palpable area of the abomasum for any roughness (peritonitis) and adhesions to the left flank; peritonitis is probably due to a perforated peptic ulcer
- **gas evacuation (optional)**:
  - evacuate abomasal gas by inserting a wide bore needle (14G), 45° to the abomasal wall firmly attached to plastic tubing (e.g. flutter valve), into the dorsocaudal part of the abomasum with the free end of the tubing held outside the animal; evacuate air passively or by attaching a vacuum
  - maintain the needle firmly in place while gently pushing the viscus ventrally with the palm of the hand
  - anticipate that the gas will be evacuated over five minutes (volume 5–15 litres) when evacuation occurs passively, until the abomasal wall is relatively flaccid and almost out of reach, low down on the left side
  - remove the needle and tubing, carefully avoiding contamination of the abdominal cavity by abomasal fluid in the tubing
  - place the palm of the left hand to the left of the omasum and gently shovel the omasum in a dorsal direction towards the accessory lobe of the liver; the abomasum is passively relocated to the right of the midline
- **repositioning without evacuation**:
  - may be attempted successfully, particularly in cows with a low rumen fill
  - place the palm of the left hand against the peritoneum of the right flank and move fully over to the left flank, beneath the rumen, remaining in contact with the abdominal wall at all times
  - when the left hand is above the displaced abomasum, place the flat palm of the hand on the distended abomasal viscus and push cranially and ventrally; gas and liquid will be heard emptying via the pylorus as the abomasum is repositioned towards the ventral midline
  - do not pull on the abomasum to reposition
- once repositioned, reach slightly cranially to the incision site and grasp the pylorus and pull it towards the incision site. Do not tug; if the pylorus does not easily move towards the bottom of the incision, check that the abomasum is fully deflated and repositioned
- pyloric region is identified visually through the right flank wound (see Figure 5.15)
- pyloric region of the abomasum: pale pink and well delineated from adjacent insertion of the greater omentum; it is firm and cannot be easily traumatised by the fingers
- if not visible through the flank incision repeat shoveling the omasum in the dorsal direction; the abomasum is easily drawn into the right flank using this technique

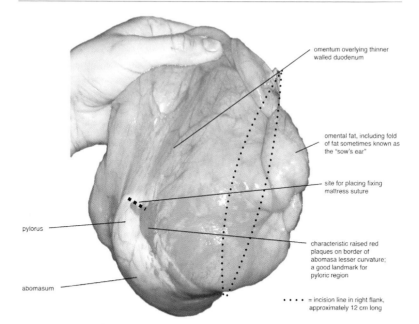

omentum overlying thinner
walled duodenum

omental fat, including fold
of fat sometimes known as
the "sow's ear"

site for placing fixing
mattress suture

pylorus

characteristic raised red
plaques on border of
abomasa lesser curvature;
a good landmark for
pyloric region

abomasum

• • • • = incision line in right flank,
approximately 12 cm long

Figure 5.15   Exteriorised pyloric region of the abomasum showing landmarks for pyloropexy.

- **omentopexy**:
  - grasp the greater omentum 5 cm caudal to the pylorus and suture the greater omentum to cranial and caudal wound edges (exit subcutaneously) with one interrupted U-shaped (mattress) suture each
  - suture the greater omentum additionally to the parietal peritoneum and transversalis muscle in closure of the ventral half of the flank incision. Pull tight and tie off U-shaped sutures under digital control before complete closure of the dorsal half of the most inner layers of the flank inicision
- **pyloropexy**:
  - using double thickness 6 metric chromic catgut, take 2 or 3 repeated bites of muscular pyloric wall (Figure 5.15) and suture with a single mattress suture tight against the body wall through the peritoneum and all muscle layers 1 cm cranial to the lower incision site. Ensure that adherence of the pylorus to the body wall is as tight as possible
- close layers of the abdominal wall in a routine manner (see Section 5.3)
- give systemic antibiotic therapy for one to three days only if an improper surgical technique was advocated or if mastitis or endometritis or any other inflammatory process is concurrently present

---

Tip

- Use as small an incision as possible to insert an arm to reduce prolapse of the omentum.
- A more ventral and cranial incision will allow easier reach to the left hand side to reposition the abomasum.

Possible complications
Post-operative complications include:

- peritonitis due to a non-sterile technique
- recurrence resulting from breakage of the omental flank pexy site suture before development of adhesion formation; less common with pyloropexy
- wound dehiscence, usually ventrally
- functional stenosis possible with a poorly executed pyloropexy, which occludes lumen (rare: the pylorus is thick and accidental entry of ligature into the lumen is unlikely)

Discussion

After successful LDA surgery, improvement is usually seen after one to three days with an increased appetite for concentrate. The 6 month post-operative survival rate ranges between 88% and 95%, irrespective of the surgical method (the 'toggle' method is slightly lower).

Left flank approach (Utrecht technique)
Though not widely practised in the UK, this (Utrecht) technique deserves greater recognition for its simplicity.

- make left flank incision (incision 2, Figure 5.6)
- explore the abdominal cavity and identity LDA
- evacuate gas from the abomasum with aneedle as previously described until the cupola of the greater curvature of the abomasum is positioned in the ventral aspect of the flank incision
- thread a 1.5–2 m length of non-absorbable suture material (polyamide polymer, 6 metric) on to a straight triangular 8 cm needle; place 5 or 6 continuous Ford interlocking sutures through the abomasal wall (avoiding the lumen), each 3 cm apart, close to the attachment of the greater omentum (see Figure 5.16). Aim to have a long length of suture material either end
- deflate the abomasum completely

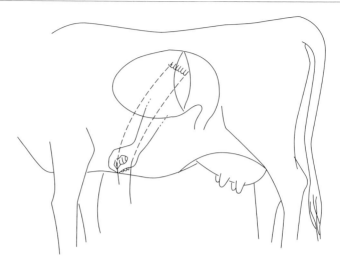

Figure 5.16 Abomasopexy from the left side using the Utrecht method. Continuous suture has been placed through the abomasal wall parallel and adjacent to the greater omentum insertion on to the abomasum. Both suture ends are then pushed through the ventral body wall just right of the midline using long straight cutting needles.

- insert the needle through the body wall slightly right of the abdominal midline, midway between the xiphisternum and umbilicus (site indicated by the assistant's finger pressure on the skin)
- ensure the needle is pulled through the skin to the exterior by the assistant, and that the end of the suture material is retained in artery forceps dangling beneath the abdominal wall
- with the second needle threaded on to the distal end of the same suture material push the needle through the ventral body wall 5 cm caudal to the first point; the assistant can again indicate the correct site
- push the semi-flaccid abomasum down towards the midline
- the assistant then ties the suture on skin of the ventral abdominal wall (placing the roll of bandage below the suture) while the surgeon ensures that the abomasum is held firmly against the ventral parietal peritoneum, so preventing interposition of the greater omentum or jejunal loops
- close the abdominal flank in a routine manner. For administration of antibiotics, see the post-operative treatment of the right flank approach
- remove the abomaso-omental skin sutures with scissors after two to three weeks, when firm adhesion of the greater omentum and abomasum to the body wall has formed
- the technique is suitable for repositioning and fixation of the displaced abomasum in cows ante partum

Left and right laparotomy approach
- really a variation on the right flank approach where a second surgical assistant pushes the abomasum down from the left side via a left flank incision to aid reposition of the primary surgeon via the right flank incision
- has the disadvantages of requiring two surgical sites to be prepared (and presumably a higher risk of infection); two surgeons; two wounds
- advantageous for ease of repositioning and for introducing more recently qualified vets to abomasal surgery

Right paramedian approach
- reposition and fixation present few difficulties with this approach
- may be performed under sedation (xylazine, i.v. or i.m.) and local analgesia, or under GA
- the animal is supported by straw bales laterally by each fore limb, and hind legs should be roped away from the operative site; plastic bags or rectal gloves on the feet may reduce site contamination. An assistant, restraining the head, is required to keep the fore legs away from the surgical field, operator's head and hands
- incision is midway between the umbilicus and xiphisternum approximately 20 cm long and 5 cm paramedian to the right, avoiding any large (mammary) vein (may spray beforehand on the standing cow)
- clip and surgically prepare the site; regional infiltration of local anaesthetic
- incise the skin, subcutaneous fat, external rectus sheath (consisting of fascia of the external oblique abdominal muscle and split fascia of the internal oblique abdominal muscle), rectus muscle (blunt dissection), internal rectus sheath (consisting of split fascia of the internal oblique abdominal muscle and fascia of the transvere abdominal muscle) and peritonum (see Figure 5.17)

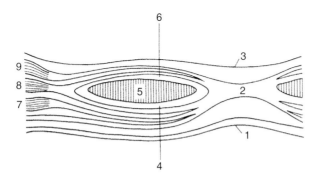

Figure 5.17 Diagrammatic cross-section of the ventral midline of the abdominal wall. 1. skin; 2. *linea alba*; 3. peritoneum; 4. external sheath of rectus muscle; 5. rectus muscle; 6. internal sheath of rectus muscle; 7. external oblique muscle; 8. internal oblique muscle; 9. transverse muscle. (From Cox, 1987.)

- note the small amount of subperitoneal fat overlying the peritoneum, which is incised and lengthened with straight scissors
- explore the abdominal cavity thoroughly
- identify the abomasum, repositioning of which has already occurred in most cases by palpating the omasum and following via the omasoabomasal fold and greater curvature of the abomasum to the pylorus
- xteriorise greater curvature of the abomasal body for identification of suture placement halfway between the omasoabomasal fold and pylorus adjacent to the attachment of the greater omentum; in deep-bodied cows with a very low rumen fill, the abomasum may need some traction to bring it up to the incision site
- suture the abomasum to the peritoneum and inner rectus sheath enclosing with each of three U-shaped (mattress) interrupted sutures about a 2 cm width of the abomasal body (using PDS or 6 metric chromic catgut). Ensure that sutures do not penetrate the lumen (danger of fistula or tearing out with the risk of fatal peritonitis) but include the serosa and muscularis
- tie up sutures that are positioned 3–4 cm apart from each other
- perform continuous suture including the peritoneum and inner rectus sheath, followed by a continuous suture including the rectus muscle
- bury this layer with a continuous layer of subcutaneous sutures of 4 metric chromic catgut or PGA
- suture the skin in a horizontal everted mattress pattern with monofilament nylon or in adapting a Ford-interlocking pattern
- for administration of antibiotics: see the post-operative treatment of the right flank approach
- remove skin sutures but not before ten days
- a potential advantage may be uterine discharge, which may easily drain during surgery
- technique is contraindicated in cows ante partum due to both the need for sedation and dorsal recumbency
- wound dehiscence may be fatal

Tip
For sedation for the right paramedial approach, chloral hydrate, though not licensed in the UK, has a distinct advantage over xylazine because the cow is less likely to lose her swallow reflex: it reduces the risk of aspirating regurgitated rumen contents.

Warning
In dorsal recumbency, large subcutaneous skin (mammary) veins can flatten and be difficult to see; cutting through a large vein may cause severe bleeding.

Percutaneous fixation (toggle or bar suture)

This is a rapid and simple technique of abomasal fixation avoiding the need for expensive laparotomy that has found widespread acceptance over the last twenty years. The steps following diagnosis of an uncomplicated LDA are:

- prepare the cow in dorsal recumbency and the surgical site as for the right paramedian approach; small blebs of local anaesthetic are required at the puncture sites; casting on the right-hand side first and rolling into sternal recumbency may aid repositioning of the abomasum
- assistant kneels in front of the udder from the left side while the surgeon confirms by auscultation the presence of the tympanitic abomasum ventrally underneath the surgical field
- trocar and cannula (Kruuse UK Ltd, Jorgensen Labs, Colorado, USA) are inserted firmly through the skin, musculature and peritoneum about a hand's-width caudal to the xiphoid and a similar distance right of the midline (see Figure 5.18)
- pull out the trocar, insert a toggle, having confirmed entry into the abomasum (gas always escapes and acidic pH can be checked with litmus paper), and pull out the cannula
- assistant holds the toggle suture with forceps
- rapidly repeat trocarisation and toggle insertion three fingers'-width caudal to the first site
- leave the cannula in place for a prolonged period in order to permit most gas to escape
- tie two sutures together allowing several centimetres of play (see Figure 5.19)
- turn the cow on to its sternum slowly and allow it to stand
- prophylactic systemic antibiotic cover is rarely used

Discussion

This percutaneous procedure requires two assistants and must be performed quickly as the abomasum can rapidly deflate once the cow is on her back. If unsuccessful, standing surgery can be done. The major hazards, apart from personal injury from poor restraint, are the risk of puncturing the rumen, fixation of the abomasum too close to the pylorus and tearing of the abomasal wall by the suture, all potentially resulting in peritonitis.

The easiest cases tend to be cows with obvious 'pings' in the left flank at the first clinical examination, since the abomasum remains gas-filled relatively longer. The technique clearly does not permit examination of other abdominal viscera for a concurrent disease (e.g. chronic adhesions, hepatic abscessation). A 60 day post-operative survival rate for this method is slightly lower than other surgical methods at 75%.

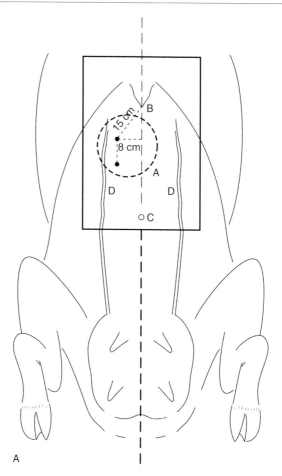

Figure 5.18 Abomasal 'toggling' procedure through the skin of the ventral cranial body wall.
A. ventral view showing puncture sites distal to the xiphisternum (B) and to the right side between the midline and right mammary vein (D).

Endoscopic LDA correction

Endoscopy can be used in a standing cow to deflate, reposition and fix an LDA. The fixation area is similar to the Utrecht, 'toggle' and paramedian approaches. It has the potential advantages of being less invasive (reduced risk of infection) whilst not requiring the cow to be placed in dorsal recumbency. Experienced operators can complete the operation in 40–45 minutes. The disadvantages include requiring specialised, relatively expensive equipment (approximately 6000 euros), but the technique is being increasingly used in Europe and North America.

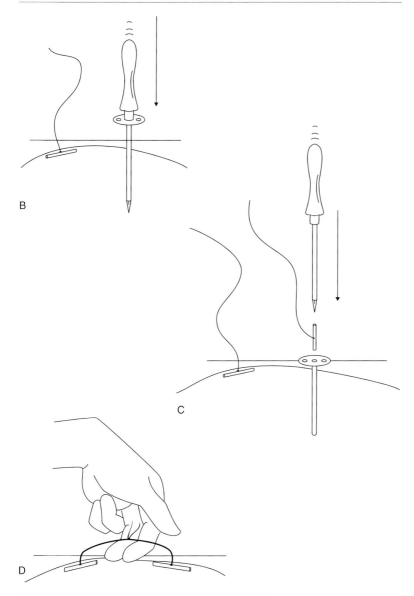

Figure 5.19   Placing sutures for the 'toggling' technique.
B. puncture by trocar and canula with first toggle in place; C. removal of trocar and insertion of toggle through canula; D. tying together of sutures from each toggle with space for insertion of two fingers.

Two-step laparoscopic toggle technique (Janowitz technique)
- this was the original endoscopic procedure, now largely replaced by the one-step technique
- **step 1** is performed with the cow fixed in a tilting table (clinic situation) in a standing position
- clip and disinfect the most dorsal third of the left flank from the 9th intercostal space to the caudal aspect of the paralumbar fossa
- after local infiltration of the anaesthetic, insert the trocar and sleeve through the stab incision for creating an optical portal in the cranial aspect of paralumbar fossa (5–10 cm ventral to transverse processes of the lumbar vertebrae and 5 cm caudal to the last rib)
- insert 0° laparoscopic optic (31 cm long; 10 mm external diameter) (Karl Storz GmbH, Germany); inspect visible structures of the left abdominal cavity
- insufflate air into the abdominal cavity until good visualisation of the abomasum is possible
- create an instrument portal in the 11th intercostal space under laparoscopic control
- insert long trocar (37 cm; Karl Storz) with a cannula through the portal into the greater curvature of the abomasum
- remove the trocar, thereby allowing the abomasum to deflate
- insert the toggle through the cannula into the abomasum before the abomasum is completely deflated
- push a double-stranded suture attached to the toggle into the abdominal cavity
- remove the instruments and portals and suture stab incisions with one simple interrupted subcutaneous suture and two simple interrupted skin sutures each
- **step 2** is performed with the cow in dorsal recumbency (using tilt table, clinic situation)
- clip and disinfect the surgical field similar to the right paramedian approach
- after local infiltration of the anaesthetic, insert the trocar and sleeve for creating an optical portal to the right and adjacent to the umbilicus; insert the optic
- inspect visible structures of the ventral abdominal cavity
- after local infiltration of the anaesthetic, insert the trocar and sleeve for creating an instrument portal about one hand's width caudal to the xyphoid and three fingers' width to the right of the midline under laparoscopic control
- insert the forceps, grasp the double-stranded suture and pull out through the instrument portal
- remove the instrumental sleeve and optic, deflate the abdominal wall and gently pull the abomasum to the ventral abdominal wall

- tie up suture strands over the gauze stent leaving space for insertion of two fingers
- suture stab incisions with a single simple interrupted subcutaneous suture and two simple interrupted skin sutures each
- tilt the table back to bring the cow to a standing position
- toggle sutures are not removed till 2 weeks after surgery in order to allow for adequate adhesion formation

One-step laparoscopic toggle technique (Christiansen technique)
- tilt table not required: cow is standing throughout
- as above to place the toggle in the abomasum
- do not push the double-stranded suture attached to the toggle into the abdominal cavity but attach it extra-abdominally to the eye at the tip of a lancet introduced into a slightly curved protecting sleeve of 100 cm length (Karl Storz)
- introduce the sleeve protecting the lancet through the instrumental portal into the abdominal cavity and push it in the ventral direction along the left abdominal wall until the tip reaches a point slightly to the right of the midline between the xyphoid and umbilicus
- penetrate the abdominal wall with the lancet tip; allow the assistant to pull the double-stranded suture through the eye; grasp the suture firmly, gently pulling the abomasum to the ventral abdominal wall; tie the suture up over a gauze stent, leaving space for insertion of two fingers
- pull the lancet tip back into the protecting sleeve and exteriorise the latter through the instrument portal
- instruments are removed and insertion sites sutured as above
- toggle sutures are not removed before at least 2 weeks after surgery in order to allow for adequate adhesion formation
- **advantages**: minimally invasive; antibiotics are not indicated by the surgical intervention; fast technique; visualisation of the abdomen (including ventral abdomen in the two-step technique); 6 month post-operative survival rate is about 90%
- **disadvantages**: not appropriate if the abomasum is not displaced at the beginning of the intervention; tilting table is very convenient but makes equipment expensive (two-step technique)

Tip

Using the one-step approach, fixation to the right of the abdomen is not always possible. Fixation slightly to the left of the midline is possible without apparent major disadvantages.

Potential complications (of all techniques)

- inability to locate or reposition the abomasum: if encountered during the right flank approach it may be necessary to perform left flank incision, especially in the case of an inexperienced surgeon
- adhesions of the abomasum to the body wall: adhesions may be out of reach in the right flank approach, again necessitating left flank laparotomy. They may be too firm to break down due to their long-standing and extensive nature. Beware of breaking down recent adhesions, which may result in exposure of abomasal lumen through a perforated ulcer. Such complications are rare (<5%)
- inability to identify the pyloric region (right flank approach): identify the caudal portion of the abomasal wall adjacent to the greater omentum, then pass a hand dorsally, and eventually the area can be identified where the abomasum is about 3 cm wide and where small lobes of greater and lesser omental fat overlap the abomasal border (known as the 'sow's ear'). The abomasum is thicker and denser at this point (pyloric antrum), which is located below rib 10, about half-way down the body wall

5.7 Right dilatation, displacement and volvulus of abomasum (RDA)

Right dilatation and displacement of the abomasum probably have a common aetiology with LDA. Incidence is lower and RDA is not so closely related to the early post-partum period. In some cases a cow may apparently have alternately LDA and RDA, the organ 'floating' from one flank to the other over a period of several days. Right dilatation occasionally occurs in younger cattle and in steers.

Signs and diagnosis of RDA

- selective anorexia and gradual weight loss
- distension of the low and mid right flank where auscultation reveals high pitched splashing and sometimes 'pinging' sounds usually extending cranially beneath the ribs
- RDA cases usually have a relatively greater abomasal distension than an LDA animal
- ballottement of the low right flank causes loud splashing sounds but rarely any pain
- cows may show profuse watery diarrhoea
- rectal examination may reveal a smooth distended viscus on the right side far cranial to the pubic brim, though only the caudal surface can be reached
- at any time an RDA can develop into a right-sided volvulus with severe compromise of the local vasculature. Few cases of RDA rapidly develop

volvulus but, once it occurs, the condition is acute and prognosis becomes guarded within hours: surgery is then an emergency
- animals with uncomplicated RDA may make spontaneous recovery but many become progressively duller, and some develop bradycardia; prognosis is then guarded.

Warning

- Exert great care diagnosing RDA using auscultation: high pitched 'pings' and sloshing sounds are common beneath the right flank and may be due to other gas/fluid interfaces, such as diarrhoeic faeces and air in the rectum.
- In cases of abomasal volvulus, the animal will be showing symptoms of shock in addition to the presence of a gas-filled viscus; it should be treated as an emergency

---

Conservative treatment of RDA

- turn the animal out to grass or into a yard for increased exercise and maintain access to bulky fodder
- some cases respond well to general symptomatic treatment: recently calved cows have been given calcium borogluconate, both i.v. and s.c.
- non-responsive cases of RDA remain at risk of developing abomasal volvulus. Many cases of volvulus have a history of chronic abomasal disease; this may justify surgery in valuable animals as soon as possible, i.e. before volvulus occurs

---

Tip

There used to be a fashion for using metoclopramide for medical treatment of RDA. Cattle do not have the necessary pyloric receptors for it to be of use; there is no strong evidence that the medication works in cattle and it is not a permitted substance for use in food-producing animals (EU). Therefore its use is not advised.

Signs of abomasal volvulus

- abdominal emergency: the cow is in shock with tachycardia; slow capillary refill time; skin tenting; mild to severe cyanosis
- weakness, possible recumbency depending on chronicity, abdominal distension, especially on the right side, with loud 'pinging' sounds on ballottement of the right flank

- abdominal pain (colic)
- rectal examination reveals large, smooth and tense-walled viscus ventrally on the right side
- (optional) abdominocentesis may reveal a large volume of reddish-brown fluid
- severe hypochloraemia and hypokalaemia, increased PCV, increased total protein
- metabolic alkalosis due to abomasal sequestration of acidic gastric secretion and later possibly metabolic acidosis
- abomasum may contain up to 50 litres of fluid
- volvulus causes severe and potentially fatal impairment of venous drainage of the abomasum, and the wall becomes ischaemic, dark red, then blue and black, at which stage rupture is likely
- differential diagnoses include caecal dilatation and dislocation, small intestinal obstruction following volvulus or invagination, functional abomasal obstruction

Discussion

In most cases of RDA and torsion, the mechanical movements initially involve dorsal displacement of the greater curvature followed by counterclockwise 180°–360° torsion of the abomasum (see Figure 5.20). Post-mortem (PM) examination reveals severe constriction of both the venous and arterial supply at the junction of the omasum and abomasum, as well as between the reticulum and omasum. The descending duodenum is completely occluded as a result of severe stenosis following external pressure and a degree of displacement. In most cases volvulus occurs in the counterclockwise direction when viewed from the right side.

Surgical treatment of RDA and abomasal volvulus

- correct right abomasal dilatation by right flank surgery after giving fluids and electrolytes (see Sections 2.1 to 2.7)
- NSAIDs, particularly with an endotoxic effect, are indicated (e.g. flunixin meglumine)
- following surgical preparation and anaesthesia, make a paracostal skin incision 20 cm long starting 10 cm below the tip of the L2 transverse process and 4 cm behind the last rib (see Figure 5.14): similar to the approach for LDA, right-sided approach
- if the general condition of the cow allows, perform a thorough exploration of the abdominal cavity

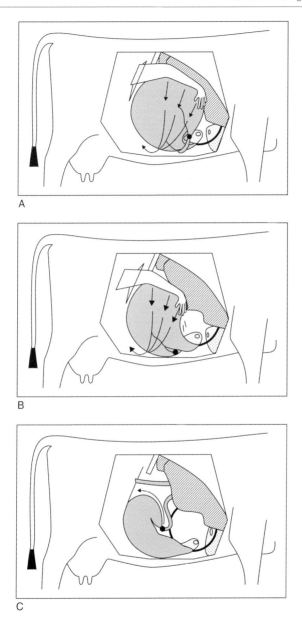

Figure 5.20 Three forms of right abomasal displacement and torsion and their manipulative correction.
A. left (anticlockwise from rear view) 360° torsion and direction of manual correction; B. left 180° anticlockwise torsion and correction; C. simple right-sided abomasal displacement (possibly with up to 90° rotation). (From Dirksen, Gründer and Stöber, 2002.)

- determine the degree of displacement and site and direction of the volvulus
- partially decompress gas from the abomasum. If necessary, especially in the case of a severe volvulus, fluid can be removed from the abomasum by first placing a 4 cm and a 7 cm diameter circular purse string suture dorsally in the serosal surface of the abomasum
- make a stab incision in the centre of the purse string and insert a stomach tube quickly in the abomasum while the inner purse string is tied up
- evacuate as much abomasal fluid as possible
- remove the tube and tie up the outer purse string suture
- oversew the site of abomasotomy by one or two mattress sutures
- examine the evacuated organ carefully for signs of abomasitis (diffuse hyperaemia) and ulceration (thickened areas, superficial fibrin deposition)
- locate the site of torsion for the final orientation
- correct the counterclockwise volvulus by pushing the greater curvature in a clockwise direction and ventrally with the flat palm of the hand or with the forearm
- confirm that the position of the pyloric region and descending duodenum are normal after complete retorsion (fundus, pyloric region, pylorus and proximal duodenum are all against the right abdominal wall)
- perform omentopexy or pyloropexy as described for the right-sided LDA approach (Section 5.6)

Discussion

Surgery of the abomasal volvulus is not indicated in cows that are unable to rise and remain standing. Such animals should be euthanased on humane grounds. They should not be slaughtered for human consumption as the animal is usually toxic. If surgery is attempted in advanced cases, i.v. fluid therapy is essential before and during surgery (see Chapter 2). Acid/base disturbances can be complicated due to massive abomasal sequestration of Cl^-, K^+ and H^+ ions, leading to metabolic alkalosis. However, metabolic acidosis can also occur due to shock. The prognosis is guarded or good in cases with a heart rate <90/min, serum urea <10 mmol/l or serum Cl^- >85 mmol/l. Cows with an abomasal volvulus of a chronic nature with a heart rate >120/min and ≥12% dehydration have a poor prognosis for survival. The sooner that an abomasal volvulus is diagnosed and surgically corrected, the better the prognosis.

> **Tip**
>
> Whilst surgery for RDA and volvulus may at first appear daunting, in fact early recognition and surgical intervention is usually rewarding: in such cases, simply gently push the dilated abomasum ventrally and slightly cranially, whereupon it will naturally have a tendency to untwist and empty.

5.8 Other abomasal conditions

Other surgical conditions of the abomasum include:

- impaction
- abomasal tympany and volvulus in calves
- ulceration (with or without perforation)

Abomasal impaction

Introduction

- may be primary, e.g. in calves following insufficient water intake
- may also be secondary to surgical correction of the abomasal volvulus or to lymphosarcoma and adhesion formation in the cranial part of the abdominal cavity

Treatment

- perform exploratory surgery through a right midflank incision
- break down the abomasal contents manually
- give liquid paraffin (5 litres, with 20 litres of water) by an orogastric tube once, or repeated 24 hours later (though this may remain in the rumen)
- some cases may slowly resolve
- abomasotomy through a right paramedian incision may be attempted in advanced cases

Abomasal tympany and volvulus in calves

Signs

- seen in calves, typically 3 weeks to 3 months old, shortly after rapid milk feeding
- signs include obvious discomfort with the head extended, colic signs and right flank tympany

- later depression and spread of tympany is found to involve the left flank
- systemic signs rapidly become severe and calves can die within a few hours
- differential diagnoses: rumen tympany (unlikely in this age group); intestinal torsion around the mesenteric root; caecal dilatation and dislocation; jejunal volvulus or intussusception

Treatment

- recumbent calves with circulatory collapse should generally be euthanased
- less severe cases: i.v. fluids, right paracostal or paramedian incision under local anaesthesia, in left lateral or dorsal recumbency
- exteriorise the abomasum, evacuate the contents by slow release of gas (tympany) or fluid (see evacuation of liquid during surgical correction of the abomasal volvulus)
- replace the organ after correction of the displacement

Abomasal ulceration

Introduction

- common condition in slaughterhouse statistics, both in calves and adults; younger cows tend to be affected within four weeks of parturition:
  - type 1: non-perforating, minimal bleeding
  - type 2: ulcer causing severe blood loss
  - type 3: perforating ulcer with acute localised peritonitis
  - type 4: perforating ulcer with diffuse peritonitis
- type 1 is often sub-clinical, while types 2, 3 and 4 usually show clinical signs and may be fatal
- in mature cows concurrent disease is often present such as mastitis, metritis and pneumonia
- abomasal ulceration tends to occur in recently calved cows (corresponding to an LDA incidence) and is related to stress, e.g. overcrowded yards and cubicle houses and/or high starch intakes relative to forage

Signs

- abdominal pain, which is not only associated with peritonitis
- calves often show perforation into the omental bursa (between the two sheets of the greater omentum), which is accompanied by protracted development of clinical signs
- melaena and pale mucous membranes (type 2)
- pyrexia and tachycardia in cases with peritonitis

- abdominocentesis (see Section 3.1) may be useful to confirm peritonitis, e.g. acute fatal cases involving a ruptured omental abscessation

Treatment

- type 2 ulcers require whole blood transfusion if the PCV drops below 15% volume (see Section 2.8)
- treatment of peritonitis requires systemic antibiotics
- i.v. fluids
- single ulcers in calves may be resected and oversewn
- correction of the primary disorder

Discussion

Abomasal ulceration in calves in the UK has been reported more frequently associated with the practice of once-a-day milk feeding. This practice is discouraged and is in any case specifically contraindicated in the first three weeks of life.

5.9 Caecal dilatation and dislocation

Definition and anatomy

- dislocation refers to any twist, torsion, volvulus or retroflexion of the caecum, which has a blunted round apex projecting caudally from the omental recess
- position varies with the volume of contents, floating dorsally if gas-filled or sinking with ample fluid contents
- a normal caecum cannot be identified on rectal palpation

Incidence and signs

- usually seen in adult dairy cows with signs rather similar to RDA for caecal dilatation and resembling an abomasal volvulus in caecal dislocation
- causes are not understood and may involve a hypocalcaemia and inhibitory effect of high volatile fatty acid concentrations in caecum on caecal motility (e.g. grazing lush pastures)
- selective anorexia (refusing concentrates) in a housed or pastured cow; more frequently seen during the production phase than in early lactation; more frequent in grazing animals

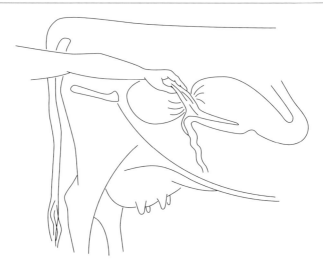

Figure 5.21   Caecal torsion and retroflexion: diagram of rectal findings. Longitudinal section through the abdomen: apex of the caecum and tense ileocaecal fold are palpable in caecal torsion.

- vague abdominal discomfort and pain, mild in caecal dilatation, severe in caecal dislocation
- some distension of the right caudal abdominal cavity, and ballottement of the upper right flank (more dorsal and caudal than in RDA and abomasal volvulus) produces sounds of fluid and gas
- faeces reduced in volume, dark, possibly covered with mucus
- rectal examination reveals little or no faeces and a mass-like end of a 'cob' loaf of bread 15–20 cm in diameter in dilatation (see Figures 5.21 and 5.22)
- position is relatively high on the right side (dilatation) or as a distended organ (retroflexed caecal body) cranially in the right ventral quadrant, or a painful palpation of the ileocaecal ligament (mainly caecal torsion)
- dislocation of the caecum produces more severe systemic signs, but disease progress is slower than in RDA or abomasal volvulus
- haematology and biochemical parameters are usually normal in caecal dilatation; in caecal dislocation the blood biochemistry is also normal or occasionally shows metabolic alkalosis with $\downarrow$Cl$^-$ and $\downarrow$K$^+$ caused by intestinal stasis
- differential diagnoses: RDA; abomasal volvulus; intestinal torsion around the mesenteric root
- confirmation of the diagnosis is done during right flank exploratory laparotomy

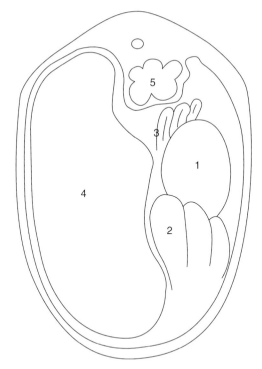

Figure 5.22   Transverse section through abdomen: 1. dilated body of caecum in case of retroflexion; 2. distended loops of spiral colon and 3. sometimes also the small intestine are palpable in caecal retroflexion; 4. rumen; 5. left kidney.

Treatment

- **medical management**: may be indicated in some cows with dilatation and duration of the disease <24 hours
- **surgical approach**: site of the incision (30 cm) is on the upper right flank, in the caudal half of the right paralumbar fossa in a slight oblique direction (from caudodorsal to cranioventral)
- exteriorise the caecum and examine it carefully for necrosis and commencing gangrene
- correct the dislocation after careful and repeated drainage at the apex (typhlotomy)
- massage firmer material out from the intra-abdominal portion of the caecum and proximal loop of the ascending colon
- inspect the caecal apex for ischaemia: the easiest surgical technique is to invert such areas into the caecal lumen and to oversew the area
- peri- and post-surgical systemic antibiotics; possibly i.v. or oral fluids

> **Tip**
>
> The caecum will usually contract as fluid is drained during a typhlotomy. Be prepared for this as it can be difficult to keep it exteriorised until the typhlotomy site is securely re-sutured.
>   Once repositioned in the abdomen, the caecum will usually refill from fluid retained proximal to the functional obstruction in distended loops of the small intestine. Repeated exteriorisation and drainage through the same typhlotomy site may be necessary until the caecum can be repositioned in its normal position without becoming grossly distended. It is unlikely, however, that all of the fluid can be drained so some remaining distention of the caecum should be expected.

Prognosis

- prognosis is good (dilatation) or guarded (dislocation)
- recurrence rate is up to 20%
- typhlectomy (partial caecectomy) is rarely indicated but is relatively simple to perform; the cow copes well with a caecum of reduced capacity

5.10 Intestinal intussusception

Introduction

- intussusception (invagination or telescoping of bowel) occasionally affects the small intestine (jejunum, ileum)
- predisposing causes are unknown but the condition is not always associated with hyperperistalsis, enteritis or diarrhoea
- any age group, from calves to older cows, may be affected, but calves appear predisposed
- complete bowel obstruction results
- rarely, a double intussusception (five layers of bowel wall superimposed on each side) develops

Signs

- sudden onset of acute abdominal pain
- groaning, kicking at belly, alternately lying and standing, paddling of hind legs
- within 12 hours acute signs are succeeded by dullness, anorexia, precipitous drop in milk yield
- initial tachycardia (heart rate 120/min) disappears, while melaena may be replaced by a total absence of faeces

- stance may be persistently abnormal after 24 hours, with the animal adopting a rocking-horse position, or may lie down and groan
- site is usually distal jejunum, or rarely the jejunoileal junction with an invaginated section (intussusceptum) passing into the caecum or into the proximal colon
- condition may last five to eight days, with slow deterioration and death from the metabolic effects of total obstruction in which plasma chloride and potassium progressively fall, with increasing metabolic shock

Diagnosis

- depends on rectal palpation of several distended small bowel loops, about 5 cm in diameter, or possibly a firm, painful and slightly mobile, fist-shaped mass relatively low on the right side or just cranial to the pelvic inlet
- in a calf, bilateral abdominal palpation may suggest a firm irregular abdominal mass
- mass may be out of reach rectally and diagnosis then depends on right-sided exploratory laparotomy
- intussusception may be detected using right abdominal ultrasonography
- differential diagnoses: intestinal volvulus or other causes of complete small intestinal obstruction; severely distended small bowel may be a case of small intestinal ileus without intussusception

Treatment

- i.v. fluids, e.g. hypertonic or isotonic saline; NSAIDs
- right flank laparotomy under paravertebral analgesia (see Section 1.9); alternatively, under GA
- standing surgery is preferable except in a calf <12 months
- exteriorise the affected bowel and attempt manual reduction in an early case
- in case of intestinal wall devitalisation, and where manual reduction is impossible, isolate with intestinal clamps, resect the bowel segment and mesentery and perform end-to-end or less optimal side-to-side anastomosis
- note that traction on the mesenteric root is very painful and may cause the animal to collapse; first infiltrate local anaesthetic into the affected segment of mesentery
- the suture technique should avoid production of bowel stenosis: keep the amount of inverted bowel wall minimal; single layers of a continuous Cushing pattern, interrupted once, or an interrupted Lembert pattern is suitable
- manage differing pre- and post-stenotic luminal diameters by a 45–60° angled incision line in the (smaller) post-stenotic bowel
- initial single sutures in the anti-mesenteric and mesenteric borders facilitate manipulation

- closure of the mesenteric defect is essential to prevent possible herniation
- preferred material is fine absorbable suture (e.g. 4 metric chromic catgut or vicryl) on a 45 mm 3/8 circle round-bodied needle or 3.5 metric PGA
- leakage at the suture line is rarely a problem
- maintain a strictly aseptic procedure; otherwise massive local peritonitis may result in multiple bowel adhesions
- wash the visceral peritoneal surface of the bowel with a copious volume of sterile isotonic saline before closing the abdominal incision
- after-care should include systemic antibiotics for five to seven days, hay and laxative feeds (e.g. bran) for one week
- successful surgery will be evident in the passage of loose dark faeces 6–24 hours later

---

Discussion

It is sometimes claimed that some cases recover spontaneously after sloughing the intussusceptum, but this has never been seen by the authors. Surgical intervention or euthanasia should be the two options considered for cases of intussusception.

Tip

Caecal invagination is a specific entity seen predominantly in younger calves. It is often reducible manually but they often recur, so caecal amputation is preferable (Section 5.9).

5.11 Other forms of intestinal obstruction

Intestinal obstruction is occasionally caused by other abdominal abnormalities including:

- large pedunculated fatty masses (lipomata)
- large intramesenteric areas of fat necrosis
- adventitious fibrous bands
- duodenal outflow obstruction
- duodenal sigmoid flexure (more acute deterioration)

Duodenal obstruction results in abomasal and rumenal fluid retention, and can present with similar signs to RDA. Surgical correction is done via a right flank approach. Manually correct any dorsiflexion or volvulus followed by manipulation of any impacted ingesta. Occasionally, if gas fails to pass into the descending duodenum, a side-to-side duodenoduodenostomy may be necessary to create a partial bypass of the sigmoid and cranial flexures.

Gall bladder displacement is occasionally described subsequent to pyloropexy or omentopexy following correction of LDA using the right flank approach. The duodenal sigmoid flexure becomes distended and dorsiflexed between the gall bladder, the right lobe of the liver and the body wall, and displaces the gall bladder caudodorsally. Manual correction by repositioning the gall bladder is usually possible via a right flank approach. The gall bladder may need decompressing first.

Incarceration in traumatised vas deferens ('gut-tie'): obstruction, rarely strangulation, may follow the passage of bowel through a tear of peritoneum between the *vas deferens* and abdominal wall, following a castration procedure in which excessive traction on, and recoil of, the spermatic cord results in adhesion of the cord or peritoneal fold around the bowel ('gut-tie'). Jejunum is usually involved and the condition develops slowly with signs related to a gradual lumenal occlusion (see Figure 5.23).

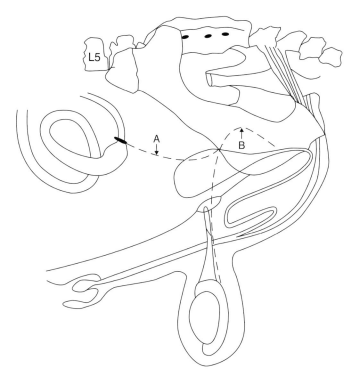

Figure 5.23 'Gut-tie' involving recoiled stump of ductus (vas) deferens adhesing around and occluding lumen of the small intestine, resulting in a bowel obstruction (compare with Figure 1.13).
A. abnormal stump of ductus (vas) deferens; B. normal position of ductus (vas) deferens.

Signs

- anorexia, dullness, reduced passage of faeces and distention of the flank
- ballottement of the flanks and palpation is inconclusive
- rectal palpation often permits easy diagnosis by recognition of the distended small intestine and one or more abnormal cord-like structures near the inguinal ring (see Figure 5.22)
- diagnosis depends on exploratory laparotomy following a suggestive history and signs
- problem is usually located near the internal inguinal ring and on the right side

Treatment

- gentle rectal traction on an adhesed spermatic cord stump may be attempted leading to rapid recovery (90% success); risk of tearing the bowel wall
- perform a right flank laparotomy in a standing or left laterally recumbent animal
- section or resect the adhesed spermatic cord or vas deferens with scissors using blind palpation
- exteriorise the bowel and check for viability
- resection and anastomosis is required in exceptional cases

5.12 Peritonitis

Introduction

- usually secondary to a diffuse or localised primary condition
- causes include perforation of an abomasal ulcer, rupture of a reticular wall or hepatic abscess, reticular perforation of a foreign body, infection following a uterine rupture or the introduction of infection at a caesarean section
- some cases follow a breakdown of surgical asepsis

Signs and diagnosis

- early cases have signs of diffuse abdominal pain and may grunt spontaneously
- acute reaction causes pyrexia (to 40.5 °C), tachycardia, arched back, anorexia and reduced ruminoreticular activity
- chronic cases, in which peritoneal exudate has organised to form extensive adhesions, are generally characterised by chronic weight loss and unthriftiness
- diagnosis is usually easy, based on history, classical signs, rectal palpation (adhesions possible; a taut rectal wall with diffuse peritonitis) and in doubtful cases abdominocentesis (see Section 3.1)

Treatment

- specific problems arise in the treatment of peritonitis due to infection in a transcellular space where antibiotics cannot reach the concentrations found in tissues and serum
- generalised purulent peritonitis has a hopeless prognosis; the animal should be euthanised
- apart from appropriate systemic antibiotics, treatment in early acute cases may include:
  - supportive i.v. fluids
  - NSAIDs to counter endotoxic shock
  - intraperitoneal antibiotics: e.g. crystalline penicillin; sulphonamides or oxytetracycline
  - intermittent peritoneal lavage (5–10 litres, t.i.d. or q.i.d.) with Hartmann's solution or 0.9% saline; dorsal flank entry port, ventral midline exit

---

Warning

Peritoneal lavage is not very effective in cattle due to blockage by fibrin clots. Prognosis is very poor.

5.13 Umbilical hernia and abscess

Introduction

- umbilical herniation is a common condition in the Holstein and other cattle breeds
- may be inherited or due to environmental factors (e.g. following umbilical abscess formation; check neonatal navel hygiene procedures on farms where hernias are prevalent)
- herniation can co-exist with umbilical abscessation

Warning

Surgery may be contra-indicated in large simple (i.e. non-infected) umbilical herniae of animals intended as breeding stock (particularly bulls), because evidence suggests the condition is inherited.

Signs

- exceptionally large umbilical hernia will be evident at birth, but the majority are first noticed a few weeks later

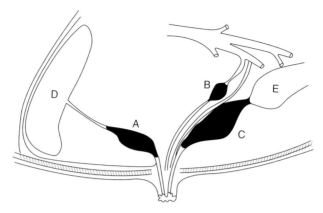

Figure 5.24   Three sites of umbilical infection with intra-abdominal involvement.
A. umbilical vein (purulent omphalophlebitis); B. umbilical artery (purulent omphaloar-
teritis). Note that there are two arteries, one either side of urachus; C. urachus (purulent
urachitis); D. liver; E. urinary bladder.

- the peritoneum-lined hernial sac may measure 3–12 cm in diameter; a
  corresponding hernial ring is typically about 1–7 cm long and 1–3 cm wide
- contents of the hernial sac are peritoneal fluid, a greater omentum and,
  in larger cases, the abomasum; a small or large intestine is sometimes
  involved.

Diagnosis

- based on history and palpation of the swelling and the adjacent ventral
  abdominal wall for signs of intra-abdominal involvement
- pain on palpation is suspicious of a septic process (see Figure 5.24) or
  incarceration
- ultrasound investigation may be considered to define the contents of an
  umbilical swelling and intra-abdominal involvement

Indications for surgery

- irreducible (incarcerated or strangulated) hernial contents irrespective of
  age, size and intended use of the calf
- increasing hernial size
- calves aged three to six months with a large hernia still present, possibly
  enlarging; even at this age, spontaneous resolution of smaller hernia
  (hernial ring ≤3 cm in diameter) is likely, though the prospect of surgery
  becomes more difficult in calves older than approximately 5–6 months.
- **Pre-operative complications**: treat discharging umbilical sinus by
  repeated local irrigation and debridement plus systemic antibiotics for

three to five days. If still not resolved, discharging an umbilical abscess cavity should be packed with swabs and overlying skin tightly sutured before starting surgery

> **Tip**
>
> - Avoid operating on calves under four weeks old unless an emergency: abscess capsule may not be thick enough for safe resection and a lower anaesthesia risk in an older patient.
> - Most hernias resolve in older calves; reserve surgery for those where they are enlarging.

Surgical technique

- reduce the ruminal volume in older calves by 24 hours of starvation (except water) to reduce post-op pressure on the surgical wound; also to reduce the degree of ruminal tympany during surgery (dorsal recumbency)
- very large hernias: withhold feed for 48 hours
- obtain deep sedation and perform local analgesic infiltration of the area with or without anterior epidural analgesia, or use GA (see Section 1.7)
- place the calf in dorsal recumbency, preferably raised from the ground, and positioned with straw bales laterally, with legs fixed cranially and caudally, and fix the tail remote from the surgical field
- in a male calf pack the preputial cavity
- clip an extensive area of the ventral abdominal wall; scrub and disinfect three times
- make an elliptical skin incision around the hernial base, continue along the midline well cranial and caudal to the limits of the hernial ring
- dissect the subcutaneous tissue bluntly to expose the hernial sac
- continue the blunt dissection down to reveal the edge of the hernial ring

Method (a): no infection or incarceration present:

- once the sac has been fully dissected away and the entire hernial ring is apparent, push the sac and contents into the abdomen without incising into the abdominal cavity
- suture the hernial ring closed using closely apposed interrupted sutures of non-absorbable/slowly absorbable material (e.g. PDS)
- far-near-near-far pulley sutures are useful to bring edges together of larger hernias, and the suture does not slip as readily as a standard suture under tension (see Figure 5.25)
- if an approximation for tying knots is difficult, pre-place sutures and secure the ends loosely with haemostatic forceps, and then use steady traction on all the sutures finally to close the ring

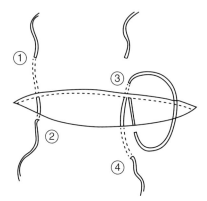

Figure 5.25 Far-near-near-far pulley suture.
Numbers 1 to 4 indicate the order of needle insertion through the body wall.

- ensure sutures are well covered by subcutaneous tissues closed by 4 metric vicryl or chromic catgut in a continuous pattern. It is essential to bury the deep suture layer and to avoid leaving potential dead space; sometimes two subcutaneous sutures are indicated
- appose the skin edges by vertical mattress sutures or a Ford-interlocking suture (monofilament nylon)
- eliminate the dead space by resecting excessive skin tissue
- give systemic antibiotics for three to five days

Method (b): infection or incarceration present:

- carefully incise the hernial sac at the junction of the body wall and sac and insert a finger into the abdominal cavity
- resect the sac and circumferentially a thin strip of the hernial ring, as long as there are no adhesions of gastrointestinal organs to the parietal peritoneum and umbilicus
- attempt gently to break down any adhesions between the hernial sac and abdominal contents. If the sac cannot be incised without damaging the contents, incise longitudinally through the *linea alba* cranial to the ring and remove the sac together with herniated viscera after any necessary enterectomy
- bring together longitudinal edges of the opening for suturing
- avoid undue tension by lengthening the ring cranially and caudally, converting the oval shape into a long ellipse
- if ring closure is likely to result in excessive suture tension, relieve the tension by making a longitudinal incision through the external rectus sheath, about 3 cm lateral to the left and right of the midline; the incision

should not extend into longitudinal muscle fibres or the internal rectus
sheath
- close the peritoneal cavity by simple interrupted sutures of a slowly
absorbable material (e.g. PDS) starting at commissures of the wound
- close the body wall and skin as in method (a)

Tip

Umbilical surgery success depends on:

- not penetrating any encapsulated infection (e.g. umbilical abscess)
- an aseptic technique
- careful haemostasis
- gentle handling of relatively friable tissues
- avoiding dead space formation
- prior starvation of the patient (empty rumen) and correct positioning
to reduce tension at the surgical site

Possible complications

- seroma formation and eventually infection of this fluid with abscessation
- haematoma: should be left untreated but if subcutaneous tissues then
become infected, drainage must be provided at once and the cavity flushed
twice daily (with saline); continue systemic antibiotics
- breakdown of hernial repair (dehiscence) with a prolapse of the omentum
to occupy a subcutaneous space: early re-operation is imperative to avoid
incarceration, adhesions and early development of diffuse peritonitis

---

Warning

Hernia repairs using a mesh are more prone to breakdown than by
apposition of hernial ring edges, even when some tension is initially
required to close the hernia. Large hernias, which truly do require a
mesh for repair, may be best referred to specialist large animal surgical
centres. Do not attempt in field conditions.

Treatment of encapsulated umbilical abscessation by surgery

- extra-capsular dissection is essential to avoid gross contamination and
peritonitis
- pre-operatively, any tract should be followed into the abdominal cavity by
palpation and/or ultrasonography to establish direction, i.e. cranially

towards the liver if the umbilical vein (septic omphalophlebitis) or caudally towards the bladder vertex (septic urachus, or septic arteritis) (see Figure 5.23)

- careful exploration with a sterile probe is often helpful
- paramedian laparotomy at the level of the umbilicus permits inspection and dissection of such infected tracts
- in most cases of septic omphaloarteriitis or septic urachitis, resection is simple under GA. Surgical excision of the infected urachus or arteries should be complete; sometimes a small area of bladder wall continuous with a pervious urachus is resected and the opening closed by two layers of continuous inverting sutures (Cushing)
- infection of the **umbilical vein** (omphalophlebitis) is potentially more serious, as sepsis may extend into the liver, permitting haematogenous spread to the heart and lungs, joints ('joint ill') and other organs; resection is then contra-indicated. If no spread has occurred, and septic omphalophlebitis does not involve the liver, the infected vein may be completely excised.
- **Marsupialisation** may be indicated in valuable stock if a single umbilical vein abscess involves the liver, without spread of the infection into the liver. The surgical treatment consists of three major steps:
  1. Extracapsularly dissect the abscess in the area of the body wall; elongate the midline incision cranially towards the xyphoid; partially exteriorise the abscess from the peritoneum and suture the abscess wall to the wound margins in the most cranial aspect of the incision; close the abdominal wall caudal to the marsupialised abscess.
  2. Three days after step 1, dissect the extra-abdominal part of the abscess 1 cm beyond the skin level. Thereafter, cautiously rinse the abscess daily until the intra-abdominal portion of the abscess is filled with granulation tissue: typically 3–5 weeks. Usually, a hernia has developed around the abscess wall at this stage.
  3. Surgical dissection of the remaining umbilical stalk outside the liver and repair of the hernia.

5.14 Alimentary conditions involving neoplasia

Alimentary tract neoplasms are, with the exception of squamous cell carcinoma, uncommon. Some are seen in the oral cavity (fibroma, sarcoma) requiring differential diagnosis from actinobacillosis and actinomycosis. Intestinal neoplasms have occasionally been incriminated in the pathogenesis of intussusception, and are then amenable to removal via bowel resection and anastomosis. Lipomata are sometimes the cause of vagal indigestion and weight loss in adult cattle, especially the Channel Island breeds, and are rarely treatable.

Squamous cell carcinoma (SCC)

- can develop in any part of the alimentary tract (oropharynx, oesophagus, oesophageal groove, rumen) as a proliferative, scirrhous, and often ulcerating series of masses, sometimes preceded by squamous papilloma
- occurrence is exclusively in upland areas where older cattle (≥8 years, usually beef types) have had prolonged exposure for several years to bracken; the toxic factor is ptaquiloside
- history of acute bracken poisoning in about 50% of cases of SCC
- its relationship to papilloma virus, which produces non-infiltrating sessile warts, is not precisely established. About one third of affected cattle have lesions of haematuria
- biopsy material may be taken for diagnostic pathology; rumenoreticular cases are almost invariably found retrospectively to have lesions in the oropharynx too
- the prognosis is hopeless and affected cattle should be slaughtered

5.15 Anal and rectal atresia

Introduction

- anal and rectal atresia (imperforate anus) in the calf are rare in comparison to lambs, anal atresia being more frequent
- inheritance of this lethal defect in cattle is not clearly established
- other defects, e.g. taillessness and spinal dysraphia may co-exist

Diagnosis

- usually made at 2–3 days old unless the stockman has made a meticulous neonatal examination
- absence of faeces draws attention to the calf, which may have a slightly distended abdomen
- perineum has a scar indicative of an anal orifice
- in anal atresia a scar may overlie a slight bulge of the subcutaneous tissues, and becomes more pronounced on increased intra-abdominal pressure, applied by pushing on the flanks or by spontaneous tenesmus
- absence of such a bulge suggests that rectal atresia may also be present
- investigation of a differential diagnosis between atresia involving the anus alone and both the anus and caudal rectum depends on surgical exploration

Surgery

- operate as soon as possible under caudal epidural analgesia (e.g. 1 ml 5% procaine without adrenaline)
- cleanse and clip an area 10 cm in diameter around the anus

- remove a 1 cm diameter circle of skin over the anal scar
- retract the skin edges with Allis forceps held by an assistant
- in anal atresia a distended blind-ended rectum is easily located by digital exploration in the pelvic midline
- attempt to suture the rectal wall to skin at this stage
- otherwise gently break down the surrounding connective tissue and attempt to exteriorise the caudal portion of the rectum
- place four stay sutures dorsally, ventrally and bilaterally into the rectum to maintain them in position and then incise this vertically for 1 cm; meconium will spurt from the lumen
- suture the rectal margin to skin in simple interrupted sutures of 4 metric chromic catgut, starting with two dorsal sutures at eleven o'clock and one o'clock positions, followed by two ventrally at seven o'clock and five o'clock
- add additional sutures laterally
- avoid as far as possible contamination of the subcutis and, more importantly, the pelvic cavity
- remove extra-rectal meconium with damp swabs; do not irrigate the wound, which could flush infection cranially
- *aftercare*: administer systemic antibiotics for five days
- maintain a lumen, minimum 2 cm diameter, which may require dilatation several weeks later as initial healing results in localised fibrosis; a cicatricial stricture is a common complication
- give a milk diet for two weeks to maintain soft faeces
- do not use for breeding

Rectal atresia treatment

- calves with additional atresia involving the rectum may prove difficult to assess and impossible to correct without the creation of a low flank caecal fistula (preternatal anus), which, though possible experimentally, cannot be justified on economic, practical and animal welfare grounds
- slight rectal atresia, with the rectum terminating 2 cm cranial to the anus, is treated by careful blunt dissection dorsally involving the mesorectum; suture to the skin as for anal atresia

Warning
Unfortunately in many cases the integrity of the blood supply is seriously impaired by inadvertent tears and stretching of the mesorectum, causing mural necrosis followed by rupture of the rectal wall and fatal faecal peritonitis extending from the pelvic cavity into the abdomen. Euthanasia is therefore advisable in cases of anal and rectal atresia that involve the absence of at least 3 cm of terminal rectum.

5.16 Rectal prolapse

Introduction

- rectal prolapse is seen in young calves and yearling cattle but rarely adults
- incomplete: prolapse of the mucosal layer only, with local oedema
- complete: total eversion of the caudal rectum with serosal rectal surfaces in contact

Aetiology and signs

- prime sign is marked tenesmus, usually as a result of severe localised pain
- severe enteritis involving passage of sloughed epithelial debris and blood, as in severe acute salmonellosis or coccidiosis
- sequel to chronic diarrhoea or chronic cough
- rarely due to other causes, e.g. urolithiasis (severe straining); severe ruminal tympany; high oestrogen intake (causing relaxation of the ischiorectal fossa); following a vaginal prolapse; rabies

Treatment

Three forms can be distinguished. All may be performed under epidural anaesthesia (see Section 1.9):

(a) Recent incomplete prolapse without mucosal injury:
- replacement and purse-string suture in subcutaneous peri-anal skin
- insert needle ventrally, emerging dorsally to expose a minimum length of non- absorbable material (e.g. sterile nylon tape) to possible contamination
- suture should be tied in a bow ventrally to permit gradual controlled slackening
- suture should permit adequate passage of faeces but prevent re-prolapse, and in a one-month-old calf should permit entry of two digits

(b) Recent incomplete prolapse with mucosal injury:
- suture tear or, if impossible, perform a rectal amputation or submucosal resection (see below)

(c) Complete prolapse:
- attempt replacement if not severely traumatised. Bathing with dilute Epsom salts, tannic acid or sugar solution may reduce the size of the oedematous mass

If replacement is impossible two procedures are available: submucosal resection or amputation.

Submucosal resection
- make two circular incisions around the circumference of the rectum, through mucosa to the submucosal tissue. The first incision is at the point where the rectum is reflected on itself, the second is about 1 cm from the mucocutaneous junction
- join two incisions by another dorsal incision at right angles, and longitudinal in direction
- dissect and remove the 'sleeve' of rectal mucosa between the two circular incisions
- effect haemostasis by swab pressure and ligation of the large vessels
- appose the mucosal edges in a row of interrupted simple sutures of 4 metric PDS, or a simple continuous row with a single interruption
- insert a purse-string suture as described above

Amputation
Two techniques are available.

Technique 1, Stairstep amputation:
- initially put a plastic syringe casing into the lumen of the rectum and insert a cross-pin fixation with two hypodermic needles to stabilise the prolapsed rectum during the suturing procedure (see Figure 5.26)
- make a circumferential incision cranial to the necrotic area, but do not cut the inner mucosa and inner submucosa
- create a stairstep and amputate 3 cm caudal to the initial circumferential incision
- use extra tissue (inner mucosal layer) to reduce the tension on the circumferential suture
- remove the hypodermic needles and syringe casing and insert a purse-string suture, as above

Technique 2, 'rectal ring' method:
- take a plastic syringe case, open at each end, or a proprietary product, and anchor with a circumpherential monofilament nylon suture at the most proximal part of the prolapse (see Figure 5.27)
- the blood supply is effectively occluded to the distal rectum, which sloughs about 10 days later

> ### Discussion
>
> A careful check must be made at frequent intervals, following technique 2, to ensure that the plastic case has not become dislodged and that defaecation can proceed normally through the lumen of the case. The method is simple but messy, and fails if the casing is dislodged, for example by contact with the pen wall or other cattle. For these reasons, technique 1 is preferable to technique 2.

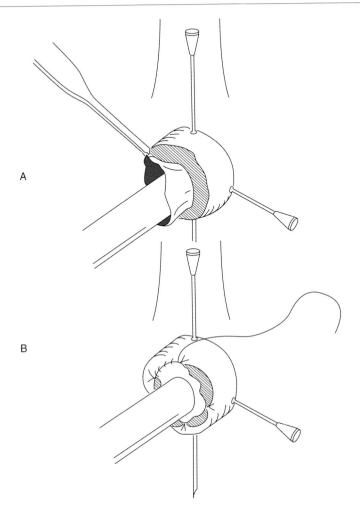

Figure 5.26   Stair-step amputation of the prolapsed rectum A and suture of mucosa B.

> **Tip**
>
> Post-operative tenesmus is delayed if the epidural block is made with a xylazine-procaine mixture (see Section 1.9) or a longer-acting analgesic drug (e.g. Bupivacaine®).

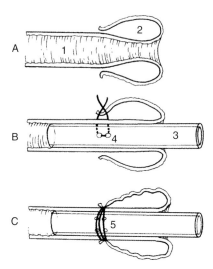

Figure 5.27 Repair of a prolapsed rectum utilising a syringe case or plastic tubing. A. 1. lumen of rectum; 2. prolapsed wall. B. Sutures are placed through skin-rectal mucosal junction and through holes (4) in the side of plastic tube (3). Second sutures are placed at 180° to first suture. C. Sutures are pulled tight over skin as tube is inserted appropriately within rectal lumen. Sutures are then tied around the circumference to occlude blood supply to prolapsed section (5). Prolapsed rectum and tube drop off some days later as a result of ischaemic necrosis.

Possible complications

- immediate excessive stenosis: resuture placing a larger diameter hollow casing into the lumen
- excessive haemorrhage: oversew the vessel including a full thickness of the wall
- severe continuous post-operative tenesmus: repeat the long-acting epidural block; produce pneumoperitoneum (insufflating through a needle placed in the left paralumbar fossa and attached to Higginson's syringe); slacken the purse-string suture
- anal stricture due to excessive fibrosis: incise the anus dorsally and ventrally through the depth of fibrous tissue, and suture the cranial commissure to the caudal commissure of the wound

CHAPTER 6

Female urinogenital surgery

6.1 Caesarean section (hysterotomy)

Indications

- relative foetal oversize: immaturity of dam, double muscling (e.g. Belgian Blue), genetic mismatching and prolonged gestation (certain sires)
- foetal deformity (e.g. *schistosoma reflexus*; ankylosis)
- relative or absolute narrowness of the pelvic canal: immaturity of the dam, traumatic pelvic deformity, e.g. fracture
- foetal emphysema with a narrow birth canal
- foetal malpresentation or posture
- irreducible uterine torsion, uterine rupture, non-complete or incomplete dilatation of the cervical os
- atresia or hypoplasia of the maternal vagina or vulva
- certain valuable pedigree breeding programmes where safe delivery of a viable foetus is paramount and where management precludes the risks associated with a natural delivery
- over-fat dam, particularly primiparous heifers, resulting in a narrow pelvic canal and a high risk of vaginal tear

Historically, hydroallantois and hydroamnion were further indications for a two-stage caesarean section (day one: slow drainage of uterine fluids; day two: caesarean section). Such cases have a better prognosis if early calving is

Bovine Surgery and Lameness, Third Edition. A. David Weaver, Owen Atkinson, Guy St. Jean and Adrian Steiner.
© 2018 John Wiley & Sons Ltd. Published 2018 by John Wiley & Sons Ltd.
Companion website: www.wiley.com/go/weaver/bovine-surgery

induced before a full-term pregnancy with corticosteroids and prostaglandins, possibly followed several days later by an i.v. oxytocin drip in non-responsive cases.

Contra-indications

The following will decrease the chance of cow survival:

- cattle in very poor bodily condition (cachectic)
- emphysematous foetus
- uterine infection

Economic factors inevitably become part of the decision-making process in many instances.

Caesarean section may still be preferable to embryotomy (fetotomy) in cases of general debility and prolonged dystocia despite the presence of a dead foetus.

Advantages of a caesarean section over embryotomy include:

- if the foetus is alive
- often faster and safer
- feasible procedure where embryotomy would be impossible (e.g. cervical non-dilatation)

Flank approach

Restraint, preparation and anaesthesia

- a standing patient is preferable: easier exteriorisation of the uterus resulting in less risk of abdominal contamination
- xylazine sedation is contra-indicated due to an induced increase of myometrial tone and uterine friability, which makes suturing more difficult; also a higher risk of sudden recumbency. However, safety considerations sometimes necessitate sedation
- a uterine relaxant (e.g. clenbuterol HCl) can be slowly injected i.v. to facilitate rotation and partial exteriorisation of the uterus (300–450 µg, depending on the size of the cow)
- administer pre-operative systemic pain relief (NSAIDs)
- if antibiotics are to be used (as is usual), administer a pre-operative systemic dose, e.g. amoxycillin or penicillin plus streptomycin i.m.
- caudal epidural anaesthesia (to reduce abdominal straining and rumen prolapsing through incision) is optional; 1 ml of local anaesthetic per 100 kg bodyweight is usually sufficient to reduce straining without increasing the risk of hind limb paresis

- local anaesthetic block: see Section 1.9. A lumbar paravertebral block is preferred (T13, L1–3)
- weak, debilitated and ataxic cattle may be cast before surgery; in such cases a cranial epidural block is a feasible alternative analgesic method (60–80 ml 2% lignocaine) or a 30 ml caudal epidural block and inverted '7' or 'L' flank analgesia
- tie the tail to the hind leg (not necessary if caudal epidural anaesthesia is used)

Discussion

The left flank site is preferred to the right flank unless a specific indication for the right side exists (e.g. over-sized foetus in the right flank with a grossly distended rumen, or previous multiple left flank incisions with excessive scar tissue). A right side incision almost inevitably results in small intestinal loops prolapsing through the wound; to avoid becoming traumatised and infected, always have a surgically prepared assistant.

Technique

- clip, scrub and disinfect the entire paralumbar fossa (last rib to hip); use of sterile drapes is optional (often difficult to use practically in a standing patient)
- make a 30–35 cm vertical incision in the middle or caudal third of the left paralumbar fossa (see Figure 5.6 (4)); incise through the skin only, using a scalpel
- muscle depth can vary considerably between patients (30 mm to >100 mm); avoid a scalpel; dissect at one point to penetrate the peritoneum (obvious influx of air into the abdominal cavity) before extending the incision ventrally and dorsally; take care not to incise the rumen wall
- haemostasis of the flank vessels is optional; sharp and blunt dissection of the muscle layers using scissors reduces bleeding
- insert a hand into the abdomen, pushing the rumen forward and feeling ventrally and caudally
- make a rapid assessment of the foetal position and the condition of the uterine wall
- bring a greater curvature of the gravid horn towards the abdominal incision by gently but firmly lifting the foetus within the uterus; this is easier if pregnancy is in the left horn
- grasp the uterine wall over the protruding part of the foetus (e.g. limb, hock in anterior presentation) and exteriorise greater curvature of the gravid

horn; if the dorsum of the foetus is towards the incision, the uterus should be rotated within the abdomen
- grasp a foetal leg just below the hock through the uterine wall and maintain firmly in a flank incision; grasp the fore limb below the carpus if the foetus is in a posterior presentation

Tip
Unless there is an intrauterine infection (e.g. a dead foetus), entry of some uterine fluid to contaminate the abdominal cavity is rarely hazardous. However, exteriorisation of the uterus prior to incision is much preferred to reduce this risk and reduce subsequent abdominal adhesions.   This depends to some extent on ensuring that the abdominal incision is the correct length and site. Assuming the calf is in an anterior presentation, a hind limb can be grasped below the hock and manipulated through the incision so that all of the limb from the foot to the point of the hock is exteriorised. The foot will be uppermost and the hock will rest on the lower part of the incision. If the incision is the correct length (just shorter than the foetus hock–foot distance), a tight fit will ensure the limb remains in place even without being held, allowing the surgeon to pick up the scissors prior to incising the uterus (Figure 6.1).

- incise the uterine wall (see Figure 6.1) along the greater curvature adjacent to the limb and towards the tip of the horn with scissors or a finger embryotomy (fetotomy) knife starting at the hock and extending towards the digits (or begin at the carpus in the fore limb, if in a posterior presentation)
- avoid incising maternal caruncles; avoid a scalpel to reduce the risk of damaging the calf
- extend the incision carefully until the limb can be exteriorised without risk of tearing the uterine wall
- manually dissect through the foetal membranes to fully exteriorise the foot; foetal fluids will begin to drain externally
- if necessary, instruct the assistant to maintain a very gentle traction on the exteriorised limb sufficient to maintain the uterine wall in the flank incision
- locate the second limb through the uterine incision and foetal membranes, which is similarly exteriorised; attachment of sterile calving ropes is optional

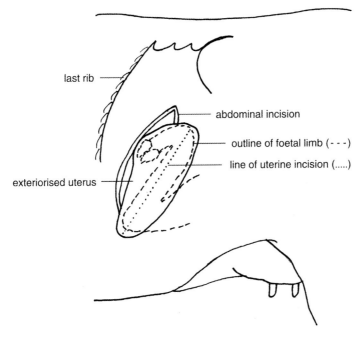

last rib

abdominal incision

outline of foetal limb (- - -)

line of uterine incision (.....)

exteriorised uterus

Figure 6.1   Exteriorised uterus and the correct line for uterine incision, between the foetal hock and foot.

- ensure that foetal traction is applied gently and in the appropriate direction, usually initially upwards, then ventrally and caudally; lengthen the uterine incision, if required, with scissors to avoid any spontaneous tearing of the uterine wall
- practise careful and slow foetal manipulation during extraction, especially in cases of *schistosoma reflexus*, muscle contracture and emphysematous calves, to avoid uterine tears
- in case of gross foetal oversize or ankylosis the skin incision may occasionally require enlargement to 40 cm
- permit the umbilical cord to rupture naturally during extraction
- after delivery hold the uterine incision in the flank wound; manually remove any loose protruding portions of the placenta, leaving the remainder in situ
- do not attempt to separate the placenta from maternal caruncles; trimming with scissors may be necessary
- non-crushing uterine clamps (vulsellum forceps) can be used to hold the uterus in position (optional)

> **Warning**
>
> Always check for a second foetus before closing the uterine incision!

- intrauterine medication is unnecessary
- while the foetus is being revived and the umbilical cord is checked, undertake uterine repair rapidly
- close the uterus with a continuous Cushing suture, followed by a continuous Lembert or a modified Cushing (Utrecht uterine suture with buried knots) (see Figure 6.2)
- sutures should incorporate serosa and muscularis, but not perforate mucosa (risk of contamination); suture knots should be buried
- suture of the uterine wall: start at the caudal ventral commissure of the wound if a single layer closure is intended or cranially if two layers are to be inserted. Suture material: either 5 or 6 metric PGA, polyglactin or 7 metric chromic catgut (see Figure 6.3)
- swab the incision after closure and check for leaks; rapid uterine contraction during suturing usually ensures a neat seal

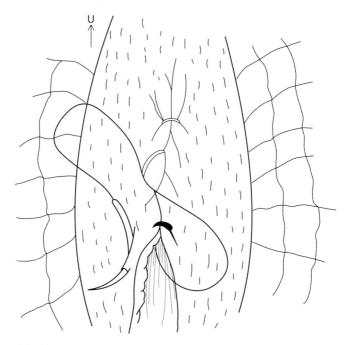

Figure 6.2   Utrecht uterine closure method with knot burial. Needle is inserted at a slight angle towards the incision and does not penetrate the uterine lumen. Sutures are placed sufficiently close to prevent leakage of uterine fluid. Care is taken to avoid the placenta.

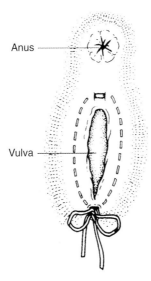

Anus

Vulva

Figure 6.3 Pattern of the Bühner suture in vulvar lips. The Gerlach-type needle, threaded with umbilical tape, is inserted below the ventral vulvar commissure, and is passed through dense fibrous tissue to emerge above the dorsal commissure. It is unthreaded and the needle alone is passed up the other side in a similar manner. It is rethreaded and the tape is pulled back ventrally. A quick release and adjustable knot is tied. Suture material is only visible at the commissures.

Tip

Removal of blood clots around the ovaries may reduce the risk of adhesions and infertility subsequently. Always check the region around the ovaries after closure of the uterus as the broad ligament of the uterus forms a natural well for blood to collect at this site.

- evacuation of foetal and other contaminating fluids from the abdominal cavity is usually unnecessary; manual removal of large blood clots may be done by scooping from the abdomen with a cupped hand
- in the case of grossly infected fluids, lavage must be attempted by irrigation with large volumes of saline (preferably), swabs and aspiration
- intra-abdominal antibiotic is not indicated
- flank wound is closed in a routine manner (see Section 5.3)
- inject oxytocin (50 i.u.) parenterally to promote uterine contraction (optional)

Post-operative care

- the calf should be given maternal colostrum as soon as possible by bottle (teat), or an oesophageal feeder if necessary
- beef dams should be encouraged to stand to permit suckling as soon as possible
- continue parenteral antibiotics for at least four days and give additional pain relief (NSAID) the following day and for longer if required
- during the following week, continue to assess patients for endotoxic shock, metritis and hypocalcaemia by following parameters: general appearance, appetite, rectal temperature, heart rate and character, colour of visible membranes, capillary refill time and willingness to attempt to stand or recumbency
- placenta is usually discharged within 24 hours of surgery and is a good prognostic sign; cases with persistent infected discharge should receive a prolonged course of systemic antibiotics

Post-operative complications

- healing of the flank wound may occur by secondary intention as a result of intraoperative contamination and excessive blood and fluid accumulation between suture layers
- avoiding deadspace on wound closure is important
- mortality following caesarean section is low (<5%, even lower if cows with poor prognosis are not operated, e.g. a dead foetus)
- mortality due to:
  - endotoxaemic shock
  - chronic severe intrauterine haemorrhage (via a massive vulval discharge)
  - septic metritis and peritonitis
- post-caesarean fertility is usually good (circa 20% of cows will be culled due to failure to conceive)

Warning

Removing a fetid or emphysematous foetus by caesarean section is a considerable challenge:

- the physical weight and size of the foetus is greater than normal
- there is usually greater adherence of the foetus to the uterus (dry; no/abnormal foetal fluids)
- friable uterus; tears easily; hard to suture; often fails to contract
- often a weak patient

The prognosis is always guarded and surgery should not be attempted on a recumbent patient or one already suffering from septicaemia; the patient is unlikely to survive and immediate euthanasia on humane grounds is indicated.

Alternative surgical techniques

1. **Lower flank incision**
   - useful for dead/emphysematous foetus to further avoid the risk of abdominal contamination
   - requires the patient to be cast in lateral recumbency
   - hind limbs are tied to a post (or other fixed object) to avoid kicking; a high dose caudal epidural block can be used (see Section 1.9) but should be avoided in endotoxic patients due to the risk of fatal hypotension
   - lower edge of the incision site is close to the ventral fold of the flank, taking care to avoid mammary veins (see Figure 5.6 (3))
   - sterile drapes can be used to pack incision edges once the uterus has been exteriorised to avoid further contamination; care should be taken so that irrigation of the uterus after wound closure does not result in fluids draining back into the abdomen
   - surgically scrubbed assistants are always required to help manipulate the uterus and avoid exteriorisation of the viscera
   - required traction may be difficult: a pulley from an overhead beam or tractor loader can be useful
2. **Midline**
   - ventral midline is a potential surgical approach in young beef heifers and in the case of a large distended and septic uterus; it requires excellent restraint involving more manpower
   - cast at an oblique angle between right lateral and dorsal recumbency and restrain the legs
   - clip and scrub the operative field from 12 cm cranial to umbilicus caudally to the udder and cover the body with a sterile drape having a 30 cm window
   - incise the skin caudally from 5–7 cm cranial to the umbilicus as required
   - incise fat, fascia, *linea alba* and peritoneum longitudinally
   - push the free edge of the greater omentum cranially and exteriorise the gravid horn by traction on the foetal limb
   - proceed then as for a flank incision; the omentum can be drawn over the uterine incision before closing the body wall
   - suture the peritoneum and *linea alba* with a simple continuous or interrupted appositional mattress eversion suture of PGA or monofilament nylon (7 metric)

- bury this suture layer with simple continuous chromic catgut
- suture skin and subcutis with monofilament nylon in an interrupted mattress pattern

6.2 Vaginal and cervical prolapse

Introduction

This condition is typically seen in late gestation or the early post-partum period in fat beef (especially Hereford and Santa Gertrudis) and dairy breeds (Holstein and Channel Island).

The chronic case, which starts about the eighth or ninth month of gestation, presents quite different problems from the post-parturient form. Salvage after parturition is the best solution, as it will recur in the succeeding gestation.

Predisposing factors

- excessive fat deposition in perivaginal connective tissue
- relaxation of sacrotuberous ligaments due to hormonal influence (endocrine imbalance)
- increased intra-abdominal pressure following greater abdominal size in late pregnancy
- high roughage intake
- severe cold weather and poor conformation (large flaccid vulva)
- severe post-partum tenesmus due to vaginal injury
- inheritance is postulated in some Hereford bloodlines, but not proven

Treatment of pre-parturient chronic case

- NSAIDs
- caudal epidural analgesia is followed by thorough cleaning and replacement of the vagina
- moderate cases of vaginal prolapse in pregnant cows not near to term (e.g. seven months gestation) are best treated by a modified Caslick's operation to close the dorsal vulvar commissure, which is then cut at parturition to avoid vulvar tears.

Severe cases near term can be managed in two ways:

Technique 1. Perivulvar suture using Bühner's method (see Figure 6.3)

- surgical scrub of the perivulvar area and careful cleansing of the exposed vagina

- place a subcutaneous suture of nylon tape in deep tissues around the vulva with a long vulvar needle (Gerlach pattern) as follows:
  - insert the needle, threaded with 45 cm sterile nylon tape (0.6 cm wide), approximately 3 cm below the ventral vulvar commissure and directed dorsally through deep connective tissue, to emerge midway between the dorsal commissure of the vulva and anus
  - leave one end of the tape hanging from the lower incision, remove the other end from the needle eye, and withdraw the needle
  - re-insert the unthreaded needle in a similar manner along the other edge of the vulvar lip, to emerge adjacent to the original exit point, re-thread and pull the tape out ventrally (see Figure 6.3)
  - tie the tape so that tension can easily be adjusted
- vulvar lumen should permit easy entry of four fingers; only about 1 cm length of tape is exposed through the vulvar skin dorsally and ventrally
- sutures may be completely buried by two 1 cm long horizontal incisions sutured in a mattress pattern, and placed dorsally and ventrally, if more than one month pre-partum. If inserted during late gestation, the suture is cut near the knot and removed at term; therefore it is vital to watch carefully for the first signs of calving
- there is commonly vulvar oedema for several days; local drainage of pus may occur
- a sphincter-like band of connective tissue occasionally results and may prevent a future prolapse, but can occasionally cause dystocia, necessitating dorsal episiotomy (see Section 6.5)

Technique 2. Transverse sutures

- an inferior modification of the above method, best avoided
- involves nylon tape, which is inserted in two or three deep horizontal mattress sutures across the vulvar lips
- produces more severe local reaction, pain and irritation, leading to continued tenesmus after analgesia wears off; inevitably an increased risk of sutures tearing through the skin
- unless a cow can be kept under close observation for calving, this pattern should not be used. A 'bootlace' suture lateral to the vulvar lips is preferable:
  - insert a needle with tape just lateral to the 'hairline' beside the vulvar lips
  - thread the suture material through or simply tie the sutures over a short length of rubber or plastic tubing, reducing the risk of suture tear-out

Treatment of post-parturient case

- technique 1 above is suitable
- initially in a recently calved cow, simple replacement under a long-acting (up to eight hours' duration) epidural block with local anaesthetic and xylazine is successful in most instances (see Section 1.9)

Technique 3. Modified Caslick's operation
- Caslick's operation is performed primarily to correct pneumovagina and is otherwise occasionally used to correct mild cases of vaginal prolapse
- in some cases the bladder must be catheterised before surgery
- after vaginal replacement the vulvar lumen is surgically occluded over its dorsal three-quarters:
  - resect the vulvar mucous membrane dorsally over an area measuring about 5 cm long and 1.5 cm wide
  - suture apposing surfaces with fine nylon or caprolactan (e.g. Vetafil), supported by two deeper mattress sutures of similar non-absorbable material
  - sutures are removed after two to three weeks
- incise the suture line shortly before imminent parturition
- success rate with Caslick's procedure is only moderate

Technique 4. Cervicopexy (see Figure 6.4)

Introduction

- a radical method for preventing further vaginal prolapse; very effective if properly performed in the valuable non-pregnant cow; two surgeons are required
- via a left-flank laparotomy incision a suture is placed through the ventral portion of the cervix and prepubic tendon just lateral to the midline

Technique

- select large full-curved cutting needle and thick, non-absorbable multi-filamentous suture material (polypropylene 7 metric)
- instruct the assistant to apply uterine vulsellum forceps to the ventral part of cervical os per vagina, pushing the forceps cranially to aid identification, which is essential for correct placement and for avoidance of the urethra and bladder; insertion of the bladder catheter is useful
- after inserting a ventral cervical suture pass a double length of suture material through the prepubic tendon 5 cm cranial and lateral to the pecten of the pubis (see Figure 6.4)
- throw knots outside the abdominal cavity and carry them along the suture material with the thumb and fingers to avoid entrapment of the small intestine
- ensure a minimum of four throws to each knot
- cut the suture material with scissors, leaving a 3 cm end
- this modified Winkler cervicopexy is easier and safer than the original vaginal approach
- many cows continue to strain following surgery

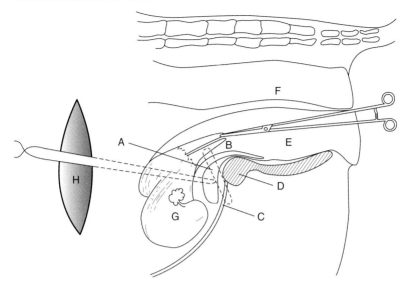

Figure 6.4 Cervicopexy through the left flank laparotomy (vertical view).
A. suture through ventral part of cervix (B) which is fixed and manipulated by assistant holding long-handled uterine forceps (E) in vagina; C. point of insertion of suture through prepubic tendon; D. pubis and ventral part of pelvis (shaded); F. rectum; G. uterus; H. flank incision and suture throw; J. bladder.

6.3 Uterine prolapse

Introduction

- occurs not infrequently (0.5% of calvings) following the third stage of labour, and usually involves complete inversion of the gravid cornu; most cases occur within two hours of parturition
- prevalent both in multiparous dairy cows in good condition (hypocalcaemia) and in cases of malnutrition and chronic disease
- aetiology of uterine inversion and prolapse appear to be associated with the onset of uterine atony during the third stage of labour; many cows also have hypocalcaemia and clinical signs of milk fever
- sometimes associated with severe dystocia and subsequent tenesmus

Treatment

Instruct the farmer to wrap the prolapsed uterus in a clean moist sheet to prevent further contamination if the cow is recumbent. If standing, and sufficient help is available, the uterus should be supported in a slightly elevated position in clean cloths until veterinary assistance arrives. The cow should be kept quiet.

- inject calcium borogluconate s.c. or i.v. as soon as possible
- induce caudal epidural analgesia (5 ml procaine 5% + 0.75 ml xylazine 2%) to eliminate straining
- NSAID will reduce post-op discomfort if given initially
- for recumbent patients: position the cow in sternal recumbency with the hind legs in caudal extension, to tilt the perineal region at an angle of 45° to the ground, a position that considerably facilitates replacement (see Figure 6.5); ropes tied to the hind feet will aid in moving and maintaining the position; a good head restraint is necessary; it is also useful to have an assistant sitting astride the cow, holding the tail and facing the prolapse
- if still standing, the cow may have replacement attempted if two farm personnel are available; otherwise it is advisable to cast and place in the appropriate position (Figure 6.5)

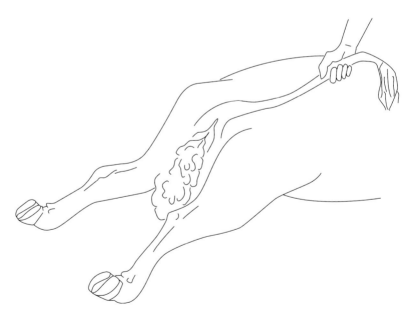

Figure 6.5 Optimal position for replacement of the prolapsed uterus. Both hind legs are extended caudally. Pelvis is tilted downwards about 30° in this position. In the standing cow a high epidural block may be given to facilitate manipulation.

> **Tip**
>
> Do not attempt to replace the prolapse without positioning the cow correctly, particularly if the cow is in lateral recumbency or her hind legs are beneath her abdomen. Excessive intra-abdominal pressure and gravity will work against you. Replacement in a standing cow is perfectly possible, but is facilitated greatly if the weight of the prolapse is taken by assistants on either side, suspending the uterus in a clean sheet.

- cleanse the viscus initially with warm water and then warm saline, and remove foetal membranes if they are already detaching spontaneously
- inspect the uterus for tears and for the possible presence, within it, of a distended bladder, which should be drained either by manual pressure through the uterine wall or by catheterisation
- place the uterus and underlying cloth on clean plastic sheeting placed across both hocks in the recumbent cow (e.g. an opened-out feed bag)
- with the organ elevated, so that its lower edge is level with the ischium, start replacement by gentle pressure, using the palms of the obstetrically lubricated hands over the areas nearest to the vulvar lips, working in a circular manner around the mass
- practise gentle massage to avoid uterine perforation!
- after the initial partial reposition, maintain the reposed part by ensuring that the remaining prolapsed uterus is kept above the vulvar lips
- progressively replace the whole organ in this manner and ensure that it moves cranial to the cervix into its normal position

> **Tip**
>
> If reposition is impossible after several minutes' manipulation, locate the opening into the non-pregnant horn (usually about level with the vulva) and insert a closed fist and apply firm pressure into the pelvic cavity. This lifts the uterus and applies a steady pressure back into the abdominal cavity. Use the other hand to feed the edges through the vulva. Care must be taken so that pressure applied with the fist does not cause a uterine tear, yet is sufficient to repel the organ.
>
> An assistant astride the cow can take some of the weight of the uterus by lifting either edge of the plastic sheet. However, in practice, lifting the uterus whilst applying a repelling pressure is most effectively achieved by placing the uterus on one's thighs and adopting a half kneeling position.

> In very difficult cases, and particularly where assistance is lacking, the hind limbs of the cow may be lifted using a rope suspended from a tractor loader, similar to the up-ending technique used in sheep.

- check there is no residual inversion of the cornu (you may use an empty bottle as an arm extension)
- if complete inversion is still impossible, fill the uterine lumen with normal saline and then siphon off through a disinfected stomach tube
- after reduction, inject oxytocin (20–50 i.u., i.m.) to speed involution, which can be checked by manual *per vaginum* examination

After care

- suture of the vulvar lips (e.g. Caslick) is not indicated
- limited vaginal trauma can be ignored, but any large deep laceration should be sutured with catgut
- cows with extensive areas of vaginal epithelial necrosis and trauma require submucosal resection, which is a haemorrhagic, slow procedure indicated only in selected cases
- a four to five day course of systemic antibiotics is indicated in all but the cleanest of cases, which is quickly replaced without trauma; repeated NSAIDs may be indicated

Complications

- recurrence of the prolapse following the return of sensation to the perineal region is uncommon, but carries a poor prognosis as it indicates a problem with uterine contracture
- the usefulness of a Bühner pattern vulvar suture (see Section 6.2) inserted for two to three days to avoid this hazard is controversial as it may induce tenesmus, and in any case is an unnecessary painful procedure for the vast majority of cases
- follow-up visit advisable 12–24 hours later to check the vagina and cervix
- other complications include haemorrhage, metritis, toxaemia, septicemia, paresis, and uterine rupture with bladder or intestinal eventration
- internal haemorrhage following tears to blood vessels in the broad ligament is a particular hazard that is difficult to assess at the time; a failure of improved demeanour in the hours following replacement should stimulate a re-examination of the patient; fluid therapy and blood transfusion (see Section 2.8) may be attempted but the prognosis is extremely unfavourable.

Prognosis for re-breeding is good and recurrence of prolapse at the next parturition is inexplicably uncommon.

Amputation of the uterus (hysterectomy)

Introduction

- major surgery is rarely indicated
- amputation is performed in cows in which the organ is so severely damaged (lacerations, necrosis, freezing, gangrene) that reposition would result in death and in cases of prolonged prolapse in which replacement proves impossible
- consider the economic cost of action! Amputation is the sole alternative to salvage. The prognosis is guarded or poor
- major problems include haemorrhage and shock; pre-operative whole blood or hypertonic (7.2%) saline may be advisable (see Section 2.8)
- surgery is performed under an epidural block

Wash and prepare the operative field. Two techniques are available. Surgical assistance is required.

Technique 1

- insert several transfixing and circumferential sutures of nylon tape just caudal to the cervix
- resect the uterus about 5–10 cm caudal to this point, placing further haemostatic sutures throughout the margin

Technique 2

- make a dorsal incision through the uterine wall to bifurcation
- identify and fan out the left and right mesometrium
- ligate vessels in series, larger vessels individually, smaller vessels in groups (chromic catgut 7 metric)
- incise the mesometrium 1 cm distal to sutures
- permit stumps to retract intra-abdominally
- insert a mattress suture line just cranial to the cervix
- amputate the uterus 1 cm distal to mattress sutures
- return the stump and vagina into the pelvic cavity
- give systemic antibiotics for three to five days; post-operative give NSAIDs for pain relief

Post-operative problems

- haemorrhage from uterine vessels; shock
- milking cows may remain profitable for one to two years as long as ovariectomy (see Section 6.6) is performed at hysterectomy.

6.4 Perineal laceration

Classification

- **first degree***:* involves mucosa of the vulva/vestibule/vagina
- **second degree***:* involves full thickness of the vulva/vestibule/vagina wall, but not the rectal wall or anus
- **third degree***:* involves full depth of the vulva/vestibule/vaginal walls, as well as rectovaginal tears, including the anal sphincter or rectovaginal fistula

This section considers primarily third degree perineal lacerations, i.e. the most severe form

Clinical signs and indication

- injury is almost always a result of damage from the foetal head or limbs at parturition
- if possible, injury can be anticipated, such as a veterinarian attending a dystocia case may perform dorsal episiotomy (10 o'clock or 2 o'clock position) to prevent such severe laceration; repair of such a surgical episiotomy wound is relatively simple (see Section 6.5)
- surgery is essential if breeding is to be resumed, since the severe ragged and irregular tear soon becomes oedematous and grossly contaminated by faeces; faeces in the vagina starts a chronic inflammatory process that soon spreads to involve the cervix
- untreated cows typically suffer from urine pooling in the cranial vagina (urovagina) and pneumovagina, particularly during oestrus

Technique

- delay surgery until the defect is completely epithelialised, possibly six weeks post-partum
- some surgeons prefer immediate surgery (not longer than four hours post-partum), but the existence of inflammation and infection often leads to failure
- keep the cow off feed for 12–24 hours (reduce faeces)
- caudal epidural analgesia (local anaesthetic, possibly with xylocaine) in a standing animal
- cleanse the surrounding area and irrigate the vagina with warm isotonic saline solution
- empty the rectum of faeces and pack rectal lumen cranial to the defect with absorbent cloths

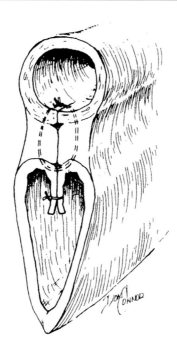

Figure 6.6 Repair of third degree perineal laceration with an interrupted modified Lembert suture in the dorsal layer (rectum to dorsal vagina) and a continuous horizontal mattress suture in the vestibular mucosa. (From Youngquist, 1997. Reproduced with permission of W.B. Saunders)

- instruct the assistant to retract the lateral borders of the cloaca to expose cranially the shelf formed by the rectal and vaginal mucosa dorsally and laterally, and supporting the underlying muscular layers
- incise transversely along the caudal edge of the rectovaginal shelf, and extend the incision laterally to the skin edge of the original dorsal vulval commissure (see Figure 6.6)
- completely separate the vaginal mucosa from the edge of this shelf to a depth of about 5 cm
- suture the musculofibrous bridge, starting cranially, in a transverse plane to appose the left and right surfaces (e.g. 5 or 6 metric PGA)
- start the suture in the vaginal lumen and also include the four edges of the vaginal mucosa
- ensure the sutures are placed tight and that their distance apart is such that it is not possible to insert a digit between them
- avoid suturing the skin edges caudally (contra-indicated) since it could increase the difficulty in defaecation
- give systemic antibiotic prophylactic cover for 5 days

Possible complications

- inadequate mucosal undermining (a technically difficult procedure) results in an inadequate thickness of bridge
- poor placement of sutures with excessive space permitting faecal material to pass into the vagina
- sutures tearing out
- inadvertent suture of the anal skin margin causing stricture
- gross wound infection
- all these problems result in partial or complete wound breakdown; such events may necessitate a second operation with a very guarded prognosis
- dystocia at any succeeding parturition does not appear to be an increased risk

6.5 Episiotomy

Indication

- when vulva and vestibule are liable to be torn at parturition due to foetal oversize, small or immature vestibular region or excessive friction resulting from inadequate lubrication of the area
- surgical incision is preferable to a ragged, uncontrolled and bruised iatrogenic tear

Technique

- caudal epidural local anaesthesia
- make a simple oblique incision at the 10 o'clock or 2 o'clock position through the skin, and also the vestibular mucosal layer if necessary
- avoid lengthening dorsally to the anal sphincter or cranially to damage caudal branches of the vaginal artery
- suture incision in two layers after delivery: continuous chromic catgut or Vicryl™ in mucosa, interrupted monofilament nylon in the skin
- antibiotics unnecessary; NSAIDs useful to limit post-operative pain and swelling
- primary healing is usual

6.6 Ovariectomy

Indications

- alleged prolongation of lactation in mature cows as well as improvement in feed efficiency compared with non-spayed heifers

- convenient husbandry measure permitting spayed heifers and cows to run within the herd with a bull without risk of pregnancy
- occasionally unilateral surgery in the case of ovarian pathology or persistent ovarian cyst
- little comparative data are available regarding lactation and feed efficiency in spayed and non-spayed cattle, and much of it is contradictory
- not widely practised in Europe, but common in parts of both South, Middle and North America where a single surgeon, working at a restraint chute with a well-organised team, can spay up to 40 heifers an hour
- operated animals should be permanently identified.

Warning

Spaying cattle for management purposes is not a permitted procedure under UK legislation (e.g. The Mutilations (Permitted Procedures) (England) Regulations 2007). The procedure could only therefore be used for individual cases with specific clinical indications.

Technique

- the site for ovariectomy in a heifer (six to twelve months old) is the flank (standing) or midline caudal abdomen (recumbent)
- in the cow it is the vagina (colpotomy) or flank (standing)
- prior to surgery starve the animal for 24 hours, with no water restriction

Flank approach

- clip the left flank, wash, scrub and disinfect the paralumbar fossa
- paravertebral analgesia (L1–2) or local infiltration ('T-block', 'reverse 7') (see Section 1.9)
- aseptic technique
- make a vertical incision 10–13 cm long in the left flank ventral to lumbar transverse processes 3–4
- separate muscles with scissors and incise peritoneum
- insert a hand to enlarge the peritoneal incision and locate the ovaries
- remove the ovaries with a small effeminator (since the ovarian pedicle is not anaesthetised by the paravertebral block, a swab soaked with a local anaesthetic solution should be applied to the pedicle for 1 minute before using effeminator). Important: do not drop either ovary into the abdominal cavity
- check that the structure removed is entirely ovarian
- suture the abdominal wall routinely
- give systemic antibiotics for one to three days

Vaginal approach (cows only) (see Figure 6.7)

- epidural anaesthesia
- make a stab incision about 5 cm long through the vaginal wall at the 10 o'clock or 2 o'clock position just caudal to the cervix with a sheathed knife (take care to avoid the aorta and rectum)
- insert two fingers to locate one ovary and draw it back into the vagina
- apply a local anaesthetic soaked swab to the pedicle for 1 minute
- insert a long-handled chain ecraseur or spaying shears and remove the ovary (no ligation required)
- repeat on the second side; no vaginal suture is required
- give systemic antibiotics for one to three days, plus an analgesic

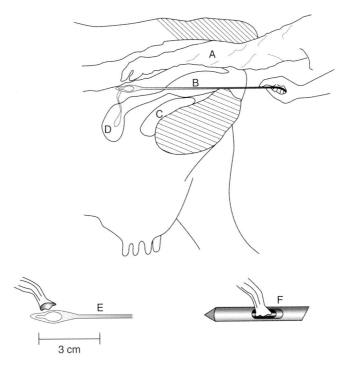

3 cm

Figure 6.7 Ovariectomy with the Willis instrument inserted through the vaginal stab wound under rectal guidance.
The ovary is manipulated through a notch for transection of the ovarian pedicle. With a K-R device the inner sleeve cuts the ovarian pedicle while retaining the ovary in the lumen (see smaller illustrations).
A. sleeved arm in rectum; B. Willis instrument directed through vaginal fornix to ovary; C. bladder; D. uterine body; E. Willis instrument and close-up; F. K-R instrument.

Possible complications

- untoward sequelae include excessive hemorrhage from the ovarian stump, especially from a granulosa cell tumour, and peritonitis
- vaginal approach carries the risk of bowel perforation

Discussion

In the USA specialised spay instruments (K-R: Jorgensen Laboratories, Loveland, CO and Willis: Willis Veterinary Supply, Prehso, SD) have been developed for the colpotomy (vaginal) technique in prepubertal heifers. Production of the K-R instrument has now ceased. The Willis technique (see Figure 6.7) involves bilateral intra-abdominal ovariectomy via a stab incision in the vaginal fornix, using rectal palpation firstly to locate the site of proposed penetration and secondly to manipulate each ovary in turn through the sharp-edged lumen of the spay device. The ovaries are left in the abdominal cavity. With the K-R (Kimberley-Rupp) instrument, the ovary is retained in its lumen until the second ovary has been removed.

6.7 Bladder eversion

Signs

- rare complication of chronic tenesmus, particularly following dystocia
- may mistake the organ for foetal membranes or a large vaginal polyp
- true eversion occurs through the urethral orifice; it will not fill with urine and its origin can be traced to the urethral opening on the floor of the vagina
- differentiate from the bladder prolapse, which occurs through a tear in the vaginal wall (post-parturient): a prolapsed bladder can fill with urine

Repair

- may be difficult due to oedema and possibly trauma to everted bladder
- severe tissue congestion may be present: the bladder may be necrotic or friable
- non-complicated eversions can be carefully replaced under caudal epidural local anaesthesia and gentle manipulation; the urethral opening will require stretching
- technique is similar to replacing a prolapsed uterus (but a much smaller organ and a smaller opening): apply firm and persistent repulsive pressure

whilst feeding edges of the bladder through the urethral opening. The whole everted part of the bladder may be gently squeezed in the palms of the hand to assist replacement

- management of a prolapsed bladder requires it first to be emptied (catheterisation or cystocentesis) and then replaced through laceration in the vaginal wall, which is repaired with a single-layer closure

Possible complications

- repeated eversion carries a poor prognosis
- subsequent bladder rupture may occur due to tissue necrosis

CHAPTER 7

Teat surgery

7.1 Introduction

- significant teat injuries commonly affect the orifice, and less commonly the teat sinus wall
- teat surgery is a demanding test of the skill of the veterinarian; practical and economic considerations must always be considered before attempt (see Discussion Box)
- economic loss results from a loss in milk yield (take care with antibiotic-treated milk); possible loss of quarter if there is a necessity to dry off

---

Discussion

Intensification of dairy farming has led to earlier culling of cows with many of the teat problems discussed in this chapter ('hard milker', see Section 7.2, and teat lacerations, see Section 7.5), which fail to respond to simple management such as a topical wound spray. In many countries treatment may be uneconomic, but in the developing world with small herds the individual cow remains a valuable resource and the owner demands maximum care and attention to teat conditions.

Bovine Surgery and Lameness, Third Edition. A. David Weaver, Owen Atkinson, Guy St. Jean and Adrian Steiner.
© 2018 John Wiley & Sons Ltd. Published 2018 by John Wiley & Sons Ltd.
Companion website: www.wiley.com/go/weaver/bovine-surgery

Restraint and anaesthesia

- particularly important for teat surgery because repairs must be meticulous. See Chapter 1, including Section 1.9, for a full description of regional local anaesthesia of teats
- adequate restraint is also required for operator safety; adequate anaesthesia and pain relief is necessary for cow welfare
- xylaxine alone is not sufficient for teat surgery and is contra-indicated in advanced gestation; possible sudden recumbency is a problem!
- using a Wopa-type crate with one leg lifted or lateral recumbency, both with local anaesthesia, are possible restraint methods
- ideally, a recumbent cow is positioned in a tilt table; a hydraulic tilting foot-paring crush may be available in the field
- local infusion of a local anaesthetic into the teat (2–5 ml) can be useful but is adequate only for very minor techniques (e.g. removal of a free-moving teat pea by gradual dilation of the teat canal) as the anaesthetic will not penetrate into the submucosa or deeper layers

Anatomy (see Figures 7.1 and 7.2)

- moving distally to proximally:
  - teat orifice or *ostium papillare*
  - streak canal, teat canal or *ductus papillaris*: lined with longitudinally folded stratified squamous epithelium; glandular function (produces a waxy teat plug)
  - Furstenberg's rosette: muscular sphincter at the distal end of the teat, proximal to the streak canal, involved in teat opening/closing and local immunity
  - teat sinus, *pars papillaris* or lactiferous sinus (teat part): superficial columnar, deeper cuboidal epithelium; below the mucosa is a layer of embryonal-type cells capable of rapid proliferation; longitudinal folds of the teat sinus allow expansion to accommodate milk volume
  - lactiferous sinus (glandular part), udder cistern, milk cistern or *pars glandularis*
- five primary layers to the lining of the teat, starting innermost:
  1. mucosa
  2. submucosa
  3. highly vascularised connective tissue layer: elastic and fibrous tissue including vessels and nerves
  4. muscularis (smooth muscle)
  5. skin
- for purposes of surgery, layers 2, 3 and 4 are considered as the 'intermediate layer'

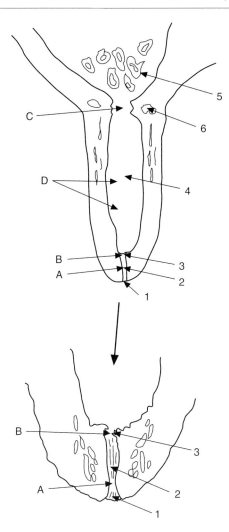

Figure 7.1 Teat anatomy and sites of stenosis.
1. teat orifice (*ostium papillare*); 2. teat or streak canal (*ductus papillaris*); 3. Fursten-berg's rosette; 4. teat sinus (*pars papillaris*); 5. lactiferous sinus or milk cistern (*pars glandularis*); 6. venous plexus.
Sites of teat obstruction: A. tight streak canal (distal obstruction); B. obstruction at Furstenberg's rosette (distal obstruction); C teat sinus obstruction (proximal obstruction); D. teat sinus obstruction (middle obstruction).

(a)

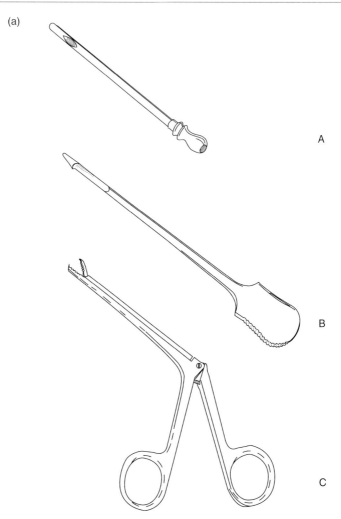

A

B

C

(a) A. milk catheter for passive milk drainage; B. Hug's teat knife, or Yankee teat bistoury, for opening or dilating the streak canal or cutting teat lumen granuloma; C. teat alligator forceps for the removal of 'milk stones', either free or attached to teat mucosa, through the streak canal.

Figure 7.2   Teat instruments.

- repairs (e.g. longitudinal lacerations) include a suturing teat in three layers: mucosa; intermediate layer; skin
- primary blood supply via the pudendal artery (inguinal canal); longitudinal arterial supply down the teat

(b)

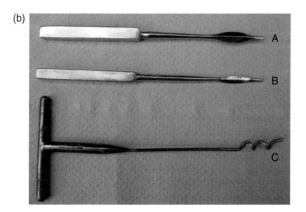

(b) A and B. Maclean's teat knives (teat bistoury) for opening or dilating streak canal; C. Hudson's teat spiral, for dilating streak canal and removal of teat granuloma. Only use teat instruments that have been sterilised prior to use.

Figure 7.2 (*Continued*)

- venous drainage via the vein encircling the teat sphincter flowing to the large venous plexus at the base of the teat, draining into the pudendal vein

7.2 Obstruction of teat orifice, streak canal or Furstenberg's rosette

Aetiology

- common problem
- partial obstruction ('hard milker') due to a local blunt (self) trauma, e.g. a crushed or trodden teat
- possibly secondary to hyperkeratosis of the teat orifice due to milking machine malfunction (e.g. excessive vacuum pressure)
- possibly secondary to microtraumatic wounds sometimes permitting the development of *Fusobacterium necrophorum* infection ('blackspot'); poor bedding hygiene may be implicated

Signs

- a quarter milks out slowly, or a 'valve' is evident, and a vicious cycle may develop as the remaining quarters tend to be over-milked, resulting in bruising and eversion of the teat orifice and development of mastitis
- some cases are inoperable.

Treatment of obstruction of streak canal

- controversial; no controlled studies on the efficacy of a method
- in mild cases consider simple temporary insertion of a wax teat plug tube
- alternatively, tense the orifice between a finger and thumb and cleanse with iodophor solution; insert Maclean's® teat knife (bistoury) once and withdraw rapidly whilst maintaining pressure of the finger and thumb at the orifice
- check the adequacy of milk flow and, if poor, re-insert the knife and rotate 90° to the original incision before once again withdrawing rapidly (to make a cross-shaped cut)
- insert a wax teat plug for five days (optional)
- ideally remove milk from the quarter every two to three hours for the first two days; important to stop stenosis by rapid healing and scar tissue
- administer prophylactic intramammary antibiotics
- instruct the stockman to roll the end of the teat regularly before applying the machine (opens incision; reduces early first intention healing)
- in the case of mastitis, treat with intramammary antibiotics before any treatment
- in the case of inflammation, perform passive milk drainage for resolution of the inflammation before attempting treatment
- in the case of 'black spot' infection, treat the teat orifice with a topical antibiotic cream to resolve infection; be aware that a milk withdrawal period will be required. No further treatment may be necessary.

Warning

Do not insert any temporary stiff cannula as the proximal end can cause severe trauma to the teat cistern mucosa, resulting in mastitis and/or later scar tissue of the teat cistern.

Treatment of obstruction in the area of Fürstenberg's rosette with theloresectoscope/thelotomy

- remove obstructing tissue in Furstenberg's rosette or proximal streak canal under visual control during thelotomy or, if available, with theloresectoscope (see Figure 7.3)
- if theloresectoscope is available, perform the lateral approach via a stab incision in the teat and remove all protruding tissue with the incorporated cautery sling; suture a stab incision with a simple suture in the intermediate layer and two simple skin sutures
- allow passive milk drainage instead of machine milking for 10 days after thelotomy or for 3 days after theloresectoscopy

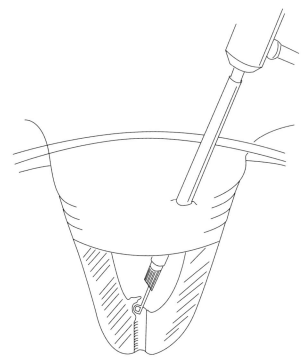

Figure 7.3   Theloresectoscopy. The scope is introduced into the teat sinus through a lateral teat wall incision. Stenotic tissue around Furstenberg's rosette is removed with the cautery sling.

- do not perform surgery as long as mastitis or teat inflammation is present
- normal machine milking returns in 75–90% of cases; the recurrence rate is lower if obstruction tissue is removed with the cautery sling instead of cutting with a scalpel

7.3 Milk stones and teat lumen granuloma

Introduction

- also known as 'pea' (free-moving object) or 'spider' (proliferation of granulation tissue near Furstenberg's rosette)
- milk stones, also known as lactoliths, are small calcium calculi, often with a small granulation tissue nidus (result of trauma)
- a true granuloma lesion is a discrete proliferation of granulation tissue covered by mucosa and caused by blunt trauma, which initially causes a submucosal haematoma projecting into the teat cistern

Signs

- often asymptomatic but can eventually cause interference with the free passage of milk
- often intermittent obstruction; usually can feel the 'pea' in the cistern or near the streak canal
- rarely pedunculated
- painless.

Treatment

- small peas can be milked out of the teat canal by high pressure produced by manual stripping of the teat
- complete removal of a true granuloma is often difficult and the recurrence rate is high
- attempted blind removal via a mosquito or long alligator forceps, teat bistoury (Hug's teat knife), or fixation and traction by Hudson's teat spiral, often causes further trauma and recurrence
- freely moving obstructions (not pedunculated):
  - carefully insert Hudson's teat spiral fully into the teat cistern by screwing through the teat canal
  - apply firm downward pressure of the pea by squeezing the teat hard in a milking action (with the base of the teat occluded by the thumb and forefinger)
  - simultaneously, gently withdraw the teat spiral to dilate the teat canal at the proximal end (not twisting); the pea should enter the teat canal and be removed by a combination of gradual withdrawal of the teat spiral and continued pressure of milk in the teat cistern
  - other teat dilator instruments are sometimes used in a similar way
  - limit repeated attempts: risk of trauma to the teat canal and subsequent stenosis
  - alternatively, surgically dilate the teat canal using a teat knife (see Section 7.2); high risk of subsequent scaring and stenosis
- in cases producing clinical signs and if mass is pedunculated, with the membrane less than 6 mm thick and coverage of the resection site with mucosa is possible:
  - open surgery (thelotomy) in lateral recumbency following a ring block
  - vertical incision in the teat wall opposite mass and resection by scalpel
  - undermine mucosa around the lesion and cover the lesion with mobilised mucosa
  - ensure adequate haemostasis before covering the defect
  - suture in three layers: mucosa with a fine continuous absorbable material, then an intermediate layer and finally skin
  - teat wound heals well after a careful, sterile technique

- milk daily using a sterile teat cannula (passive milk drainage)
- return to machine milking of a quarter on day 11
- drying off the quarter is advisable with pedunculated peas with a granulo-matous membrane > 5 mm, or with peas that cannot easily be removed by the methods described above

7.4 Teat base membrane obstruction

- congenital form in heifers; acquired form in cows
- usually at the start of a new lactation
- aetiology unknown, possibly inflammation of the basal annular membrane; anecdotally linked to a previous mycoplasma infection in heifers
- teat lance or Hug's knife (see Figure 7.2a) is inserted in an attempt to break down the annular membrane
- prognosis is very poor and treatment usually hopeless; allowing the quarter to remain dry is the only option

7.5 Traumatic lacerations of teat

Introduction

- factors affecting the outcome and prognosis include:
  - involvement of the streak canal worsens the prognosis for return to a normal milk flow
  - direction of wound: longitudinal wounds heal better than transverse ones
  - integrity of the blood supply to the distal wound margin may be minimal in the case of a distal horizontal wound
  - degree of wound contamination and the presence of infection
  - amount of skin loss
- always consider a conservative treatment by drying off the quarter; surgery is not always the best option

Treatment

Non-perforating horizontal lacerations with skin flaps
- skin flaps, usually located at the level of the streak canal, may be carefully removed with a scalpel, as dehiscence after suturing is very likely to occur
- cover the wound over with a waterproof film (e.g. Opsite® Smith & Nephew) followed by a teat bandage (e.g. Leukopor®) to keep the wound clean, and limit teat swelling
- secondary intention healing will occur, which usually results in a perfectly functional teat and is much preferable to a permanent skin flap

Non-perforating longitudinal teat lacerations (not involving teat sinus)

- basic surgical principles apply and all wounds must be regarded as contaminated
- thorough gentle cleansing with non-irritant dilute antiseptic, e.g. povidone-iodine or chlorhexidine, or saline
- suture the submucosa and skin in two layers after cleansing, irrigation and meticulous debridement; preserve all non-affected tissue
- insert a continuous suture into the muscle layer with monofilament 2 metric absorbable suture material; simple skin sutures using interrupted 2 metric polypropylene or skin staples
- *alternatively*: do not suture; allow healing by secondary intension
- cover the wound over with a waterproof film (e.g. Opsite Smith & Nephew) followed by a teat bandage (e.g. Leukopor tape) to keep the wound clean, and limit teat swelling
- use NSAIDs to reduce pain and inflammation; swelling of the teat is common and can lead to wound breakdown
- allow passive milk drainage every milking; a shortened period of machine milking may be possible depending on the degree of discomfort, which does not appear to impede healing (leave the teat bandage in place)
- potential problems include:
  - excessive suture tension, which causes puckering and skin necrosis
  - poor healing resulting from inadequate debridement or cleansing of the lesion
  - severe teat swelling resulting in excessive suture tension and wound breakdown
  - clinical mastitis (treat appropriately)

Perforating teat lacerations (involving teat sinus)

- will always require suturing in three layers if the teat is to be salvaged (see Figure 7.4)
- these lacerations should be treated as an emergency
- carries a poor prognosis: if healing does occur, a milk fistula is common
- better to dry off the quarter if the lesion is not fresh (>12 hours) or grossly contaminated; may be possible to effect a surgical repair later (e.g. at drying off)
- work in good operating facilities, with adequate light, cleanliness and efficient analgesia
- ensure the stockman understands post-operative care

Surgical technique

- cleanse with copious sterile isotonic saline
- trim off the devitalised skin, intermediate layer and mucosa

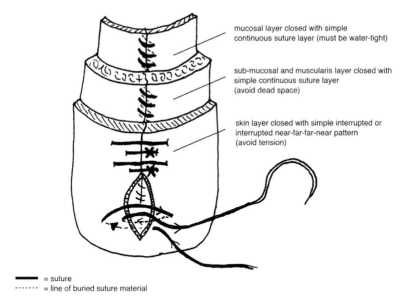

mucosal layer closed with simple
continuous suture layer (must be water-tight)

sub-mucosal and muscularis layer closed with
simple continuous suture layer
(avoid dead space)

skin layer closed with simple interrupted or
interrupted near-far-far-near pattern
(avoid tension)

▬▬▬ = suture
------- = line of buried suture material

Figure 7.4 Suturing longitudinal teat lacerations that penetrate the teat sinus in three layers.

- control the haemorrhage using clamps or a tourniquet on the teat base and swabbing with sterile gauze (do this after trimming in order to assess tissue vitality)
- remove all blood clots including clots in the teat lumen: these will prevent healing
- close the mucosal layer using a continuous layer; use a round-bodied swaged-on needle and 1 or 1.5 metric polyglactin 910 (Vicryl®)
- insert a teat cannula to carefully check the integrity of the suture line: any milk leakage will prevent healing and a sinus or complete wound break-down will result
- close the intermediate layer (including submucosa and muscularis) using a simple continuous pattern and 1.5 metric polyglactin 910
- suture the skin using simple interrupted sutures of 3 metric polygactin 10, or a synthetic non-absorbable suture; ensure the dead space is closed; a near-far-far-near pattern may be used to reduce tension on the sutures
- cover the wound over with a waterproof film (e.g. Opsite Smith & Nephew) followed by a teat bandage (e.g. Leukopor tape) to keep the wound clean, and limit teat swelling
- use NSAIDs to reduce pain and inflammation
- prophylactic intramammary antibiotics is a sensible precaution; an aque-ous solution of crystalline penicillin may be preferable to using non-aqueous intramammary preparations, which can impede healing

- allow passive milk drainage or (preferably) machine milking using a reduced period, leaving the teat bandage in place; avoid hand stripping, which is more likely to cause wound breakdown
- remove the skin sutures after 10–14 days
- possible causes of breakdown:
  - severe post-operative oedema
  - poor suture technique
  - infection
  - excessive suture tension
  - necrosis of wound edges
  - leakage of milk through the mucosa layer

7.6 Imperforate teat

- aetiology is congenital in heifers, or acquired as a result of trauma in adult cattle
- assess whether milk is present in the teat sinus and if Fürstenberg's rosette is present
- surgery is only indicated in positive cases
- perforate at the expected site of the streak canal and introduce a temporary teat plug for 10 days
- hard milking, milk leakage and mastitis are frequent complications

7.7 Incompetent teat sphincter

- aetiology is invariably traumatic in the case of a single teat, which constantly or intermittently leaks milk
- treatment is difficult and indicated only in chronic case (>3 weeks) as fibrosis of granulation tissue repair may correct the condition spontaneously
- inject a minute volume of teflon or irritant drug (e.g. sterile Lugol's iodine) with tuberculin or insulin syringe around the teat orifice (e.g. 4 × 0.1 ml) to stimulate discrete circumferential fibrosis
- technique is hazardous and results unpredictable

7.8 Teat amputation

Supernumerary teats

- congenital and inherited condition
- the teats tend to be small, are commonly caudal, but sometimes are attached to the normal teat
- remove when one to nine months old; never within one month of parturition (oedema, wound breakdown, infection, mastitis)

- up to three months old, removal may be performed by an unqualified but trained person, but under anaesthesia
- UK law requires that surgery in calves over three months old be performed by a veterinary surgeon under anaesthesia; Swiss law requires all ruminant surgical procedures to be performed by a veterinarian under anaesthesia; many countries have no such legislation to cover this, or other specific procedures

Technique

- carefully identify supernumerary teats: always turn over small calves for good visualisation
- small calves: resect with scissors
- older calf: crush at the base with a small Burdizzo® (emasculator) and resect with a knife along the inner edge of the blades
- line of section should be cranial to caudal, not transverse, so that subsequent scar merges into natural folds of udder skin
- suture only if the wound edges separate

Amputation due to disease (cows)

- indicated in severe purulent or gangrenous mastitis of one quarter to permit drainage
- also after irreversible teat damage

Technique

- local analgesia of the teat base and application of a good restraint
- place the teat clamp (Burdizzo) at the proximal aspect of the teat; amputate with a scalpel at the junction between the proximal and middle third of the teat
- ligate the vessels if necessary: significant bleeding is likely
- retain the teat lumen by continuous sutures in the wall (skin to mucosa) using a Ford-interlocking suture to maintain drainage
- irrigation with copious amounts of tap water may be useful
- the quarter will eventually dry off as a result of secondary infection and mastitis

Amputation due to injury

- teat amputation may also be indicated in cows with severe teat damage where reconstructive surgery and return to normal function cannot be expected, e.g. loss of the distal portion of the teat, or long, oblique or transverse tears into the teat canal
- amputation and closure of the teat sinus is only successful in the absence of infection

- alternatively, an open sinus is an acceptable option for distal teat lacerations, though significant milk leakage can be expected

Technique

- amputation site is 1–2 cm distal to the udder–teat junction
- transect the teat by scalpel, resecting the mucous membrane 1 cm below the cut surface
- ligate bleeding vessels
- invert the mucosa by continuous suture in the deep intermediate layer (see Figure 7.5)

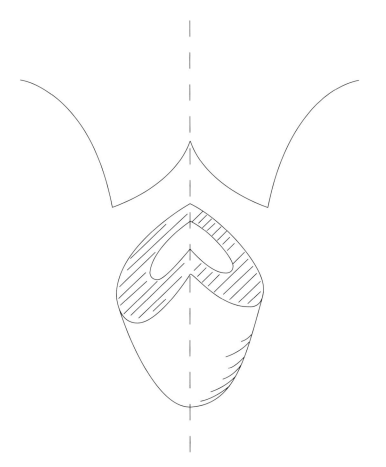

Figure 7.5 Teat amputation with primary closure: cut surfaces for closed teat amputation.

- insert horizontal mattress sutures to close the superficial intermediate layer
- appose skin edges with simple sutures or metal clips (staples)
- infuse antibiotics into the quarter before final sutures are placed (optional)

Discussion
Meticulous care to details of the technique is vital in surgical repair of traumatic teat lesions. A multiplicity of suture patterns that may be recommended illustrates the unsatisfactory results commonly obtained, but this is more likely to be a result of deficiencies and breakdown in basic surgical principles than to any defect in the suture configuration. Dedicated after-care by the stockman and veterinarian is of major importance for success. Apart from wound breakdown and local infection, mastitis remains the major hazard, and up to 40% of teat-traumatised cows are culled for mastitis within, or at the end of, that particular lactation.

CHAPTER 8

Male urinogenital surgery

8.1 Preputial prolapse or eversion

Introduction

- a mild degree of intermittent preputial prolapse or eversion is considered normal in some breeds, notably the polled Hereford and Aberdeen Angus in the UK and the Brahman and Santa Gertrudis breeds (*Bos indicus*) in North America
- prolapse develops during a normal non-erectile movement of the penis within the preputial cavity
- pathological prolapse is more likely in individuals exposed to preputial trauma

Predisposing factors

- pendulous and long sheath
- large preputial orifice with a limited ability to contract
- poor development of the preputial and retractor penis muscles in some polled breeds (see above)

Bovine Surgery and Lameness, Third Edition. A. David Weaver, Owen Atkinson, Guy St. Jean and Adrian Steiner.
© 2018 John Wiley & Sons Ltd. Published 2018 by John Wiley & Sons Ltd.
Companion website: www.wiley.com/go/weaver/bovine-surgery

Preputial trauma

- pathological prolapse is more likely in bulls at range or pasture exposed to trauma, which includes irritation from foreign bodies (vegetation, dust or earth), or which are secondary to penile injury
- common site of injury is the mucosa adjacent to the skin–prepuce junction
- frostbite can cause major problems in certain areas in the winter
- all cases of preputial prolapse should have a complete physical examination of the external genitalia
- sequence of events following injury is:
  - severe localised oedema and hyperaemic congestion
  - extensive fibrosis with secondarily infected fissures and cracks
  - areas of granulation tissue develop in the cracks with secondary infection and possible abscessation
  - as a result, penile erection may be abnormal, with only the glans tip passing through this damaged region or a complete inability to extend the penis (paraphimosis)
- an alternative common site of preputial trauma leading to prolapse is the reflection of the parietal prepuce on to the body of the penis; may be sustained during artificial collection of semen or as an injury at natural service

Conservative treatment

- recent injury to the prolapsed mucosa may be treated conservatively (most economical):
  - carefully cleanse the area with a non-irritant dilute antiseptic solution (povidone-iodine)
  - soak the damaged prepuce in swabs containing 25% magnesium sulfate solution to reduce oedema
  - apply emollient dressing (e.g. zinc and castor oil ointment) and replace the prolapse
  - place a purse-string suture in the preputial orifice or, if the prepuce is too oedematous to be reduced, a polyvinyl or rubber tube (2.5 cm diameter and 15 cm long) is placed in the preputial lumen and wrapped firmly with elastic tape
  - tape is applied directly to the tube and the skin on the sheath, beginning at the preputial orifice and extending towards the abdominal wall
  - placement of tube decreases oedema and permits escape of the urine
  - administer systemic antibiotics and anti-inflammatory drugs for five days, as well as local antibiotic irrigation
  - dress any prolapsed preputial mucosa with lanolin-based ointment and keep covered with stockinette to prevent further trauma

- snuggly wrap any prolapsed prepuce within stockinette in an adhesive bandage, which attaches to the sheath to act as a pressure bandage; change daily whilst the prolapse is monitored for reduction in size
- check for urine pooling in the sheath and preputial cavity, which will exacerbate inflammation

Surgical treatment: circumcision

- cases with secondary diffuse fibrosis and excoriation or recurrent and chronic cases require surgery in lateral recumbency
- attempt reduction in oedema pre-surgery using pressure bandages as described above
- sedation and ring block local analgesic infiltration, or general anaesthesia (see Chapter 1)
- a rubber-band tourniquet may be applied proximally to decrease haemorrhage
- two circumcision techniques are used commonly in bulls:
  - resection and anastomosis, also known as posthioplasty or reefing;
  - surgical amputation, resulting in the loss of equal amounts of external and internal lining of the prolapsed portion of prepuce, performed using a suture or ring technique
- four potential post-operative complications must be recognised before surgery is attempted:
  i. prepuce can be made too short for breeding: it depends on the breed but, as a general rule, the usable prepuce must be twice as long as the free portion of the penis; particularly a problem for *Bos taurus*
  ii. the surgeon should remove only the diseased portion of the prepuce
  iii. circumferential scar (cicatrix) contraction can result in phimosis
  iv. post-operative haemorrhage can cause dehiscence and infection

---

Warning

Consider if there is an economic justification for circumcision surgery; the risks of complications resulting in loss of use for breeding are considerable.

---

1. Resection and anastomosis technique (performed with the penis extended)
- close clip and shave the hair from the distal portion of the sheath and preputial orifice
- if penile extension is possible, place towel forceps in the apical ligament or alternatively have an assistant hold the penis

- scrub and prepare the prepuce and penis
- place two marking sutures proximal and distal to the area of prepuce to be removed to ensure that the prepuce is aligned anatomically when sutured
- examine the prepuce and make a circular incision through the epithelium of the prepuce proximal to the area to be resected
- deepen this incision until normal tissue is observed
- make a second circular incision distal to the area to be removed; in *Bos indicus* bulls, it is usually necessary to resect at least 15 cm of prepuce to prevent recurrence of the prolapse; in *Bos taurus* bulls, as much prepuce as possible should be retained
- connect these two circular incisions and then with two longitudinal incisions
- remove the pathological portion of prepuce by sharp dissection. It is important to control any haemorrhage, because even small haematomas could induce wound dehiscence
- ligate any large veins or arteries
- lavage the surgical site copiously with saline solution
- extend and retract the penis until the two incisions are in apposition, thus ensuring that the penis is freely movable; the two marking sutures should also be aligned
- if the elastic tissue has been incised appose it using interrupted absorbable sutures
- close the epithelium with a simple interrupted pattern
- suture a 4 cm diameter Penrose drain to the free portion of the penis with three or four interrupted absorbable sutures; place sutures superficially to avoid the urethra. The Penrose drain will direct urine away from the incision line during the healing period
- insert a gas-sterilised 15 cm section of 2.5 cm polyvinyl or rubber tube into the prepuce with the Penrose drain through it
- attach the tube to the sheath with elastic adhesive tape and completely enclose the incision. The adhesive tape can be sutured to the skin to prevent premature dislodgement of the tube; presence of the tube decreases oedema formation and aids in the prevention of stenosis

After-care:
- administer systemic antibiotics for a minimum of five days after surgery
- remove the bandage and tube five to seven days after surgery
- replace the tube and bandage if a penile prolapse occurs; vigorous attempts to extend the penis and inspect the surgical site should not be made until three weeks after surgery
- do not remove the preputial sutures because such attempts may damage the surgical wound
- keep the bull from breeding for at least 60 days when, if possible, the animal should be evaluated to make sure the penis is extendable without

restriction of the prepuce. Oedema of the prepuce usually persists for ten days after surgery. NSAIDs and diuretic agents can be used if oedema is excessive

Technique of surgical amputation (penis not extended)

- may be performed when penile extension is not possible because of phimosis or adhesions
- clip and prepare aseptically the area of the end of the sheath
- attach two Backhaus towel clamps to the distal end of the prepuce and extend fully from the sheath
- place a finger inside the prepuce
- insert horizontal mattress sutures for the full thickness through the prepuce immediately proximal to the area of amputation: these mattress sutures should overlap one another through both layers of the prepuce, but not the lumen, to control bleeding (see Figure 8.1a); tie tightly
- amputate the prepuce through an oblique line to create an oval orifice (see Figure 8.1b)
- appose the edges of the prepuce with a simple interrupted pattern
- suture a Penrose drain to the penis and insert a tube into the prepuce and attach with elastic tape
- the post-operative management is similar to the first technique

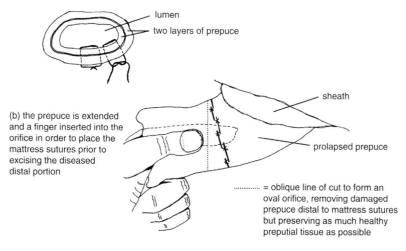

(a) tight mattress sutures passed through both layers of prolapsed prepuce to reduce bleeding. Afterwards, the cut edges of the prepuce are sutured together using a simple continuous suture.

lumen

two layers of prepuce

sheath

(b) the prepuce is extended and a finger inserted into the orifice in order to place the mattress sutures prior to excising the diseased distal portion

prolapsed prepuce

.... = oblique line of cut to form an oval orifice, removing damaged prepuce distal to mattress sutures but preserving as much healthy preputial tissue as possible

Figure 8.1   Surgical amputation of the preputial prolapse using method 2 (penis not extended).

- a V-shaped incision at the ventral aspect of the preputial orifice can be made to reduce the risk of phimosis
- a modification of the amputation technique has been described in which as much as possible of the unaffected inner aspect of the prolapsed prepuce is left and only the external aspect affected by the inflammatory process is removed; this is especially crucial in *Bos taurus* breeds

Preputial amputation with ring (penis not extended)
- preputial amputation using the ring technique involves the insertion of a plastic ring into the preputial cavity
- this technique can be advantageous to the practitioner with limited facilities; it is primarily a salvage procedure
- the ring and sutures act as a tourniquet, and the prepuce distal to the ring will slough due to ischaemic necrosis in about 14 days
- the ring is made from a tube 5 cm long and 4 cm in diameter with 1 mm holes drilled through the wall spaced 5 mm apart at the midpoint; the ends of the tube should be smooth and the tube should be sterilised
- place the bull in lateral recumbency
- place the plastic ring into the preputial cavity so that the holes are located at the desired point of amputation
- put a ligating suture pattern around the prepuce through the holes in the ring using a non-absorbable suture material and tie every suture tightly
- amputate the prepuce 5 mm distal to the suture line. Minimal haemorrhage is observed if all sutures have been tightened sufficiently
- extend the penis through the plastic ring and suture a Penrose drain to it
- return the penis, prepuce and ring to the preputial cavity and place a purse-string suture at the preputial orifice to prevent prolapse

After-care:
- after two weeks remove the purse-string suture and pull the ring out; necrotic tissue and sutures are often still attached to the ring; the ring may slough spontaneously during this period
- sexual rest is recommended for 60 days after treatment
- prognosis for a return to breeding is only fair

Intrapreputial adhesions

- present problems in penile exposure, evaluation and management
- exposure may be very difficult and accompanied by tearing of the adjacent preputial mucosa
- degree of mechanical hindrance caused by the adhesions may be hard to evaluate since, though some adhesions will be palpable, others will not
- adhesions are frequently obliquely longitudinal rather than circumferential

Surgery:
- remove the mucosa overlying the adhesions between circumferential incisions
- resect all fibrotic adhesions down to the *tunica albuginea*
- carefully appose mucosal edges, as in the first circumcision technique (see above)

After-care:
- the bull should be rested for two to three weeks, depending on the degree of post-operative oedema, and can then be teased with increasing frequency (initially every three days, later daily) to prevent recurrence of fibrosis and adhesions
- prognosis is guarded or poor depending on the area resected

8.2 Penile haematoma

Introduction

- more accurately termed rupture of the *corpus cavernosum penis* (CCP) following a rent in the *tunica albuginea* (TA) (see Figure 8.2)
- blood explodes into the surrounding tissues forming a large haematoma
- less commonly, some major vessels dorsal to the TA are ruptured without involvement of the TA itself

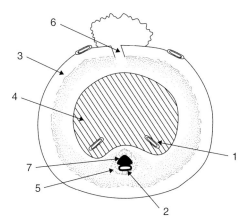

Figure 8.2 Cross-section of the penis just distal to distal flexure (sigmoid) to show the haematoma site.
1. deep veins of penis; 2. artery of penis; 3. *tunica albuginea*; 4. *corpus cavernosum penis*; 5. *corpus cavernosum urethrae*; 6. usual site of penile haematoma, with blood from *corpus cavernosum penis* escaping through dorsal tear in *tunica albuginea*; 7. urethra

- occurs during vigorous, over-enthusiastic thrusting at intromission, or possibly spontaneously during masturbation
- penis may undergo severe downward bending leading to a tear in *tunica albuginea* (TA)
- a relatively commonly encountered penile injury; alleged to have a higher incidence in horned English breeds (e.g. Hereford)

Signs and pathology

- the site of the rupture is immediately cranial to the scrotal and usually dorsal, close to insertion of the retractor penis muscles near the distal flexure of the sigmoid
- rupture of the CCP causes an immediate haematoma, which may grow over a few days to a variable extent as a result of slow leakage
- a lesion may be strictly localised or relatively diffuse; initially the lesion may be missed unless careful clinical examination is made including palpation of the area cranial to the scrotum
- the bull will show signs of pain and discomfort
- the deeper the site of the rupture, the poorer is the prognosis
- important to assess the degree of possible extension of the penis after the rupture:
  - if good extension is still possible on manipulation, then the prognosis is good
  - the inability to extend the penis has a very poor prognosis
- secondary preputial oedema and preputial prolapse may occur, rarely with some penile protrusion
- compression of lymphatic and venous drainage may cause secondary preputial prolapse

---

Warning

The natural course of a penile haematoma is gradual reduction of the swelling, as oedema disappears and the haematoma is slowly organised into fibrous tissue. A significant proportion of cases of penile haematoma, however, develop the serious complication of an abscess at the site (often *Trueperella pyogenes*) with a fibrous adhesion; the prognosis is then grave.

Abscessation usually leads to a fluctuating swelling to one side of the penis, separate from the penile body. Avoid exploratory paracentesis, which can result in iatrogenic infection of a sterile haematoma.

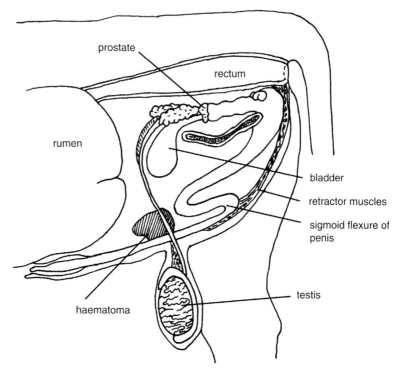

Figure 8.3   Anatomy of bovine penis showing the sigmoid flexure, retractor muscles and site of haematoma following a rupture of the *corpus cavernosum penis.*

Differential diagnosis

- preputial prolapse of primary origin
- penile injury of other aetiology
- urethral rupture due to occlusion by calculus

Conservative treatment

- small haematoma rapidly shrinks, is often hard to detect ten days later and requires no treatment; good prognosis
- a larger haematoma may resolve following medical treatment:
  - remove the bull from the herd and ensure sexual rest for 60 days
  - give systemic antibiotics for seven days and NSAID pain relief
  - apply hot packs, cold water sprays or possibly ultrasound; all these methods lack controlled studies but have allegedly reduced the healing period, but also increase the degree of fibrosis

- after 30 days manually extend the penis and check the sensation of the free portion; lack of sensation indicates bilateral nerve damage and the bull will neither breed nor ejaculate into an artificial vagina

Surgical treatment (see Figure 8.4)

- due to the possibility of infection entering the haematoma and causing abscessation, surgery is advisable for all cases where economically justifiable, except for smaller haematomata (<20 cm) that rapidly resolve
- delay surgery until 7–10 days after the accident
- place the bull on systemic antibiotics as soon as possible following injury
- note that long-term systemic antibiotic therapy (oxytetracyclines, sulphonamides) may temporarily adversely affect fertility
- operate with an aseptic technique under GA (sedation and local infiltration analgesia are not recommended); may require referral to University clinic
- starve for 48 hours and no water for 24 hours
- place the bull in lateral recumbency
- aseptic preparation of the affected area, which should be draped throughout surgery
- incise laterally through the skin of the sheath into lateral aspect of CCP over haematoma
- carefully evacuate the haematoma of all clotted blood by blunt dissection with fingers and gentle curettage
- exteriorise the penis proximal to the haematoma to inspect the distal part of sigmoid flexure, where the source of the haemorrhage may sometimes be identified

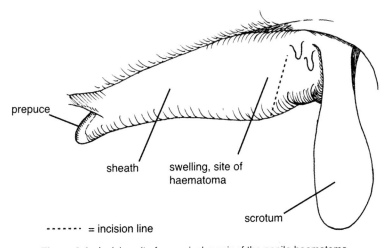

Figure 8.4 Incision site for surgical repair of the penile haematoma.

- remove any superficial blood clots; bluntly dissect through the elastic tissue to identify the rent
- if possible, suture the tear in TA, after debridement of edges, with simple interrupted sutures of 5 metric PGA
- cautiously try to break down any adhesions around the penis that have formed since the accident
- irrigate the haematoma cavity with three mega crystalline penicillin G dissolved in 20 ml of normal saline, and try to appose the wall of the haematoma cavity
- similarly, close the subcutaneous tissues in a simple continuous pattern with PGA after the assistant has grasped and extended the penis to the maximum extent
- close the skin incision with interrupted non-absorbable simple or mattress sutures
- maintain the bull on systemic antibiotics for a further five days after surgery
- avoid insertion of drains in an attempt to reduce the post-operative accumulation of serum

After-care

- four days after surgery tranquillise the bull and assess the potential degree of penile protrusion and break down any small adhesions
- tease the bull after three weeks to discourage development of scar tissue and adhesions of subcutaneous tissues to the penile body
- the bull may be returned to service after 60 days
- prognosis is guarded, but about 75% return to natural breeding following surgery

Possible complications

- temporary seroma formation, abscessation, adhesions to the sheath, nerve damage (with desensitisation of the glans penis)
- vascular shunt formation, recurrence of injury and preputial injury from secondary prolapse

8.3 Urolithiasis

Introduction

- calculus is a clinical problem in entire but more frequently in castrated male cattle
- triple phosphate calculi are found in cattle on concentrate feed
- silica calculi in cattle on high silica pasture grass or hay (e.g. North America)

- not a problem in female cattle due to their relatively larger urethral diameter, though severe cystitis occasionally develops from a bladder packed with calculi

Clinical signs

- initial straining with partial or complete urinary obstruction
- clinical cases are dull and feed intake is reduced
- after the initial 24 hours of obstruction tenesmus ceases
- blockage can be at a proximal or distal part of the sigmoid flexure, distal 30 cm of the penis, or over the ischial arch
- later pressure necrosis of urethral mucosa and eventual urethral rupture with seepage of urine into subcutaneous tissues of the ventral body wall and possibly scrotum is possible in untreated cases: obvious ventral oedema
- rupture of bladder, often in the dorsal cranial part of the fundus but occasionally near the bladder neck, and gradual accumulation of intra-abdominal urine is another possibility ('water belly'); diagnosis with ultrasound; consider paracentesis (see Section 3.1)
- subcutaneous accumulation of urine can be treated by longitudinal skin incisions to allow drainage; eventually results in skin slough as the blood supply is impaired, leaving a moist area of granulating tissue (30–40 cm diameter) in which the penis may be identified and from which urine drips (mild uraemia)
- following complete urinary obstruction and bladder rupture, cattle may remain comparatively bright; blood urea increases after three days at a rate of about 10 mmol/litre/day, with death from uraemia and associated metabolic problems after seven to ten days

Treatment

- surgery to allow urine drainage in cases of ruptured urethra may be undertaken in uraemic cattle, with the aim of economic salvage several weeks later when there is no metabolic abnormality and the surgical wounds have healed
- urethrostomy is a relatively simple procedure that will usually salvage non-breeding bulls and bullocks (see below)

Urethrotomy

- in rare cases an attempt can be made to preserve the breeding capacity of a valuable bull by urethrotomy to remove calculi, but surgery is seldom successful for several reasons:
  - precise location of one or more calculi may be difficult to establish
  - several calculi may necessitate multiple incisions

  - closure of the urethral wall is awkward, as attempts at simple apposition, with minimal stenosis, frequently result in urinary seepage through the incision
  - fibrosis and chronic stenosis are common sequelae, eventually leading to recurrence of blockage by several smaller calculi
- intraurethral insertion of a polypropylene catheter to a site proximal to the incision and protruding through the glans can be attempted; in this technique urethral sutures pass through the muscularis and outer serosal layers only. The catheter is removed five to seven days later
- urethral obstruction caused by one or more calculi lodged in the sigmoid region should be relieved by a midline incision in the caudal dorsal aspect of the scrotum, i.e. the ventral perineal region. The relatively mobile sigmoid may be exteriorised for palpation and surgery

Urethrostomy

- urethrostomy, i.e. a permanent urethral fistula, is indicated in complete urethral obstruction at the level of, or distal to, the ischial arch; a salvage operation
- caudal epidural analgesia (see Section 1.9)
- routine skin preparation from the anus to the scrotal neck and about 10 cm to each side of the midline
- blunt dissection around the distal part of the root and proximal body of the penis; the crura are surrounded by the ischiocavernosus muscles, which meet in a midline *raphé* (see Figure 8.5)
- pull the penis to the skin incision (see Figure 8.6)
- incise the penis longitudinally, precisely in the midline (otherwise the urethra will be bypassed), separating the bulbourethral and ischiocavernosus muscles
- enter the urethral lumen 0.5–1.5 cm deep to the muscular surface, after incising the surrounding *corpus cavernosum urethrae* (Figure 8.5 (3)). Inevitably some haemorrhage occurs from the related venous bed. Cattle with a grossly distended bladder and a patent pelvic urethra void urine through the incision at this point
- extend the incision distally by 2–6 cm, depending on the patient size
- suture the urethral mucosa and minimal depth of fibrous tissue component of erectile tissue to skin with 5 metric PGA attached to the swaged-on needle
- place initial sutures dorsally and ventrally and then continue the suture laterally
- place an in-dwelling catheter (flexible polypropylene with a large lumen, 5–10 mm external diameter) into the bladder and suture to the skin with encircling tape; the catheter keeps the lumen patent
- flush the bladder via the catheter daily with saline (optional) and remove the catheter after three days

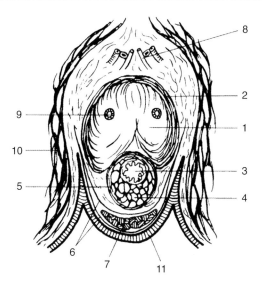

Figure 8.5 Horizontal section through the perineal region of a steer to indicate the structures in the perineal urethro(s)tomy.
1. *corpus cavernosum*; 2. *tunica albuginea*; 3. *urethra*; 4. *corpus spongiosum*; 5. *tunica albuginea of corpus spongiosum*; 6. perineal fascia; 7. retractor penis muscle; 8. dorsal artery, vein and nerve of penis; 9. deep artery of penis; 10. medial muscles of thigh; 11. skin.

- the size of urethrostomy should prevent significant stenosis due to scar tissue contraction; ensure the longitudinal incision in the penis and urethra is at least 2–3 cm long

---

Discussion

A more dorsal incision site avoids the problem of the catheter tip impinging on distal orifices of the ducts of the bulbourethral glands, which lie dorsolaterally in the urethral mucosa. It is also easier to locate the penis with a more dorsal incision, and the incision is almost certainly likely to be proximal to the obstruction.

A more ventral incision, closer to the scrotal neck, will be in the region of the distal bend of the sigmoid flexure, which is a common site for the calculus to cause an obstruction. At this site, part of the obstruction may be proximal to the incision but calculi can usually be flushed out using a catheter. The main advantage of the more ventral incision is that urine scalding of the perineum and inner thighs is less likely to be a problem as the urine tends to be directed more caudally.

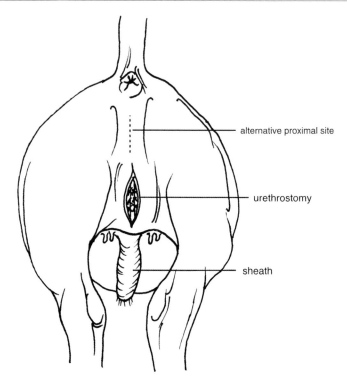

Figure 8.6   Urethrostomy: two alternative sites in the perineum region. Surgery is easier to perform on proximal sites (sigmoid flexure of the penis is easier to locate) but have a greater risk of urine scalding, causing problems.

Penile amputation

- involves creation of a permanent perineal urethrostomy in the proximal part of the transected penis; a salvage operation where damage to the penis is extensive after a uthethral rupture, so the urethrostomy technique described above is not possible
- distal penis is resected
- caudal epidural analgesia, and prepare skin as for the previous technique
- skin incision 15–30 cm long, midway between the caudal aspect of the scrotal neck and ischium
- isolate the penis from surrounding structures, pulling penis forcibly through the skin incision
- identify the fine pink retractor penis muscles (Figures 8.3 and 8.5 (7)), clamp proximally with artery forceps and then section distally
- continue an upward direction of traction on the penis and use blunt dissection with fingers around the sigmoid flexure to facilitate easy

exteriorisation of this portion; the penis still remains attached to the prepuce
- either continue the traction to tear down the preputial attachment to the skin at the preputial orifice or incise the preputial tissues with scalpel and scissors just caudal to the skin–preputial junction; leave the preputial orifice unsutured
- transect completely the exteriorised penis after ligation at a point estimated to permit about a 10 cm protrusion of the penile stump through the skin wound
- ligate the dorsal artery and vein of the remaining penis, situated cranially in the stump, with 7 metric chromic catgut
- incise the urethra proximally from the cut end for 3 cm to produce a flared spatulate end to reduce the stenosis risk
- place PGA sutures through each side from the external fibrous coat into the urethral mucosa for haemostasis
- suture the penis into the skin edges so that the stump protrudes about 5 cm at an angle of 30° to horizontal
- appose the remaining subcutaneous tissues and skin by monofilament nylon sutures
- massage petrolatum jelly into the skin to reduce skin scald
- give systemic antibiotics for five days; clean the penile stump twice daily for three days

Possible complications

- continued haemorrhage occasionally requires additional ligation
- urine scalding of perineal skin and escutcheon
- urethral stricture
- ventral abdominal subcutaneous accumulation of urine resulting from urethral rupture; can be drained via multiple longitudinal stab incisions, but the skin is likely to slough eventually

8.4 Ruptured bladder

Introduction

- usually as a sequel to urolithiasis and urethral obstruction in male cattle
- diagnosis is based on:
  - rectal palpation; bladder cannot be detected
  - abdominal ballottement for fluid thrill
  - abdominal paracentesis ventral midline (see Section 3.1)
  - ultrasound examination
- usually the most pragmatic decision is to slaughter the animal as surgical repair carries a very poor prognosis

Treatment

- as a first step the abdominal urine is drained slowly (approximately 2 litres/5 minutes) via a ventral abdominal cannula attached externally to wide-bore tubing and screw clips (to adjust the flow rate)
- drainage may start before preparation for laparotomy
- rapid reduction of intra-abdominal pressure imposes unnecessary cardiovascular stress as the abdominal venous bed distends

Surgical repair of bladder

- if the general condition permits, left flank laparotomy is done standing, or otherwise in right lateral recumbency
- paravertebral analgesia L1–3 (see Section 1.9)
- vertical left flank incision 20–30 cm long in the caudal paralumbar fossa
- grasp the bladder with the right hand and explore the surface with the left hand; a rupture is frequently found dorsal and cranial
- rupture more caudally, involving the bladder neck and trigone area, is extremely difficult to repair surgically
- evert the bladder and examine the mucosa, especially of neck, to assess the severity of cystitis and to remove any calculi; any detected in the peritoneal cavity are harmless
- confirm the patency of a distal urinary tract (urethra) by flushing saline via a catheter inserted through the bladder neck, around the ischial arch; in case of a urethral obstruction, further surgery is indicated (see above)
- place a continuous inversion suture (Lembert or Cushing pattern) in the bladder wall closure using 7 metric chromic catgut
- close the body wall routinely disregarding residual abdominal urine

Alternative salvage technique relying on spontaneous healing

- may be suitable for a steer or bull with a dorsal and cranial bladder rupture (see Figure 8.7)
- perform right flank laparotomy
- pass a mushroom-headed rubber (Foley) catheter through the ventral body wall, following a stab incision through the skin to grasp the catheter tip with forceps within the abdomen
- make a stab incision in the vertex of the bladder
- insert a catheter through the stab incision and inflate the balloon with 15 ml of saline to keep the catheter in place
- ensure that the catheter is slightly curved within the abdominal cavity to avoid possible displacement during movement, such as standing up, and to allow for some growth

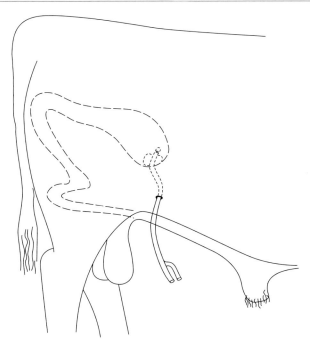

Figure 8.7   Implantation of a Foley catheter into teh urinary bladder for temporary drainage in urolithiasis in male cattle. Catheter exits the abdominal cavity to the right of the prepuce.

- anchor the catheter to skin
- remove the catheter only if normal urine later passes through the urethra; otherwise leave in place until salvage some weeks later
- give systemic antibiotics to all cases following a ruptured bladder; cases benefit from i.v. fluids

Possible complications of bladder surgery

- death from circulatory failure and metabolic disturbance (uraemia)
- bladder wall breakdown (poor surgical technique or poor access to the bladder)
- severe chronic haemorrhagic cystitis
- blood-borne or ascending infection leading to pyelonephritis
- urethral stenosis and renewed bladder rupture
- bladder atony
- diffuse peritonitis

Warning

Consider the welfare of the patient: a ruptured bladder always carries a poor prognosis so euthanasia is the recommended ethical step in all but exceptional circumstances, irrespective of economic considerations.

8.5 Prevention of intromission

Introduction

- various methods have been developed to prevent intromission (insertion of the penis into the vulva and vagina of the female) in cattle in preparation of a teaser bull
- penile translocation is outlined as a possible surgical technique (see below)
- several techniques may be unlawful in some countries; there are ethical considerations in any case (see Discussion Text Box)
- other potential surgical techniques that have been used historically to prevent intromission include:
  - penectomy: penis transected and exposed in the perineum
  - phallectomy: penis shortened by removing the distal extremity, but the organ remains in the preputial cavity
  - penopexy: penis transfixed to the abdominal wall ventrally or to the ventral perineum via sigmoid flexure
  - preputial obstruction: prosthetic device is fixed in the orifice, preventing extrusion of the penis, or insertion of a purse-string suture at the preputial orifice with creation of a preputial fistula ventrally for the urine to escape

Discussion

Surgery to prevent intromission, by itself, does not eliminate the risk of pregnancy. Combining the surgery with vasectomy or epididymectomy to render the animal sterile is the usual precaution.

The advantage of surgery that prevents intromission is to reduce the possible hazards of venereal disease. However, the surgical options are all mutilations that are questionable ethically. All such penile mutilations for the purposes of breeding management are forbidden in the UK by legislation.

Penile–prepuce translocation

- surgery should be done well before the breeding season in animals ideally 250–300 kg bodyweight, aged 6–12 months

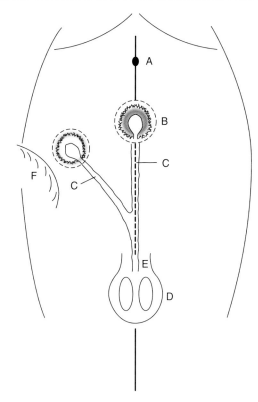

Figure 8.8 Penile and preputial translocation in a young bull ('teaser bull'), ventral view. Lines of skin incisions around the prepuce, penis and new body wall site are shown as interrupted lines (--------).
A. umbilicus; B. skin–prepuce junction in midline; C. penis; D. scrotum; E. level of sigmoid flexure; F. fold of right flank.

- the operation creates a new preputial opening into which the penis and prepuce are sutured
- surgery is performed in dorsal recumbency under GA or deep sedation with local analgesia
- the aim is to redirect the preputial orifice and penis 30° laterally, usually to the right
- mark the proposed site on the skin in the standing bull, usually at the level of the fold of the flank (see Figure 8.8)
- clip and disinfect the new site and the preputial region for an aseptic procedure
- irrigate the preputial cavity with dilute (1%) povidone-iodine solution and close the orifice with a purse-string suture (infection risk!)

- remove an 8 cm diameter circle of skin from the new site and cover temporarily with a moist sterile swab
- make a corresponding incision around the preputial orifice, having marked (e.g. with temporary suture) a cranial midline point, and continue dissection close to the midline caudally
- elevate the preputial coat from the body wall and carefully ligate the extensive vascular supply
- stop dissection at the distal part of the sigmoid flexure; this tunnel may be advantageously started with long-handled straight scissors
- cover the prepuce with a sterile glove before pushing it into the subcutis
- carefully avoiding any torsion on the penis or prepuce and noting the cranial midline point previously marked, place preputial skin into the new site and, using blunt dissection, move the penis into the appropriate position along the abdominal wall (see Figure 8.8c)
- insert a series of interrupted chromic catgut sutures in the subcutaneous tissues
- suture the skin with simple interrupted sutures of monofilament nylon
- close the midline skin defect similarly, but include several deeper sutures into the *linea alba* and rectus sheath to avoid leaving a potential dead space
- carry out a five-day course of systemic antibiotics
- perform epididymectomy (Section 8.7) or vasectomy (Section 8.6)
- three weeks after surgery several ejaculates (approximately three) should be evaluated to ensure that the bull is safe for use as a 'teaser'

8.6 Vasectomy

Introduction

- a portion of *ductus deferens* is removed from the spermatic cord on the cranial aspect of the scrotal neck (see Figure 8.9)
- the technique is practised to produce a teaser bull, to aid oestrus detection
- intromission is unaffected, allowing the risk of transmission of venereal disease
- surgery may be attempted in the standing animal, but is easier if the bull is dorsally recumbent with the hind legs extended caudally or in lateral recumbency with the upper hind leg held well forward

Restraint and anaesthesia

Standing method

- xylazine sedation (low dose range, i.e. 0.1–0.15 mg/kg i.m.) followed by local infiltration with 10 ml local anaesthetic injected subcutaneously

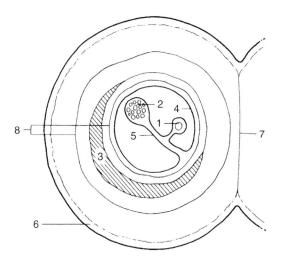

Figure 8.9 Diagrammatic cross-section of the scrotal neck (left side) showing the relationship of *vas deferens*, vascular supply including pampiniform plexus, and cremaster muscle, to vaginal tunics.
1. *vas deferens* enclosed in internal *tunica vaginalis*; 2. vasculature (pampiniform plexus and spermatic artery) in internal *tunica vaginalis*; 3. cremaster muscle; 4. external *tunica vaginalis*; 5. internal *tunica vaginalis*; 6. skin; 7. scrotal septum (*tunica dartos*); 8. internal and external spermatic fascia.

around the proposed incision site, carefully avoiding possible injection into the pampiniform plexus

Recumbent method
- the risks of GA in bulls should be borne in mind
- xylazine sedation (high dose range, i.e. 0.2 mg/kg i.m.) supplemented by local infiltration of local anaesthetic is the usual option

---

Warning

If heavy sedation is used for recumbent method, ensure legs are well secured to a fixed object with rope as being kicked in the face during surgery is a real risk.

Surgical technique

- clip hair from the entire upper half of the scrotum and scrotal neck
- scrub and thoroughly prepare the scrotum and adjacent skin for aseptic surgery

- make a vertical incision 2–5 cm long on the caudolateral (if standing) or craniomedial (recumbent) aspect of the lower part of the scrotal neck over tensed cord structures; in the standing position the skin must be rotated through 90°
- grasp the spermatic cord between the thumb and first two fingers and gently rotate to identify *ductus deferens* as a very firm 'thick string' or wire-like structure about 4 mm in diameter (it is the hardest structure in the cord)
- carefully make a small nick in the vaginal tunic over the *ductus deferens* and either place a hook beneath it or grasp it in Allis tissue forceps
- bring the ductus through the skin incision and clamp across with two pairs of artery forceps about 5 cm apart (see Figure 8.10 (B))

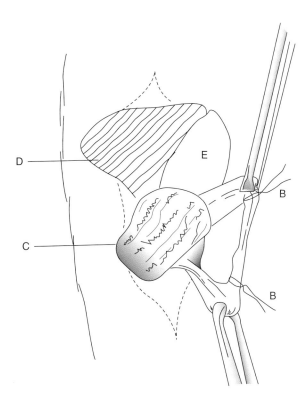

Figure 8.10 Vasectomy in recumbent bull. Vertical incision in the lower scrotal neck and cord structures elevated by scissors (see also Figure 8.9).
A. cord-like *ductus (vas) deferens* in internal *tunica vaginalis*, held by Allis forceps; B. non-absorbable sutures ligating ductus before resection of 5 cm; C. adjacent pampiniform plexus; D. cremaster muscle; E. fold of *external tunica* vaginalis incised to expose A and C.

- resect the intervening section of the ductus with scissors and place silk ligatures (3 metric) below each forceps: ligature avoids possible re-anastomosis
- release the forceps
- return the cut ends of the ductus into the spermatic cord
- close the skin incision with interrupted horizontal mattress sutures of monofilament nylon
- repeat the surgery through a second incision on the other side; it is possible to access both spermatic cords through a single midline incision but there is more sub-cutaneous fascia to bluntly dissect and is not recommended

Post-op care

- give systemic antibiotics for five days
- check the bull for absence of semen by teasing once weekly for three weeks
- remove the skin sutures after 10–14 days
- mild scrotal oedema can occur
- wound breakdown is rare

Tip

Always retain the resected ductus for identification (e.g. examine for semen), and preferably histopathology, to confirm the correct tissue has been removed. Under a dissecting microscope, the vas canal has a characteristic star shape. Fix in formaldehyde and retain for the lifetime of the bull in case of the need of further evidence.

The surgeon may face litigation if the bull is subsequently claimed to be still fertile. The precautions described (remove at least 5 cm of each *vas deferens*; ligate both cut ends; check post-surgery for correct tissue identification; wait at least three weeks and check for the absence of semen by artificial collection) will all reduce the risk of later fertility. The owner should nevertheless be made aware that on very rare occasions a bull can still become fertile due to re-anastomosis of the *vas deferens*.

8.7 Epididymectomy

Introduction

- alternative procedure for production of teaser bulls to identify females in oestrus
- also called caudal epididymectomy
- tail of the epididymis is resected

Restraint and anaesthesia

- surgery can be done in a standing bull under xylazine sedation and local infiltration
- strict asepsis is essential

Technique

- clip, wash and disinfect the entire scrotal surface; dry and repeat disinfection
- push the testicle distally with one hand so that the epididymal tail is readily identifiable
- incise into the epididymis at the most ventral point, avoiding the testicular substance (see Figure 8.11)
- continue the blunt dissection of the tail from the body of the testis carefully
- grasp a large portion of the tail with Allis forceps and place large artery forceps transversely proximal to this tissue, which is then resected
- resected tissue must be checked for semen, since inadvertently only fat and connective tissue may be removed
- place a firm absorbable suture (e.g. vicryl® 7 metric) proximal to the artery forceps, which is then removed
- insert two or three horizontal mattress sutures to appose the skin edges
- give systemic antibiotics for five days
- remove the sutures in 10–14 days
- tease the bull weekly for three weeks when no live sperm should be seen and the bull is then suitable for work as a 'teaser'
- check for removal of the correct tissue and retain in formaldehyde, as for vasectomy (see above)

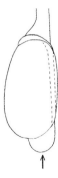

Figure 8.11 Location of head, body and tail of the epididymis in relation to the testicle. Arrow indicates the direction and site of the incision in epididymectomy.

Discussion

Whether to opt for vasectomy or epididymectomy is a personal choice. With experience, both are relatively straightforward options, though in less experienced hands the identification of the correct tissue can sometimes be surprisingly difficult, particularly in fat animals where the *vas deferens* can be surrounded by fat.

The spermatic cord and epididymis are both very vascular tissues, as of course are the testes. Vasectomy is possibly less likely to result in inadvertent copious haemorrhage than epididymectomy, which can affect visualisation for accurate ligation.

8.8 Congenital penile abnormalities

Corkscrew penis or spiral penis

Introduction

- congenital defect, involving the dorsal apical ligament, occurring in bulls older than one year
- many affected bulls are known to have served successfully and have sired progeny
- any breed can be affected, but polled breeds such as polled Hereford have a higher incidence
- inheritance is questionable; presumably otherwise it is acquired after trauma
- economic cost of the procedure is a major factor in considering possible surgery

Signs

- seen just before or immediately following extrusion of the penis from the sheath
- in severe cases the penile tip is caught in the distal part of the preputial cavity and may only be extruded naturally with some difficulty
- extruded penis spirals to the left or right through a 30° angle, viewed from the right side, and 180–270° when viewed (theoretically) from the rear
- glans penis tends to hit the right perineal region of the cow, about 20–30 cm from the vulva
- spiralling action may be variable in degree; in intermittent cases bulls may maintain a low level of fertility in the field

- in normal bulls, occurrence of deviation and complete spiralling after intromission increases the contact area between the penis and vagina, and may therefore increase tactile stimuli and so promote ejaculation
- in affected bulls the deviation or complete spiralling occurs prior to intromission and prevents coitus
- anatomical explanation involves slipping of the dorsal apical ligament across to the left and ventrally; the penile integument in affected bulls is then fully stretched over the penis and produces spiralling early in the process of copulation
- as long as the inheritance remains questionable, surgery should only be undertaken after ethical considerations, and then reserved for valuable bulls required for natural service

Surgical repair

- two techniques are given, one using penile *tunica albuginea* (TA) and the other with *fascia lata* from the thigh region

Technique 1. Penile tunica albuginea *(see Figure 8.12)*

- GA, lateral or dorsal recumbency
- extend penis, avoiding accidental spiral rotation, and apply a rubber tourniquet at the base
- grasp the glans with forceps or tie with a bandage, and maintain the penis in full extension
- make a dorsal midline incision through the penile mucosa from just cranial to reflection of the prepuce forwards to just caudal to the glans
- expose the underlying dorsal ligament of the penis
- incise longitudinally through the middle of the ligament into the TA
- incise 3 mm laterally to the left and right, parallel to previous incisions
- incise transversely and distally across the distal end of the previous three incisions, so creating two strips (2 mm wide) of ligament and TA
- resect about 1 cm of strip length and re-attach strips to the distal end of the dorsal ligament with alternate sutures of 6 metric chromic catgut and 3 metric stainless steel (respectively to provoke a tissue reaction and for strength)
- the strip is tacked on to an underlying fibrous coat with interrupted sutures every 6–7 mm, ensuring firm contact and deep insertion into the TA
- close the penile epithelium with 4 metric chromic catgut interrupted sutures
- irrigate the wound with an aqueous solution of penicillin G and release the tourniquet

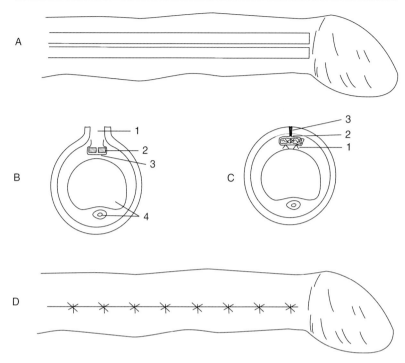

Figure 8.12 Surgical correction of spiral deviation of the penis ('corkscrew penis'). A. dorsal surface of penis with epithelium incised and two strips (each 10 cm × 2 mm) of apical ligament freed from *tunica albuginea* (TA) except proximally; B. cross-section of penis showing (from dorsal): 1. incision through penile epithelium; 2. two sections of dorsal ligament (shaded); 3. incision in TA; 4. *corpus cavernosum penis* and urethra ventrally; C. enlarged cross-section showing position of sutures fixing strips of apical ligament to TA; 1. sutures from strips to TA; 2. suture closing TA over strips; 3. closure of penile epithelium; D. interrupted sutures closing the penile epithelium.

- give antibiotics systemically for five days
- close the preputial orifice temporarily by encircling a muslin bandage for some hours until the bull has recovered from anaesthesia and can retain the penis in the preputial cavity
- irrigate the preputial cavity daily with oleaginous antibiotic preparation from day four to day ten
- allow sexual rest for eight weeks and then tease the bull to ascertain a new position of erect penis

Technique 2. Fascia lata graft
- GA, right lateral recumbency
- first collect the *fascia lata* graft as follows:
  - clip and prepare a liberal area from the proximal tibia to the *tuber coxae* for surgery
  - make an incision beginning 8 cm dorsolateral to the patella and continued for 20 cm towards the *tuber coxae*; continue the incision to the *fascia lata* of the *vastus lateralis* muscle
  - collect a 3 cm wide and 20 cm long rectangular strip of the deep *fascia lata*; remove connective tissue from this strip and keep the graft in saline (homogenic *fascia lata* preserved in 70% ethyl alcohol also has been used successfully to reduce surgical time and avoid a second incision on the patient)
  - close the fascial layers in a simple continuous pattern and appose the skin with non-absorbable suture material in a routine fashion
- extend the penis manually and prepare the penis and prepuce for aseptic surgery
- make a 20 cm skin incision on the dorsum of the penis starting about 2.5 cm proximal to the tip
- deepen the incision to the white fibrous apical ligament
- reflect the apical ligament laterally in both directions, exposing the TA
- do not incise the two veins on the right ventral aspect between the ligament and the TA
- place the *fascia lata* graft between the apical ligament and the TA on the dorsum of the penis
- insert four interrupted sutures of 2 metric polyglactin 910 (vicryl™) through the *fascia lata* and into the TA under the ligament, near its origin
- then place interrupted sutures along the lateral margin of the graft at 2.5 cm intervals to stretch the implant
- trim the implant to fit the distal end of the penis and suture under tension in an interrupted pattern
- return the apical ligament over the implant and suture it with a simple interrupted pattern of the same material; the thickest portion of the ligament should be on the dorsum of the penis
- close the last layer with 3 metric vicryl
- insert a tube into the preputial cavity and secure to the sheath with elastic tape to maintain the penis in a retracted position

After-care

- give systemic antibiotic agents for three to five days
- allow sexual rest for 60 days

- sometimes (resulting from over- or under-correction) a second operation is required
- prognosis remains guarded

Persistent frenulum

Introduction

- a band of fibrous tissue running from close to the penile tip to near the junction of the penile part of the prepuce and sheath, causing a marked ventral deviation of the erect penis
- prevents intromission
- congenital anomaly
- persistence of the embryonic ectodermal lamella connects the penis to the penile part of the prepuce, which usually separates slowly, starting cranially, after the calf is two months old; its completion is hormone-dependent, but may be delayed until eight months. This ventral surface is the last to separate
- excessive thickness of the ventral bridge (= frenulum), perhaps containing blood vessels, may be an aetiological factor
- in the USA it is most common in Aberdeen Angus and Shorthorn bulls, but has a low incidence

Surgical treatment

- investigate and operate with the bull restrained in the crush/chute
- in case of a very thick frenulum, the dorsal nerve of the penis may be blocked before ligation
- ligate blood vessels in the frenulum and section fibrous structure with scissors
- good prognosis
- as the condition is possibly inherited, the ethics of surgery are dubious in any other than terminal sire bulls

Other congenital anomalies of bovine penis

- these include:
  - short penis (infantile)
  - short retractor penis muscle
  - tight penile adnexa
- all three congenital conditions have a low incidence; the main sign is that the penis fails to reach the vulva despite a normal erection
- no surgical correction possible

8.9 Penile neoplasia

Penile tumours occur in two forms, papillomatosis or fibropapilloma and malignant squamous cell carcinoma.

Papillomatosis

- occurs in young bulls, reared in groups
- caused by a host-specific Papovavirus (BPV1)

Signs

- haemorrhage from the penis, often on turning out to cows or at breeding examination
- located on free portion of the penis
- generally multiple and sessile, but chronic cases may have a pedunculated mass
- phimosis or paraphimosis is possible

Treatment

- slow spontaneous regression can occur
- autogenous wart vaccine is usually unsuccessful
- surgical removal (knife or Burdizzo®), electrocautery or cryosurgery
- unless a simple procedure, the patient should be in lateral recumbency to facilitate precision
- sedation with xylazine; analgesia by local infiltration of dorsal nerves of the penis (see Section 1.9) or a ring block of the penis
- care is required not to incise the urethra (potential fistula formation)
- ligate or cauterise significant bleeding vessels
- close the epithelial defect with 4 or 5 metric chromic catgut or vicryl (optional)
- prognosis is good

Malignant squamous cell carcinoma

- a rare condition in adult bulls
- usually rapidly invasive and involves multiple ulcerating and proliferating masses
- biopsy and histopathology can confirm the diagnosis
- surgery is usually impossible and prognosis therefore poor

8.10 Castration

Introduction

- need for castration ('testectomy' or orchidectomy) is increasingly questioned on scientific, economic and humanitarian grounds
- usually for pasture-finished beef animals where safety and public liability considerations of keeping adult bulls at pasture is the main concern
- two basic forms of castration are possible: bloodless and open surgical (scalpel)

Warning

The legislation covering castration of bulls in the UK is twofold:

- **Anaesthesia legislation**:
  - anaesthesia is legally required for all bulls over two months of age
  - an elastrator ring may only be used in bull calves 0–7 days old
- **Veterinary Surgeons Act**:
  - castration may only be carried out by a veterinary surgeon, by whatever method, if the bull is older than two months of age

---

Discussion

Analgesia and anaesthesia during castration

Whatever the legislation, whichever method of castration and whatever the age of the bull, the use of anaesthesia and analgesia is recommended by the authors in every case of castration. An intratesticular block is the most commonly used local anaesthesia (see Section 1.9), but this is ineffective in anaesthetising the scrotal skin so a 2 ml subcutaneous deposit of local anaesthetic should also be used.

An alternative technique involves subcutaneous infiltration at the scrotal neck and injection of a further 3–5 ml into each cord. One author (AS) believes that intratesticular injection is painful and minimally effective and should therefore be avoided.Administration of NSAIDs at the time of castration has been demonstrated to reduce a potential growth check and treated calves demonstrate less signs of pain and abnormal behaviour during the following 48 hours. The authors recommend the routine use of NSAIDs administered immediately prior to castration.

Bloodless methods

Rubber ring (elastrator) method
- application of a tight-fitting rubber ring to the scrotal neck in calves
- causes considerable post-operative discomfort and marked setback to growth
- not a recommended technique, but commonly used by farmers
- in the UK, only legally permitted in the first week of life (see Warning Text Box)
- illegal without anaesthetic in some countries (e.g. Germany, Switzerland)
- sepsis is not uncommon at the site following skin necrosis
- careless application can fail to position both testes below the rubber ring, resulting in induced (iatrogenic) inguinal cryptorchidism
- carries a risk of tetanus, probably as the duration of pressure necrosis is much longer than in other bloodless methods
- in the USA, a rubber band tubing method has been used even for large feedlot bulls, but the authors do not advise this on animal welfare grounds

Burdizzo method
- the Burdizzo emasculatome instrument achieves bloodless castration by crushing the spermatic cord through the scrotal skin; testes undergo atrophy due to a disrupted blood supply
- suitable for calves one to twelve weeks old, depending on the breed and development
- the calf must be in standing position
- the surgeon stands beside or directly behind the calf (beware of kicks; keep the head up and stand tight in behind the patient), keeping the hindquarters against a suitable pen wall with the head placed and tied or held in a corner by an assistant
- local and systemic analgesia, as described in Discussion Text Box and Section 1.9
- the surgeon controls the correct application of the Burdizzo (see Figure 8.13): the instrument is applied laterally on to the scrotal neck by an assistant behind the calf
- cord is held tight laterally in the scrotal neck by the first finger and thumb of the surgeon
- the second hand controls the position of the jaws; instruct the assistant initially to close the jaws slowly until they are about 8–10 mm apart and are about to clamp skin and cord firmly; alternatively, if assistance is unavailable, use the knee and elbow to partially close the jaws
- with the cord palpably and precisely located between the jaws, order a rapid full closure by the assistant or transfer both hands to handles to close the jaws fully, but without allowing the spermatic cord to slip from its position

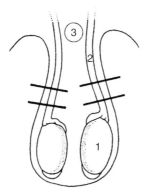

Figure 8.13 Diagram of a vertical section through the scrotum, showing the correct position for application of the Burdizzo (bloodless) emasculator. Cord is pushed laterally to produce minimal skin trauma. Area of undamaged skin is left in midline and maintains blood supply to the ventral part of the scrotal skin. The instrument is applied remote from the penis.
1. testicle; 2. spermatic cord; 3. penis.

- maintain the jaws closed for 5–10 seconds, during which the operator checks that the cord is correctly crushed
- a characteristic crunching sound/feel accompanies the closure
- lateral cord-stops on the emasculator blades help to prevent displacement of the cord during closure
- slightly separate the jaws and then slide them 1 cm distally, and close a second time on the same side (in contrast to the first crushing, any pain reaction is minimal)
- repeat the procedure on the second side
- ensure that the crushed lines in the skin are offset (see Figure 8.13) and do not form a continuous band around the scrotal neck, which could otherwise lead to skin necrosis with infection
- do not crush the median (scrotal) raphé
- check after four weeks (young calf) or six weeks (older calf) for a palpable atrophy of the testicular tissue, which forms a fibrous knob or knot-like structure approximately the size of the diameter of the spermatic cord

---

Tip

A certain dexterity is definitely required for successful use of Burdizzo castrators. There are various tips to aid their use:

- initially at least, use alongside a more experienced operator
- a second assistant can be invaluable to close the jaws fully

- one model has been designed with a knee grip to assist single-operator use
- always check for correct cord position when the jaws are fully closed
- only use well-maintained equipment: the instrument should be capable of cutting a piece of string or straw inserted between two pieces of card or paper, without tearing the card/paper when functioning normally
- always store the Burdizzo in the open-jaw position to avoid slack jaws
- avoid clamping the penis!

Possible complications of the Burdizzo method:
- inadvertent crushing of the penis by an inexperienced operator if the jaws are applied too high; causes urethral blockage and rupture with urine seepage. A salvage procedure may be possible but euthanasia is more common
- gross bruising of the scrotal tissues due to slackness of the jaws
- oedema of the caudal abdominal wall and scrotum due to slack jaws
- failure to cause testicular atrophy due to slack jaws, incomplete jaw closure or not waiting at least 5-10 seconds when the jaws are closed
- unilateral absence of testicular atrophy, as the cord was inadvertently completely or partially missed
- scrotal necrosis due to not staggering the clamping positions (ischaemia of scrotal skin)
- tetanus; tetanus prophylais is advisable
- severe testicular and scrotal oedema if bulls are too large/old; may result in rupture of scrotal skin and partial prolapse of testes, requiring surgical removal

Surgical (scalpel) method

Involves removal of the testicles and haemostasis of the spermatic cord vessels by:

- traction on the spermatic cord or
- torsion and traction on the spermatic cord or
- crushing using an emasculator or
- crushing and ligation of the spermatic cord

Technique
- perform surgery in a standing position with the stockman restraining the head and hindquarters and holding the tail laterally

- local and systemic analgesia, as described in Discussion Text Box and Section 1.9
- wash and cleanse the scrotal skin with dilute (0.5%) povidone-iodine solution; preferably wear disposable gloves
- stand or crouch behind the calf to grasp the neck of the scrotum with the non-dominant hand, ensuring both testes are within the scrotum, squeezed tight against the scrotal skin distally
- make two vertical incisions using a scalpel held in the dominant hand through the lateral scrotal skin (both sides) into the testicular substance, keeping the testicles tensed and pulled distally, and continue the incision along the distal, i.e. ventral, border of the scrotum (ensuring subsequent drainage); aim for a 'J-shaped' incision
- scrotal incisions should be slightly shorter than the testicular length
- squeeze one testicle at a time through the scrotum so it prolapses through the skin wound and then through the parietal vaginal tunic; lengthen and deepen the incision in the parietal layer of the vaginal tunic if necessary to exteriorise the testis, but try and avoid excessive prolapse of the testicular tissue through the visceral layer of the vaginal tunic
- the testicle is grasped in a non-dominant hand (not sterile) and vascular and non-vascular portions of the cord are identified (vascular: cranial including the pampiniform plexus and vas deferens)
- insert the first finger of the dominant hand (sterile) through the vaginal tunic proximal to the epididymis in order to break the connection of the tail of the epididymis to the parietal vaginal tunic
- the testis should now hang freely from the scrotum with the tail of the epididymis lowermost

Technique now varies depending on the method of haemostasis:
- small calf (one week to two months): torsion or traction alone are both possibilities
- large calf (two to six months): emasculator, torsion or traction in descending order of preference; torsion alone may be excessively painful
- small bull: emasculator, preferably with ligation

Emasculator method
- apply after separating the vascular and non-vascular parts of the cord
- brief period (10 seconds) to crush the non-vascular position just proximal to the epididymis
- longer period (20–120 seconds depending on the size of the cord and the age of the animal), crushing the proximal part of the vascular portion of the cord, using traction on distal structures to separate them from the jaws of the instrument

Torsion method
- break down the non-vascular part of the cord by traction
- twist the vascular portion several (five or six) times in the proximal part of the cord and then use gentle traction to break the cord distal to the torsion point

Traction method
- break down the non-vascular part and then grasp the vascular portion proximally, increasing steady traction until the cord ruptures and undergoes considerable elastic recoil
- replace any tissue protruding from the wound by pulling the scrotal skin ventrally; rarely, resection of any protruding section of *ductus deferens* is required
- do not handle tissue unnecessarily
- do not become involved in calf restraint (contamination risk!)
- maintain the scalpel and emasculator in a bucket with antiseptic and have a second bucket of antiseptic solution for washing the scrotum
- local medication is unnecessary but tetanus prophylaxis is advised; application of topical antibiotic spray to the scrotal wound may reduce the risk of local infection
- consider fly control and avoid open castration in the fly season

Newberry castration technique
- the initial scrotal incision may be made with a Newberry® knife (Newberry castrating knife, Jorgensen Labs, Loveland, CO, USA)
- this is a 24.5 cm long instrument with a steel-bladed clamp, which is placed transversely across the base of the scrotum, closed and immediately pulled ventrally to open both scrotal sacs without removal of any scrotal tissue (see Figure 8.14). Both testicles may then be removed with the emasculator.

Technique for small bull
- emasculator and ligation; see Figure 8.15
- strict aseptic precautions and antiseptic preparation of the skin are essential; use a sterile emasculator and suture material
- incise as above, caudally, into the substance of the scrotum, continuing incision distally
- apply the emasculator to a non-vascular part of the cord, then to the vascular portion, close tightly and remove the testis
- leave the instrument in place for a minimum of 1 minute
- place a circumferential ligature around the cord 1 cm proximal to the blade, as extra security against haemorrhage is essential

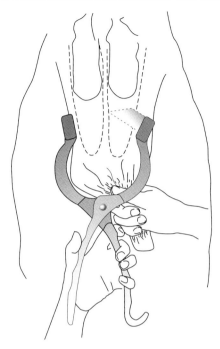

Figure 8.14 Newberry castration technique. View from rear, showing testes pushed upwards, scrotum pulled down by right hand and a Newberry knife being applied across the scrotum for transverse incision, before being pulled quickly downwards. Dotted lines represent the position of the *tunica vaginalis*, through which the testes are then extracted.

- place the artery forceps on the edge of the cord proximal to the ligature but not across the cord, remove the emasculator and check carefully for haemorrhage
- release the artery forceps
- ensure clean bedding; some exercise is advisable for one week

Possible complications of surgical methods
- scrotal infection: improve drainage by ensuring the apex of the scrotum is open and irrigate the scrotum with water; systemic antibiotics
- immediate massive scrotal haemorrhage: pack the scrotum with cotton wool or sterile gauze, attempt to identify the source and grasp with forceps; apply a mass ligature (catgut) to the area
- testicular tissue prolapses from the wound (usually *tunica vaginalis* and fat): resect tissue by pulling the scrotal skin ventrally; sutures should not be necessary

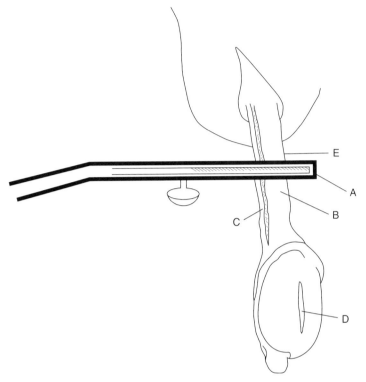

Figure 8.15   Emasculator castration (diagrammatic). Scrotum has been incised distally into the testis (D), which has then been expressed from the scrotum. Parietal *tunica vaginalis* has been sectioned by scalpel and has retracted into the scrotum.
A. Emasculator placed across cord structures with the cutting edge of the blade distal and the crushing edge proximal ('nut' to 'nut'); B. *pampiniform plexus* and spermatic artery; C. *ductus deferens*; D. testicular incision; E. site for application of artery forceps to retain the stump for an inspection of a few seconds if warranted.

- 'gut tie' is a very rare sequel to haemostasis by torsion, where the intestine becomes incarcerated by a traumatised recoiled *vas deferens;* see Figure 5.23 and Section 5.11

Tip
Usually, surgical castration is performed on a batch of calves and maintaining surgical sterility can be challenging, but it is still necessary to reduce the risk of infection.   It should be possible to have a sterile hand (dominant hand) and a non-sterile hand (non-dominant hand). Thus a right-handed operator

will grasp the scrotum with the left hand and hold the scalpel in the right hand (dominant hand). Then the left hand is used to grasp the prolapsed testicle, whilst avoiding touching the parietal vaginal tunic. Once the scalpel has been replaced in the bucket of disinfectant, the sterile right hand can be used to gently peel back the parietal vaginal tunic, if necessary, and break down its attachment with the epididymis. It should be possible to complete the technique without handling any tissue that will remain in the animal.

Warning

Personal safety is an important consideration during surgical castration. As well as the possibility of being kicked (reduced by good restraint), it is not uncommon for self-inflicted cuts, including potentially to the major blood vessels of the wrist. The following precautions are useful:

- use a handle with the scalpel (not blade only)
- replace blades frequently so they are always sharp
- do not have cotton wool in the bucket of disinfectant used for the scalpel as it will be obscured; use two buckets (one for scalpel, one for disinfecting skin)
- when making scrotal incisions, hold the neck of the scrotum in the non-dominant hand with the palm facing *away*; this ensures that a slip of the blade cannot result in severing the arteries or veins on the wrist.

8.11 Cryptorchidism and ectopic testicle

Introduction

- true cryptorchidism with retention of a testicle either intra-abdominally or in the inguinal region is rare in calves
- an ectopic testicle is far more usual, where the testis can be located subcutaneously in a parapenile position, often as far cranially as the prepuce
- cryptorchidism or ectopic testes are usually unilateral, commonly on the left side
- incompletely descended testicle of young bulls (up to 2 months of age) will generally descend into the scrotum within a few months, so delayed surgery may be advisable

Ectopic testicle

- when only one testicle can be located in the scrotum, always next palpate subcutaneously on either side of the sheath on the ventral abdomen to locate an ectopic testicle
- ectopic testicle, which is usually slightly smaller than a normally descended one, can be very easily removed surgically at the same time as castration
- tense the testicle against the skin; insert a local anaesthetic; incise on to the testicle and remove as described for a normal surgical castration
- usually no requirement for skin sutures

Cryptorchidectomy

- in the rare case of a true cryptorchid testis, management depends on its position
- if determined in a calf to be inguinal, surgical removal is best done under local analgesia, the calf restrained in lateral or dorsal recumbency
- if not detected in the inguinum, an abdominal approach under deep sedation and paravertebral analgesia, or GA, is indicated
- the calf should be prepared for sterile surgery, including drapes, to avoid any risk of the development of peritonitis

Inguinal testicle

- inguinal testis should be removed before the contralateral (normally descended) testis
- disinfection of the surrounding skin followed by local infiltration of the skin and subcutis over and around the testis, which is tensed firmly in the hand
- incision over the testis, through the *tunica vaginalis* to expose the body
- isolate the spermatic cord and ligate or apply an emasculatror to the vascular pedicle
- cut through the non-vascular part and remove the testicle

Abdominal testicle

- before exploratory laparotomy, make a final digital exploration of the area immediately external to the external inguinal ring and the parapenile tissues
- incise cranially to the external inguinal ring to permit entry of two digits
- testis is usually adjacent to the inguinal canal and is easily exteriorised for routine removal
- give antibiotic cover for 3 days

CHAPTER 9

Musculoskeletal conditions and lameness

9.1 Introduction and welfare

Cattle lameness is hugely detrimental to both the economic success and the welfare of dairy cows. In the UK, independent studies have estimated the mean prevalence of lame cows in dairy herds to be between 32 and 36%, but with a wide range. Some herds have no lame cows whilst others have greater than 50% prevalence. Approximately 10% of dairy cows

Bovine Surgery and Lameness, Third Edition. A. David Weaver, Owen Atkinson, Guy St. Jean and Adrian Steiner.
© 2018 John Wiley & Sons Ltd. Published 2018 by John Wiley & Sons Ltd.
Companion website: www.wiley.com/go/weaver/bovine-surgery

are severely lame (mobility score 3) – in other words are unable to walk at a brisk human pace or normally to keep up with the herd.

The subject of bovine lameness is too vast for this text. This chapter focuses on treatment of individual cases, with only brief reference to herd level control and lameness epidemiology.

The poor welfare of lame cows is obvious. This is on a herd level, with too high lameness prevalence, and on an individual level, particularly when chronically lame cows are left to suffer for long periods of time, sometimes for years. This is particularly true for deep sepsis lesions, which resolve into a chronic 'club foot' and severe bony changes, or for cows that have a necrotic toe. The surgery sections of this chapter give clear treatment alternatives should the cow be retained in the herd. **Conservative treatments for these cases are rarely acceptable** due to the chronic pain the cow will endure.

Economic effects

- not always easily apparent; lame cows continue to produce saleable milk
- however, reduced yield over a long time span, reduced fertility and an increased risk of premature culling (as a low value cull cow) all contribute to make lameness one of the costliest production diseases of the dairy industry
- in the UK, lameness is estimated to cost the average herd 4.1 pence per litre
- not all of this cost is likely to be recoverable unless lameness is eliminated, but it is a very reasonable ambition to at least halve it
- put in context, the mean cost of lameness is approximately 15% of the overall cost of milk production

9.2 Mobility (lameness) scoring

- mobility scoring (MS) is a simple system of inspection of herd individuals designed to record the prevalence of lameness and the individual severity of locomotor impairment
- the MS system adopted in the UK is the AHDB Dairy four-point system, 0, 1, 2 and 3 (see Table 9.1)
- MS 0 and 1 are considered 'not lame'; MS 2 and 3 are considered 'lame'
- most MS 3 cows begin as a less severe lameness (MS 2) before progressing to a more advanced lesion
- treatment of lesions of MS 3 cows is less likely to result in a full resolution, or at least take a long time to recover
- MS 2 cows are lame and almost inevitably have a lesion that is visible on close inspection of the foot, but they will not have an altered walking speed and will be embedded within the herd; it is important to actively seek these

Table 9.1   The AHDB Dairy (DairyCo) Mobility Score System.

Score	Description	Findings
0	Walks with even weight bearing and rhythm on all four feet, with a flat back. Long, fluid strides possible.	Not lame. Unlikely to have a lesion.
1	Steps uneven (rhythm or weight bearing) or strides shortened. The affected limb or limbs are not immediately identifiable.	Not lame. Unlikely to have a visible lesion, but may be recovering or in very early stages of pathology.
2	Uneven weight bearing on a limb that is immediately identifiable and/or obviously shorted strides. There is usually, but not necessarily, an arch to the centre of the back when walking.	Lame. There is a very strong likelihood of a painful foot lesion, which will be visible on inspection of the foot and benefit from treatment.
3	Unable to walk as fast as a brisk human pace and cannot normally keep up with the healthy herd. The cow will also have the signs of lameness of score 2 animals.	Lame. Inspection of the foot will usually result in identification of an obvious painful lesion.

cows for treatment, which usually involves mobility scoring the herd on a regular basis
• other lameness scoring systems can be used (e.g. Sprecher 5-point system commonly adopted in the USA)

Discussion

• Most reasons for lameness are due to lesions of the foot, rather than upper limb lameness.
• Being a prey animal, cows have evolved to mask lameness well, and this creates a considerable challenge in our ability to detect early cases for treatment.

Tip

Mobility scoring is useful to:

1. identify lesions for early treatment
2. measure lameness in a herd

Lameness incidence versus prevalence

- compared to other clinical disorders, such as mastitis or retained placenta, recording lameness incidence is particularly difficult
- a single lameness incident often has an ill-defined start and end point, and may endure over a protracted period
- recording prevalence (versus incidence) using periodic herd mobility scoring (e.g. weekly) is a more practical way of recording lameness
- however, mobility scoring gives no indications to the cause of lameness or lesions present

9.3 Functional foot anatomy

- the hoof capsule consists of four distinct types of horn, all produced from different regions of germinal epithelial cells (pododerm) (see Table 9.2 and Figure 9.6)
- the junction between the different horn types can be natural weak points; e.g. leading to white line disease
- the junction between the horn and underlying corium (soft tissue) can also be a weakness and fluid accumulation (e.g. pus in a white line abscess) can lead to separation of the horn from the corium
- within the hoof capsule is the pedal bone (P3) and the navicular bone
- phalanges, P1, P2 and P3, are directly comparable to the phalanges of the middle two human fingers
- the accessary digits have no phalanges and are vestiges of digits 2 and 5 (see Figures 9.1 and 9.2)

Table 9.2   Four principle horn types.

Horn	Description	Physical properties
Wall horn	Akin to the fingernail or nail of a dog's paw	Hard. Strong. Under normal circumstances, this should be the main weight-bearing horn
Sole horn	Akin to the pad of a dog's paw	Slightly pliable; like plastic. Becomes the main weight-bearing horn when the wall wears, for example on concrete
White line horn	The 'glue' forming the junction between the wall and sole	Structurally weak, in order to allow sole and wall horn to move in relation to each other
Perioplic horn	Akin to the hardened skin at the nail bed, forming the 'cuticle'	Rubbery. Its greatest importance in the bovine hoof is that it makes up the soft heel bulb

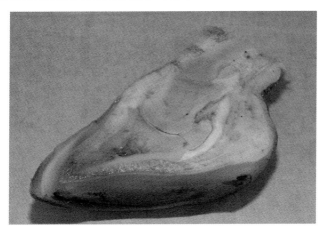

Figure 9.1   Cross-section of a bovine digit.

- P3 is suspended within the hoof capsule by firm attachments to the hoof wall via the laminae, and resting on the digital cushion, which to a large extent protects the sole corium from concussive forces (see Figures 9.3 to 9.6)
- when the laminar connections are weakened, the downwards pressure of the pedal bone on the sole corium leads to concussive damage responsible for sole bruising and sole ulcers
- laminae, normally forming a strong bond suspending the pedal bone within the hoof capsule, are a line of least resistance for pus to travel along, for

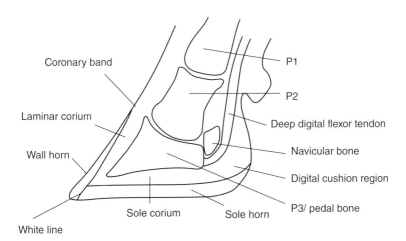

Figure 9.2   Labelled diagram of cross-section of the foot.

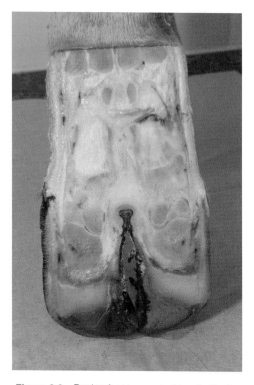

Figure 9.3   Bovine foot transected longitudinally.

example in a white line abscess where pus under-runs the wall to burst at the coronary band (see Figures 9.5 and 9.6)

- in thin cows, cows undergoing weight loss and older cows, the protective shock-absorbing properties of the digital cushion are reduced, leading to more contusion of the sole corium

9.4 Main foot lesions: terminology and summary

In the intensive cattle enterprises common in western Europe and North America:

- 95% of lame cattle are dairy breeds
- 80–90% of cases involve the digits
- 80% of digital lameness is located in the hind limbs
- 50% of digital lameness involves the horny tissue and 50% the skin, mostly digital dermatitis
- 70% of the horny lesions involve the outer claw

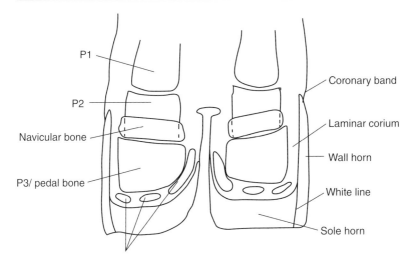

Digital cushions, extending distally towards toe from heel.

Figure 9.4 Labelled diagram of the foot transected longitudinally.

The three major digital lameness problems with rather similar incidence rates (UK) are digital dermatitis, sole ulcer and white line disease.

Lesions are classified into two broad categories:

1. infectious diseases, or lesions of the **skin**
2. non-infectious diseases, or **claw horn lesions**

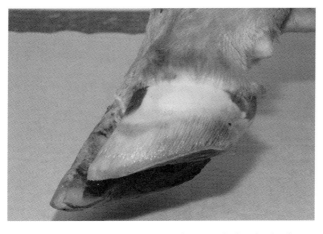

Figure 9.5 Bovine digit with the hoof removed, showing laminae.

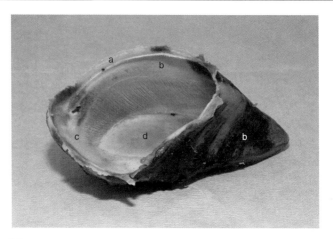

Figure 9.6   A hoof capsule, showing laminar attachments on the inner surface of the wall, and labelled to show different horn types.
a = perioplic horn; b = wall horn; c = bulb of heel, d = sole horn.

Discussion

- Many primary non-infectious (claw horn) lesions become infected, and some of the most severe lesions of the foot are mixed lesions, particularly where digital dermatitis bacteria have invaded the underlying corium after an initial claw horn insult.
- Confusion arises over different terminology applied to lesions, depending on the geographical region, understanding of the lesion and opinion. The main terminology used in this text is consistent with the ICAR claw health atlas, 2015 (ICAR – International Committee for Animal Recording).
- Descriptive terms are commonly used, such as 'wall ulcer', 'under-run sole' or 'foot abscess'. Whilst these may be useful to describe the lesion, they are not useful to describe the underlying cause – not always obvious to the untrained eye.

There are three main infectious (skin) lesions and three main claw horn lesions (see Tables 9.3 and 9.4). The usual locations of the most important conditions of the foot are shown in Figure 9.7.

Lesions and infectious diseases of digital skin

- three broad lesions: digital dermatitis (treponemes); interdigital phlegmon/foul of the foot (*Fusiformis necrophorus*); heel horn erosion/interdigital dermatitis (*Dichelobacter nodosus*)

Table 9.3   The main infectious agents causing foot lesions.

Infectious bacteria	UK lesion name	Alternative terminology	Latin nomenclature
Treponemes	Digital dermatitis*	Mortellaro disease Hairy warts Strawberry disease	*dermatitis digitalis* *dermatitis verrucosa* *(verrucose form)*
Dichelobacter nodosus (formerly *Bacteroides nodosus*)	Heel horn erosion*	Slurry heel Interdigital dermatitis* Scald	*dermatitis interdigitalis;* *erosio ungulae*
Fusiformis necrophorus	Foul of the foot	Foot rot (US) Interdigital necrobacillosis Luer (SW England) Interdigital phlegmon*	*phlegmona interdigitalis*

* = ICAR preferred term

Table 9.4   The three main claw horn lesions.

Lesion (UK name)	Alternative nomenclature	Latin nomenclature
Sole haemorrhage*	Sole bruising Laminitis (colloquial, not technical term)	*pododermatitis aseptica diffusa*
White line disease*	White line separation	*pododermatitis septica diffusa*
Ulcer*	Rusterholz disease Sole ulcer	*pododermatitis circumscripta septica*

* = ICAR preferred term

- it is an over-simplification to consider single pathogen species/groups for the three main skin lesions; mixed infections are common, even in the case of digital dermatitis where treponemes account for only one part of the microflora found in these lesions
- heel horn erosion is likely to involve chemical degradation of the horn in addition to pathogens
- useful to consider interdigital hyperplasia (growths, or 'tylomas') alongside the infectious/skin lesions. The precise aetiology is uncertain, but it likely that interdigital hyperplasia is often the result of one or more infectious agents causing chronic irritation to the interdigital skin. Certain breeds have a predisposition (e.g. Hereford cattle). Chronic traumatic irritation is also a possible cause

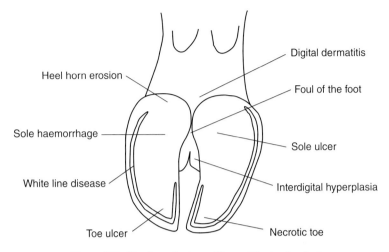

Figure 9.7   The important conditions of the bovine foot.

Claw horn lesions

- three primary lesions are described, though the distinction is blurred: sole haemorrhage; ulcer; white line disease (see Table 9.4)
- lesions are inter-related: sole haemorrhage is recognised as a precursor to sole ulcers
- aetiology related to contusion of the solar corium: pressure from the pedal bone above is likely to result in ulcers on the typical site, in zone 4 of the sole (see Figures 9.7 and 9.8)
- cows with thin soles are more likely to have lesions in zone 5, probably due to contusion from an uneven ground surface (e.g. toe ulcer, Figure 9.7)

Discussion

Risk factors for sole haemorrhage and sole ulcer include:

- long toes, increasing the weight born at the rear of the sole
- poor cow comfort, and/or long milking times resulting in long standing times
- early *post partum*, due to natural weakening of the laminar attachment leading to sinking of the pedal bone
- heifers, who naturally have thinner or less dense digital cushions
- thin cows, those losing weight quickly and old cows, which have thinner, less dense or more fibrous digital cushions

Risk factors for white line disease include:

- shearing (sideways) forces on the feet
- poor cow flow: affected by stockmanship and/or facility design (e.g. narrow passageways)
- thin soles
- long walking distances
- soft horn (e.g. wet conditions; biotin deficiency)
- stoney walkways
- slippery floors
- overcrowding
- over-zealous oestrus and mounting behaviour (e.g. breeding bulls; cystic cows)

Additional claw horn lesions include traumatic lesions and descriptive terms for findings on various parts of the hoof. These are listed in Table 9.5.

Claw zones

- 12 zones of the hooves and surrounding skin
- aid accurate lesion recording (see Figure 9.8)

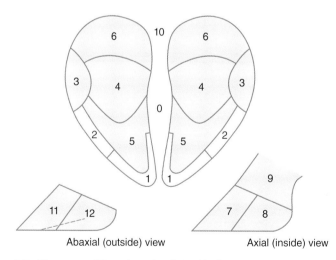

Abaxial (outside) view   Axial (inside) view

Figure 9.8   The zones of the sole and wall. 1. white line zone at toe; 2 and 3. abaxial white line zones; 4. main sole ulcer site; 5. apex of sole; 6. bulb (heel); 7 and 8. axial wall including white line and axial groove; 11 and 12. abaxial wall. Zones 0, 9 and 10 are skin zones; 9. includes the skin on the dorsal aspect of the foot, which can be a site for digital dermatitis, though the main site is 10, at the heel.

Table 9.5 Less common claw horn lesions.

Lesion (UK name)	Alternative description	Latin nomenclature
Punctured sole	Stone penetration	*pododermatitis septica traumatica*
Vertical horn fissure* (longitudinal)	Split wall Sand crack	*fissura ungulae longitudinalis*
Horizontal horn fissure* (transverse)	Hardship groove	*fissura ungulae transversalis*
Toe ulcer*		
Bulb ulcer*	Heel ulcer; sole fissure; cracked sole	
Toe necrosis*	Rotten toe; hollow toe	*apicalis necrotica*
Axial horn fissure*	White line disease of medial wall	
Corkscrew claw*		

* = ICAR preferred term

9.5 Hoof trimming technique: corrective (therapeutic) and preventive trims

The Dutch five-step method, initially published by Dr Toussaint Raven in 1985, is still the recognised approach, albeit that minor variations have evolved. It is important to recognise the difference between 'steps' and 'cuts': some steps involve more than one cut.

A summary of the five-step method is described here (for hind feet) followed by some of the main variations around the theme.

Discussion

Toe length: cut 1 of steps 1 and 2 determine the toe length. It is important that the correct length is chosen as this will also determine the thickness of sole, which remains once the trimming is complete. Toussaint Raven's original recommendation was 75 mm, but recent research suggests this is too short for the majority of cows today. For most Holsteins, the appropriate length to trim to is 85 mm (90 mm if trimming to a point using the 'white line' method). A slightly shorter length may be appropriate for younger Holsteins (e.g. parity 1 and 2). Less experienced trimmers should err on the safer side and trim to 85–90 mm as a minimum, measured from the most proximal part of the dorsal hoof wall at the coronet.

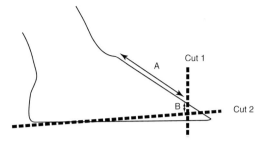

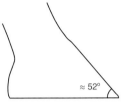

A more upright stance is achieved by cut 1 and cut 2, such that the dorsal wall angle is approximately 52° (55° hind foot, 50° front foot).
Step 1 achieves this in inner claw, whilst step 2 achieves this for the outer claw.

Figure 9.9   Cut 1 and cut 2 used in steps 1 and 2.

Step 1:
- inner (medial) claw
- **cut one**: toe length (A, on Figure 9.9) 75–95 mm (depending on the breed/size of the cow)
- **cut two**: depth of sole (B, on Figure 9.9) 7 mm; the horn is removed from the sole towards the toe only
- heel spared (see Figure 9.9)

Warning
There is often no need to remove any horn at all from the inner claw during step 1: if the toe length is correct, do not remove the horn unnecessarily to avoid thin soles. It is important to maintain a weight-bearing surface on the inner claw to off-load the outer claw in step 4.

Step 2:
- outer (lateral) claw
- **cut one**: toe length (A) 75–95 mm (depending on the breed/size of the cow)
- **cut two**: depth of the sole (B) 7 mm; the sole horn is likely to be removed from the heel to the toe
- key objective is to level the weight bearing between the medial and lateral claws (see Figure 9.10)

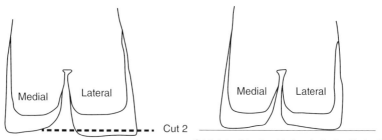

Cut 2 of step 2 has the objective of not only achieving the correct dorsal wall angle, but also to ensure the lateral and medial claws become evenly weight bearing.

Figure 9.10   Step 2: cut 2 must level the weight-bearing between the medial and lateral claws.

Discussion

Foot trimming equipment

A basic equipment list is suggested:
- right-handed and left-handed hoof knives (use both, whichever your dominant hand is)
- good quality hardened steel hoof pincers (e.g. Diamond™ brand)
- hoof-testing pliers
- neoprene wrist protectors
- thick latex gloves
- protective canvas or PVC apron with leg straps (waist height)

Operators using a rotary rasp should use an alloy or titanium cutting-type rasp with adjustable blades (e.g. Wopa™ WG 2060). Abrasive-type discs, although considerably cheaper, can generate excessive heat, and are far less effective. It is imperative to wear suitable personal protective equipment particularly when using mechanical rasps.

Further images and descriptions of trimming equipment can be found on the companion website for this book.

Step 3:
- both claws are modelled to remove the pressure from the usual sole ulcer site
- rear 2/3 of the sole area
- avoid all wall horn entirely
- slightly wider lateral claw has a shallower, wider hollow created (see Figure 9.11). This is the claw where sole bruising and sole ulcers are most commonly found

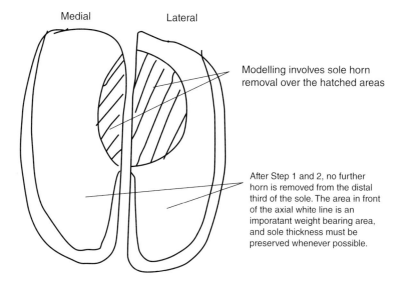

Medial   Lateral

Modelling involves sole horn removal over the hatched areas

After Step 1 and 2, no further horn is removed from the distal third of the sole. The area in front of the axial white line is an imporatant weight bearing area, and sole thickness must be preserved whenever possible.

Figure 9.11   Modelling in step 3.

Step 4:
- for a preventive trim, it may not be necessary to progress beyond step 3
- steps 4 and 5 are therapeutic steps: to relieve weight bearing from a claw horn lesion (step 4) or to treat a skin lesion (step 5)
- if claw horn lesions are commonplace in a herd, step 4 may be used as a preventive measure, in the absence of a lesion, in order to further offload the weight to pre-empt a lesion occurring
- step 4 is removal of the additional sole horn from the rear 2/3 of the sole (i.e. behind the axial white) (see Figure 9.12)
- the axial wall and toe region of the sole are preserved as important weight-bearing surfaces
- step 4 should increase the weight borne by the medial claw in comparison to the lateral claw

Step 5:
- loose horn is removed from the heel bulbs during the final step
- erosions and pits, which are part of heel horn erosion, should be opened up, whilst avoiding cutting into the sensitive deeper tissues (avoid bleeding)
- this final step should also be used to check for and treat any further skin lesions, such as digital dermatitis

Trimming variations

- **Front feet**: the description above is for the **hind feet**. The medial claw is the larger claw of the **front feet** and will need additional horn removed

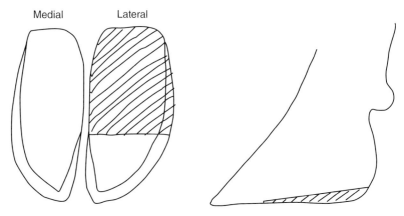

Medial   Lateral

Figure 9.12 Additional horn removal in step 4. The hatched area shows where additional horn is removed to reduce weight bearing on the rear 2/3 of the lateral claw in step 4.

during step 4. Step 1 for the **front feet** is for the **lateral claw** and step 2 for the **medial claw**.

- Alternative toe lengths: originally 75 mm was the proposed toe length. In reality, different breeds, and even animals within a breed, have naturally different toe lengths; 80–85 mm is probably appropriate for most of today's Holstein breed
- The interpretation of step 5 is open to debate. When the original Dutch method was first described, digital dermatitis was not prevalent; now it seems sensible to include digital dermatitis treatment into step 5 as well as heel horn erosion.
- The **'Dairyland' method** practised by some operators, mainly in the USA, includes seven steps. The principle differences are a greater degree of modelling in the lateral claw and a step that 'removes the buckle' of the dorsal wall, if present (i.e. to make the dorsal wall flat before measuring the toe length). Grinding the dorsal wall could be detrimental (see key principles). The 'Dairyland' method places a greater emphasis on measuring the dorsal wall angle.
- The **'Kansas' method** differs from the standard Dutch method as the correct sole thickness is gauged by sole horn dehydration/natural flaking, and a greater flexibility is allowed on toe length. The sole is trimmed with a slight slope inwards in the axial-abaxial plane (whilst the foot is non-weight-bearing).
- The **'white line' method** differs very slightly from the Dutch method as the toe length is cut 5 mm longer, but the correct sole depth is gauged by trimming the sole until the white line is seen at the toe. The resulting trimmed claw does not have a blunt-ended dorsal wall at the toe.

- The functional difference in the above method variations is likely to be minimal.

Discussion

The key principles of routine trimming

- Achieve a dorsal wall angle of $\approx$ 52°.
- Balance weight bearing between the lateral and medial claws.
- Always measure toe length of both claws: this cannot be guessed and cut 1 of steps 1 and 2 determines the sole thickness.
- Off-load claw horn lesions, either by step 4 alone or in combination with blocking the contra-lateral claw. There is good evidence that blocking speeds recovery from claw horn lesions.
- Avoid removing the dorsal and lateral wall horn except from the bottom surface in contact with the floor. A common bad habit is shaping the outer wall, particularly with a grinder, in order to achieve the correct wall angle without using steps 1 and 2. The wall is the strength of the hoof.
- Preserve the axial wall. Another bad habit often seen is thinning of the axial wall by vertical knife strokes or grinding between the toes. The wall is the strength of the hoof, and in normal circumstances the bottom edge of the wall is the main weight-bearing surface.
- Relieve pressure over the main sole ulcer site: modelling.
- Avoid thin soles: knowing when **not** to trim is important. Thin soles occur with over-wear and over-trimming.
- Correct heel depth (30–40 mm). Low heels can result in too shallow a dorsal wall angle and stretched flexor tendons. High heels can occur with painful digital dermatitis lesions where animals walk on 'tip-toes', leading to excess wear and thin soles at the toe. The original Dutch five-step method is not always easy to interpret for animals with a high heel depth as the toe length may already be short. In such instances, the dorsal wall angle is the best guide for horn removal at the rear of the hoof.

9.6 Therapeutic trimming of claw horn lesions

The objectives of therapeutic trims can be summarised thus:

1. Remove weight from the lesion. Use a block.
2. Remove all under-run horn to the point of attachment.
3. Avoid bleeding.

> **Tip**
>
> - Fixing a block or orthopaedic shoe to the non-diseased claw (usually the medial claw on the hind feet) will reduce weight bearing over a claw horn lesion over trimming alone; this is likely to significantly reduce the recovery time for most claw horn lesions as well as reducing discomfort.
> - Routine use of NSAIDs in addition to a therapeutic trim has been found to improve the recovery rate and reduce the recurrence rate when used in early treatment of claw horn lesions.

As claw horn lesions can vary enormously in severity, it can be difficult to know exactly how much horn to remove. The three principles provide a useful guide. However, removal of unattached horn whilst avoiding bleeding (trauma to the underlying corium) requires patience, skill and very sharp knives.

Complicated claw horn lesions

- claw horn lesions often become infected
- digital dermatitis treponemes have been associated with 'non-healing' lesions
- to facilitate treatment of an infected corium and reduce the likelihood of digital dermatitis infections further eroding the horn–corium junction, it is particularly important to follow the second principle of removing under-run horn to the point of attachment

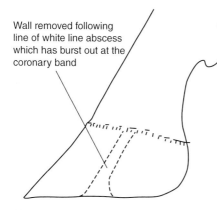

Wall removed following line of white line abscess which has burst out at the coronary band

It is not necessary to leave a bridge of horn (contra-indicated) or to create a prosthetic bridge in an attempt to stabilise the horn at the coronary band.

As long as the underlying laminar corium is not damaged by aggressive use of the knife and infection is controlled, a healthy granulation bed will produce new keratinised tissue to fill in the wall horn deficit

The partner digit should be blocked whilst healing occurs, which may take several months.

Figure 9.13 Wall resection with a white line abscess extending to the coronary band.

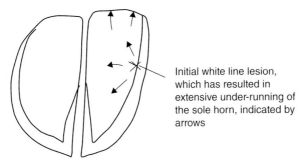

Initial white line lesion, which has resulted in extensive under-running of the sole horn, indicated by arrows

Figure 9.14 Under-run sole often occurs as a consequence of a white line lesion. An under-run sole can lead to a 'double sole' – sometimes more than one.

- for example, white line abscesses that have continued to the coronary band require the wall to be removed along the whole length of the lesion (see Figure 9.13)
- abscesses that have under-run the sole, commonly bursting at the heel bulb, require all the sole to be removed to the point of attachment (see Figures 9.14, 9.15 and 9.16)
- an under-run sole may require extensive sole horn to be removed, towards the toe and also towards the heel
- in the absence of infection, new sole horn will very quickly form, resulting in a recovery time of 3–6 weeks
- the partner digit should be blocked for this period

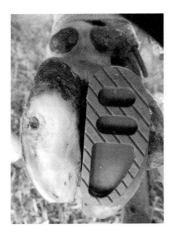

Under-run horn has been removed to the point of firm attachment between the sole horn and the underlying corium. Lateral wall has also been removed to some extent, again until its firm attachment can be seen with the underlying laminar corium.

An orthopaedic shoe has been fixed to the partner claw to remove weight from the lesion and aid recovery.

Administering NSAIDs to the cow will speed recovery time and reduce the risk of relapse.

Figure 9.15 A pared sole with a small area of under-running following a white line lesion.

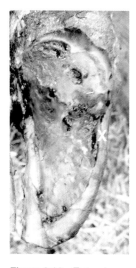

The initial white line lesion marked with X has become infected, possibly with digital dermatitis treponemes, with the consequence of extensive under-running of the entire sole. This has been removed exposing the underlying corium.Once infection is controlled, the sole corium can be expected to produce a new sole horn in a matter of weeks.

Figure 9.16 Extensive removal of the sole horn following infection, which has caused the whole sole to become under-run.

Applying orthopaedic hoof blocks

Types of orthopaedic hoof blocks

- a wide choice of blocks and adhesives are available (see Figure 9.17)
- some blocks can be used with different adhesives, for example wooden or plastic blocks can be used with either two-part polyurethane tube adhesives or powder/liquid polyacrylate resin adhesives. Some blocks are designed to use with a specific glue type, for example the expanded foam blocks with cyanoacrylate adhesive ('super glue')
- the correct block shapes and sizes should be chosen to suit the specific circumstances
- it is imperative that the overall length of the toe is not altered by the block, to avoid rapid wear at the rear of the block leading to stretched flexor tendons; achieved by setting blocks further back on the sole (surmounting the bulb of the heel by 1 cm) or by using a shoe-type block with a stepped toe area
- wedge-shaped blocks have been proposed to reduce the strain on the flexor tendon; may be beneficial in some circumstances such as prolonged periods of blocking
- blocks wear at different rates depending on the floor surface and the distance of cow travel, but the block material greatly influences the useful life-span of the block; harder, solid plastic blocks are the longest wearing, whilst expanded foam blocks wear in the shortest time

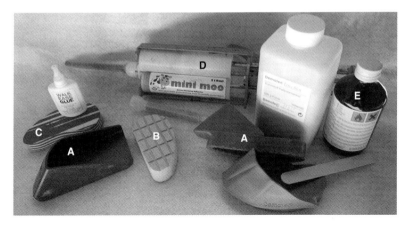

Figure 9.17 A range of orthopaedic blocks and adhesive.
A = orthopaedic shoe (e.g. Cowslips® and Easy Bloc®); B = wooden block; C = expanded foam block and cyanoacrylate adhesive (e.g. Walkease®); D = epoxy, or polyurethane adhesive (e.g. Moo Gloo®, Bovibond®); E = polyacrylate 2-part adhesive resin (e.g. Demotec 95®)

- long-lasting blocks are useful for severe claw horn lesions requiring a longer recovery time
- all blocks need checking regularly and removed or replaced if uneven wear is evident

Applying a block successfully
- applied to the healthy digit, i.e. the partner digit to the digit with the claw horn lesion, usually the medial hind claw or lateral front claw
- the digit to be blocked should be trimmed as per the Dutch method and tested for soundness, using hoof testing pliers
- should not be necessary to over-trim the digit to be blocked although loose horn and dirt must be removed from the entire sole surface, which might otherwise have been left alone after the Dutch method
- **Polyacrylate resin and polyurethane adhesives:**
  - The digit should be absolutely dry and dirt-free (e.g. use a hot air blower or pour methylated spirit over the digit and allow it to air-dry); re-clean the digit after drying
  - mix glue according to the instructions; with resin powder/liquid glues, mix the powder into the liquid (versus liquid into powder) to avoid dry powder pockets remaining
  - place the glue on the block; apply the block firmly to the hoof, **but do not squeeze too much glue from beneath the block**. Aim for a glue

thickness of ≈ 3 mm for polyurethane adhesive and ≈ 5–6 mm for poly-acrylate resin adhesive
- ensure the block is level: check for slope front to back and axial to abaxial
- remove any glue that has spilled into the interdigital area (axial edge of the block), as this can cause a hard ridge; ensure there is no glue under the bulb of the heel (only likely with resin glues and shoe-type blocks) to reduce the risk of heel bruising
- allow glue to thoroughly dry; in cold weather, pre-warming the adhesive and block is more useful than applying heat directly to a block and glue once in position. For polyacrylate resin glues, warming the liquid before-hand in a jug of hot water is usually sufficient
- **Cyanoacrylate adhesive:**
  - works best if the horn is not over-dry, so do not dry the horn with spirit or hot air
  - the bond is strongest when the adhesive layer is very thin: apply continuous very hard pressure to the block, followed by rapid lowering of the foot once the block has firmly adhered, so the cow's weight further compresses the block; lifting the contralateral leg may be of benefit
  - thin layer requires an absolutely flat smooth sole surface beneath the block

Block removal
- check blocks weekly and remove if wear is uneven or the cow shows signs of pain
- most blocks should be good for 5–6 weeks if applied properly
- removing blocks should be done with a hammer and blunt chisel; apply the chisel blade on the glue between the sole horn and the block at the rear of the hoof and give a sharp, hard tap with the hammer. The block should come off cleanly
- wooden blocks can be split in two, lengthwise, with a chisel at the rear of the block and this may facilitate removal
- avoid twisting and pulling forces (likely if removal is attempted using a hoof pincer)

Warning

Do not allow a cow to walk on a block that has worn at the heel such that her flexor tendons are stretched.

9.7 Interdigital phlegmon (foul of the foot)

Synonyms

- interdigital necrobacillosis, *phlegmona interdigitalis*, foul-in-the-foot, 'clit ill', 'foot rot', 'luer', interdigital pododermatitis
- peracute form, 'superfoul', sometimes encountered.

Signs

- acute inflammation of subcutaneous tissues of the interdigital space and adjacent coronary band, spreading to the dermis and epidermis
- sudden onset of mild to severe lameness (MS 2–3)
- all ages
- interdigital swelling, later involving the coronary band and bilateral swelling of the entire foot
- toes spread apart due to interdigital swelling, initially with unbroken skin for the first 24 hours of lameness
- sometimes a more proximal spread and commonly a secondary interdigital necrosis
- little pus but characteristic foul smell and pain with a split in the interdigital skin
- often limited to an individual but small herd outbreaks can occur

Aetiology and pathology

- interdigital trauma, and infection with *Fusobacterium necrophorum* and other organisms, including *Prevotella* (formerly *Bacteroides) melaninogenicus*
- straw, thorns and stones are often involved in the initial trauma
- cellulitis and liquefactive necrosis of interdigital skin, with fissure formation and later, if untreated, development of granulation tissue, eventually resulting in interdigital hyperplasia
- advanced cases can develop digital septic arthritis and other deeper complications
- the disease course is rapid in 'superfoul' where cows may have to be culled 48–72 hours after disease onset, due to the extent of destructive changes; 'superfoul' may involve more pathogenic strains of the same bacteria or a cocktail of several pathogens

Differential diagnosis

- due to the degree of swelling and acute pain, the main differential diagnosis (without lifting the foot) is likely to be distal interphalangeal (DIP) joint infection, usually as a sequel to a sole ulcer or white line disease

- DIP joint infection: swelling is more obviously around one of the digits rather than bilateral
- other differentials include an interdigital foreign body, sole penetration by a foreign body, severe interdigital dermatitis, interdigital changes from BVD/MD, FMD and a distal phalangeal fracture

Treatment

- systemic antibiotics; *Fusobacterium necrophorum* is a gram-negative anaerobe, and penicillin, cephalosporins, tetracycline and sulphonamides would all be suitable choices
- cleaning (debriding) the lesion and topical application of an antibiotic (e.g. oxytetracycline spray) may speed resolution
- do **not** bandage
- house on a dry floor/environment to reduce spread
- severe cases ('superfoul') require immediate attention but respond to protracted high doses of systemic antibiotics, as well as meticulous debridement under analgesia and local amoxicillin powder
- NSAIDs speed recovery in all cases; particularly helpful in severe lesions

Prophylaxis

- prompt treatment of cases will reduce spread
- if recurrent problem, address underlying trauma, e.g. hard straw; wet and unhygienic underfoot conditions; stoney tracks/gateways/areas around water troughs
- regular footbaths of zinc sulphate (5–10%), copper sulphate (5%) or formalin (4%) may help to control it within a herd

Discussion

- This is a frequent cause of lameness on some farms, implicated in up to 15% of all lameness cases.
- It is easy to diagnose and treat; prompt attention limits the economic consequences.
- Where poorly controlled, a high incidence of interdigital hyperplasia may occur, with greater economic consequences.

9.8 Digital dermatitis

Synonyms

- *dermatitis digitalis*, 'hairy warts', PDD, papillomatous digital dermatitis, foot warts, Mortellaro disease

Signs and incidence

- circumscribed superficial ulceration of the skin, usually along the coronary margin at the heels, but occasionally more dorsally
- lesions cause obvious lameness
- can develop into a mass of verrucose fronds ('hairy wart')
- known to also infect exposed corium, leading to 'non-healing' claw horn lesions
- involved in the aetiology of toe necrosis
- rarely implicated in non-digital infections, such as the udder skin
- high incidence: widespread in many dairy farms throughout Europe and North America, where incidence can reach 100% and prevalence 20%
- often the major lameness problem in dairy herds in particular
- probably worldwide, with reported cases also from Africa, China, Chile, Australasia and India

Lesion classification

- physical characteristics are classified by different stages of infection, summarised in Table 9.6

Table 9.6   Wisconsin classification of digital dermatitis lesions.

Lesion classification	Description
M0	Normal: no lesion
M1	Small (<2 cm), circumscribed red or grey erosion (focal bacterial keratolysis)
M2	Acute ulcerative or granulomatous lesion >2 cm diameter
M3	Healing scab, for example following topical treatment within 1–2 days
M4	Chronic dyskeratotic, or proliferative lesion (e.g. verrucose fronds)
M4.1	Chronic lesion with an additional subacute component
Corium infection	DD infection on the corium, associated with non-healing claw horn lesions

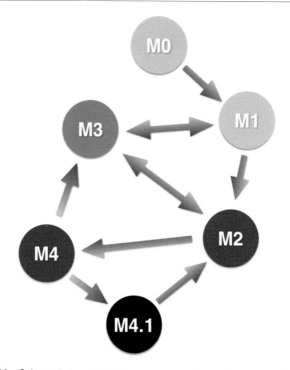

Figure 9.18   Schematic representation of the dynamics of different physical manifestations of digital dermatitis lesions, as proposed by Döpfer, Wisconsin, USA.
M0 = no lesion; M1 = new lesion; M2 = acute active lesion; M3 = healing scab; M4 = chronic proliferative lesion; M4.1 = chronic lesion with additional subacute component.

- lesions evolve through stages M1, M2, M3, M4 and M4.1 and complicate the herd population dynamics (see Figure 9.18)
- once infected with DD, a cow may at best remain a chronic carrier (M3 lesion) and at worst always have either an active M2 or M4 lesion. These carrier cows are the main reservoir of infection within a herd. Alterations in the cow's immunity as well as control methods (e.g. footbathing) are likely to be largely responsible for which lesion stage is evident.

Discussion

- Individuals within a herd can alternate between different lesion types and hence degrees of lameness and infectivity.
- Immunity, foot hygiene and control measures, such as blitz treatment or regular foot bathing, will govern the prevalence of each lesion type.

- The objective of herd control should be to reduce as far as possible the occurrence of new lesions (M1) and convert active lesions (M1, M2, M4, M4.1) to healed lesions (M3).
- DD bacteria seem to have a dormancy phase (M3), and it is debatable if full bacteriological cure is ever possible.

Bacteriology

- *Treponema* bacteria are almost certainly involved in the aetiology
- three distinct phylogroups have repeatedly been associated with digital dermatitis lesions in the UK:
  1. *Treponema medium*/*Treponema vincentii*-like spirochaetes
  2. *Treponema phagedenis*-like spirochaetes
  3. *Treponema pedis*-like spirochaetes
- culture of swabs from digital dermatitis lesions typically yield mixed bacterial infections, but the precise symbiotic nature of the various pathogens is not yet fully established
- *In vitro* culture of DD treponemes is very difficult, so PCR is usually used to confirm the presence of treponeme DNA

Differential diagnosis

- lesions are usually very characteristic
- mild forms (M1) may be indistinguishable from interdigital dermatitis lesions supposedly caused by *Dichelobacter nodosus*
- there is some debate as to whether these are in fact two distinct lesion entities

Treatment

- topical treatment with antibiotics after lifting the foot and cleaning lesions with cotton-wool gives a good immediate resolution, at least of active M2 and M4 lesions
- no known resistance to the major antibiotic classes
- aerosol sprays containing either tetracycline or thiamphenicol antibiotics or chelated copper/zinc are licensed in the EU for topical treatments
- other topical antiseptics may be effective but licensed products should be used preferentially
- successful topical treatment of severe lesions with salicylic acid crystals held in place with a bandage has been reported
- systemic antibiotics are indicated for deep infections, recurrent infections and those with extensive secondary bacterial infection

- severe proliferating lesions: surgically resect through the epidermis (not subcutis) under local anaesthesia (e.g. IVRA) in a crush/chute prior to antibiotic therapy

---

Discussion

There is a dispute as to whether bandaging lesions is beneficial to treatment. Advocates of bandaging claim that the topical antibiotic or antiseptic can be held in place for longer, but opponents claim that bandages are likely to lead to the moist anaerobic conditions and hygroscopic skin damage that is precisely necessary for DD infection to take hold. Certainly, if used, bandages should be removed after a maximum of 48 hours and are not used where this cannot be assured.

Prevention

- whereas slurry has sometimes been considered to be the natural reservoir of DD bacteria, it is more likely that carrier cows are the main reservoir and slurry is a fomite; reducing slurry build-up and slurry contamination of heels is an important control measure
- DD only develops when the skin is exposed to prolonged wetness and increased skin pH caused by urine and faeces, resulting in the breakdown of the outermost layer of skin; the normal pH of skin ≈ 5.5.
- exposure to hydrogen sulphide and ammonia from slurry raises the pH; keeping feet as dry as possible is important in prevention, again by reducing slurry, but also by encouraging longer lying times and paying attention to ventilation in housing. Slatted floors can help keep feet dry, but ammonia can still be a risk
- regular (at least twice per week) foot bathing is an accepted control measure for DD, but it must be done effectively; grossly contaminated baths, whereby the antiseptic is likely to be inactivated, may be counterproductive
- a rule of thumb is to permit no more than one cow passage per litre of solution in the bath
- some chemicals are harmful to skin integrity (e.g. formaldehyde) and so the beneficial antibacterial properties must outweigh any skin-damaging properties
- formaldehyde (2–5%), copper sulphate (2.5–5%), zinc sulphate (2-5%), glutaraldehyde (2–5%) and peracetic acid (5%) are all suitable footbath solutions, though some chemicals are human health hazards (formaldeyde and glutaraldeyde are carcinogens) and others are environmental hazards (copper sulphate)
- antibiotic footbaths are neither licensed nor allowed, even under cascade regulations in the EU; although anecdotally antibiotic footbaths can reduce the severity of lesions and dampen herd infections, they have little justification given that non-antibiotic footbaths can do a similar job

- where herd prevalence is high a blitz approach of individual treatments is likely to result in a better outcome than footbaths alone
- isolate newly purchased heifers/cows for three weeks, check for overt digital dermatitis lesions and treat or cull if affected. Even where DD already exists in a herd, biosecurity is important to prevent the introduction of new more pathogenic strains
- disinfect all foot paring instruments (knives, clippers, crush/chute) after working with an infected herd and between animals. DD treponemes have been found (using PCR) on foot paring equipment including knives and trimming discs, so this is a potential route of spread between individuals, even if probably not the predominant route
- maintaining a healthy herd and reducing stress leading to immune-compromise appears to be very important in reducing DD prevalence. Higher yielding herds and freshly calved cows are most at risk; prophylactic regular (weekly) footbathing of dry cows and in-calf heifers is advocated

9.9 Interdigital hyperplasia

Synonyms

- hyperplasia interdigitalis, corn, interdigital granuloma, interdigital vegetative dermatitis, fibroma, tyloma

Signs and pathology

- proliferative reaction of interdigital skin and/or subcutaneous tissues to form a firm mass
- skin hyperplasia with secondary ulceration
- variable degree of hyperkeratosis (misnamed papillomatosis)
- inherited in some breeds (e.g. Hereford)
- severe interdigital dermatitis or chronic *F. necrophorum* infection may precede involvement of single or bilateral limbs
- associated with poor conformation, e.g. splayed toes with a wide interdigital space
- lameness can be a variable feature, often depending on secondary infection on the mass, for example digital dermatitis, as well as size
- a single abaxial hind limb involvement suggests a secondary response to an existing insult involving interdigital swelling and sometimes a sole ulcer

Treatment

- none if small and asymptomatic
- local topical treatment (e.g. oxytetracycline spray) if small and causing lameness due to secondary infection or pressure necrosis

- some clinical cases require resection by knife surgery, electrocautery or cryosurgery: in a crush using IVRA (intravenous regional analgesia)
- surgical excision should include any fat that prolapses through the wound once a fibrous mass is removed; a narrow margin of the skin is left for re-epithelialisation of the wound
- topical application of the antibiotic is required; possibly systemic if *F. necrophorum* is suspected; remove the bandage after 2 days, if used for haemostasis
- digits may be wired together to reduce the chance of relapse, but are always trimmed to prevent splayed toes

Prevention

- uncertainty as to exact aetiology and clinical significance
- breeding policy: alter to reduce the risk of inheritance where multilimb hyperplasia is prevalent
- improved underfoot hygiene and an effective footbath strategy usually reduces the prevalence in most dairy herds
- prevention is better than cure: surgical removal often results in a relapse; if underfoot conditions do not improve, new cases will continue to occur, as well as these relapses
- removal of interdigital masses is an act of veterinary surgery (UK legislation) and requires anaesthesia. Illegal removal by lay trimmers and farmers by 'a flick of the knife' should be strongly discouraged on a welfare basis, as well as being an ineffective approach

9.10 Sole ulcer

Synonyms

- sol(e)ar ulceration; Rusterholz ulcer; *pododermatitis circumscripta*
- heel ulcer and toe ulcer are related conditions, but occur in different regions of the sole and may have subtle differences in aetiology

Signs

- a circumscribed limited reaction of the pododerm (deep sensitive tissues) often characterised by an erosive defect typically at the sole–heel junction of the lateral hind claw
- ulcers occur from the corium outwards, and are **not** due to penetration injury or ingress of foreign material (contrast a penetration injury or white line abscess)

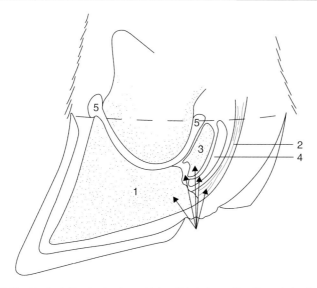

Figure 9.19 Typical site of sole ulcer of lateral hind claw with adjacent structures that may be affected by deep sepsis.
1. pedal bone/distal phalanx; 2. deep digital flexor tendon; 3. navicular bone (distal sesamoid); 4. navicular bursa; 5. distal interphalangeal joint.

- a moderate degree of lameness (hesitant, wary gait, slightly arched back, MS 2 or 3) typically up to three months post-partum, masking the frequently bilateral nature of the lesions, i.e. the lateral claw of both hind legs, one more painful than the other
- severe lameness (MS 3) when granulation tissue protrudes and in the presence of deeper purulent infection (osteomyelitis, septic navicular bursa and septic arthritis) (see Figure 9.19)
- an under-run heel horn exposes the sensitive corium, which may be secondarily infected, sometimes with DD treponemes, causing further under-running
- likely to be bilateral: always check for similar changes in the contralateral foot
- granulation tissue may protrude through the undermined horn
- under-running commonly extends cranially and peripherally to the abaxial white line
- often impacted material, including stones, are found in the damaged horn. Note that these are secondary and should not be confused with foreign body penetration
- **incidence:** high; major cause of lameness

- **differential diagnosis:** solar abscessation following a true foreign body penetration injury

Aetiology

- contusion of the corium at the sole ulcer site results in initial haemorrhage (sole bruising) followed by failure of normal keratinisation of epithelial keratinocytes, and a horn deficit; there are many risk factors for the initial contusion and physical traumatic damage to the corium
- the usual sole ulcer site is below the deep digital flexor tendon tuberosity on the pedal bone, forming a natural pressure point
- previous traumatic insults (and sole ulcer episodes) lead to additional bony proliferation of the pedal bone and a more significant pressure point
- long toes lead to greater weight borne at the rear of the foot, again leading to greater pressure at the predisposition site
- sinking or rotation of the pedal bone in relation to the hoof capsule is likely to increase pressure on the solar corium; circumstances include around calving, under hormonal influence (oestrogen and relaxin – relaxation of the connective tissue support); possibly metabolic insults, including toxaemia and ruminal acidosis, which may lead to metalloproteinases weakening the support at the laminae (true laminitis)
- thin cows and cows losing weight rapidly have less thick and/or dense digital cushion fat pads; the digital cushion runs in three main pillows under the proximal half of the pedal bone, supporting the pedal bone and dissipating concussive forces on the corium
- cows with a lower body condition score at drying off and calving are known to have a higher incidence of claw horn lesions in the following lactation; it is highly probable that digital cushion support and thickness are influenced by genetics, leading to speculation that certain breeds and individuals within breeds are liable to be more prone to claw horn lesions. Cows maintaining a good body condition score and hence digital cushion thickness is now an established plank of lameness prevention
- long standing times due to poor cow comfort and/or long milking or lock-up times lead to greater overall contusion at the sole corium and a higher risk for sole ulcers; loose housing, pasture and deep bedded cubicles/free stalls are associated with longer lying times and reduced claw horn lesions

Complicated sole ulcers

Two types of secondary infection are common:

1. **Deep sepsis**, including infection of the navicular bursa, deep flexor tendon and distal interphalangeal joint. A number of pathogens can be involved,

but often thick white pus can be seen at the centre of the ulcer, marking a sinus to a deeper pocket of infection, usually the distal interphalangeal joint. *Trueperella pyogenes* is likely to be implicated in such cases as an opportunistic pathogen. The foot is very painful and swollen (unilateral around the affected claw), particularly around the coronary band and heel. Flexing the foot whilst pressing on the heel bulb will compress the joint space and if infection is into the joint, pus will be seen at the centre of the ulcer site via the sinus. The toe is often over-extended due to complete or partial disruption of the insertion of the flexor tendon on the pedal bone. Conservative treatment will not be effective at this stage (see surgical treatments).

2. **Digital dermatitis infection** of the exposed corium (see Figure 9.20). More extensive under-running of the sole horn than is usual with a simple non-infected sole ulcer is likely, possibly leading to a discharging sinus at the heel. These cases respond well to treatment as long as all unattached horn is removed and the DD infection is treated (topically) on the exposed corium. Untreated DD infection of the corium can lead to non-healing sole ulcers, despite following the usual steps to treat claw horn lesions (see Section 9.6, key principles for treating claw horn lesions).

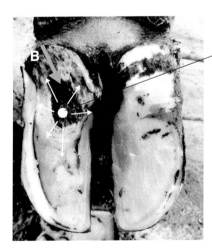

original sole ulcer lesion

White arrows indicate pus/serum fluid from sole ulcer, causing extensive under-running until bursting at the heel (B).

The grey arrow indicates entry of DD bacteria, infecting the corium, extending the lesion and possibly producing further pus which increases the extent of the under-running of the sole.

Figure 9.20   Infected sole ulcer – type 2: digital dermatitis infection of corium leading to extensive under-running of the sole. In this case the entire sole surface has been removed, exposing a new sole horn beneath. Sometimes, several layers of under-run soles can be removed where the process of under-running, separating new sole from the corium below, has repeated itself consecutively.

Treatment

- follow the Dutch five-step approach (Section 9.5) and the key principles for treating claw horn lesions (Section 9.6); apply a block to partner digit
- IVRA is useful for careful removal of all under-run horn near sensitive tissues
- protruding granulation tissue may be left alone (avoids bleeding); once pressure is removed from the site and secondary infection is controlled, a new sole will form and the granulation tissue will shrink and disappear
- avoid topical application of caustic chemicals, which will impede new horn growth by a recovering corium: although copper sulphate is commonly bandaged on to these lesions, this will impede recovery. If possible, avoid bandaging (leave open) and apply a topical antibiotic, such as oxytetracycline spray or povidone-iodine antiseptic. If a bandage is used, remove after a maximum of 48 hours
- broad-spectrum systemic antibiotics are indicated when there is sepsis, although deep sepsis (distal interphalangeal joint infection) will require surgical treatment, or the animal should be culled
- conservative treatment of deep sepsis of the distal interphalangeal joint will involve chronic pain and is unacceptable from a cow welfare perspective
- NSAIDs are indicated and will speed recovery time
- the cow should be housed where she can get up and lie down without difficulty: for example loose housing or over-sized deep bedded cubicles

Prevention

- reduce the risk factors outlined in 'aetiology'
- avoid thin cows and rapid weight loss
- ensure lying times are 12 hours or more per day (good cow comfort and suitable time budget, such as minimal milking times); this is particularly important during the calving and early lactation period
- avoid long toes: a pre-dry-off routine trim (including heifers 6–8 weeks prior to calving) may ensure cows calve with a correct hoof length and shape
- larger herds often institute a routine early-lactation trim to prevent sole ulcers and off-load the lateral hind digits by following the Dutch five-step method. The best time is debated, but a trim at around 40 days post-partum usually precedes sole ulcer formation; effectiveness of prophylactic routine trimming during lactation may depend on specific farm circumstances

- early detection and treatment of new lesions (sole haemorrhage) carries a much better prognosis than treatment of more severe lesions; mobility scoring to detect early mild lameness is important
- accustom heifers to concrete and cubicles/free stalls prior to calving (at least 3 weeks)
- cull cows that have had previous sole ulcers: they are at high risk of relapse in following lactations

9.11 White line disease

Synonyms

- white line separation; white line abscess; wall ulcer (when the wall has been removed by trimming); *pododermatitis septica diffusa;* axial wall lesion

Signs

- abaxial, or less commonly axial, wall separation from the laminar corium at a sole–wall junction
- very diverse spectrum of severity, from mild bruising at the white line, through to slight separation with some impaction of mud or faeces, to development of an abscess with a cavity that may extend under the entire sole, or under the wall horn, or both
- secondary infection with DD treponemes can lead to 'non-healing' lesions and extensive under-running
- abscessation often presents as acute onset lameness (MS 2 or MS 3)
- a black mark is usually present at the white line, which may be very small and difficult to see; hoof testing pliers are invaluable to localise the site of abscess without paring the sole unnecessarily
- abscesses may burst out at the heels or coronary band, having tracked up along the wall laminae
- advanced/chronic cases are obvious, including large wall defects ± protruding granulation tissue (previous treatment) or supracoronary septic sinus discharge
- occasionally, infection extends to the distal interphalangeal joint: the cow is very lame (MS 3) and the digit is swollen; a bead of white pus is seen from the discharging sinus to the joint if the joint space is compressed (see infected sole ulcer)
- **Incidence:** major cause of lameness; main lesion in extensive grazing herds (thin soles and walking long distances)
- **Differential diagnosis:** true foreign body penetration; small coronary vertical fissure; fractured pedal bone (where acute pain is localised to a single digit but a white line abscess is absent)

Aetiology and risk factors

- some similarity to other claw horn disorders, such as sole ulcer aetiology
- contusion of corium responsible for white line formation leads to a white line haemorrhage and probably a greater risk of white line separation
- shearing (sideways) forces cause sole–wall separation, followed by ingress of a foreign material and possibly abscess formation or infection of the corium by DD treponemes
- thin soles (over-wear; over-trimming) and wet (soft) horn predispose cows to the problem, due to a weaker sole–wall junction; wet tracks in grazing systems are a particular risk
- biotin deficiency (more likely in high-yielding herds with acidic rumen conditions) results in a weaker horn; biotin supplementation can reduce white line disease incidence
- possibly other mineral deficiencies (e.g. zinc) may contribute to a weaker horn
- specific risks include poor cow flow: for example, overcrowding, narrow passageways, sharp turns; stockmanship has a large influence; cows that are rushed or herded aggressively (e.g. sticks, dogs, quad-bikes) are at greater risk; unskilled use of backing gates in collection yards and over-stocking collection yards also increase shearing forces on the feet
- mounting behaviour (e.g. stock bull; cows in oestrus; cystic nymphomaniac cows) increases shearing forces and sole wear
- small grit particles (e.g. stony tracks; tracks with road planings) increases the risk of foreign material entry and abscessation
- the floor surface influences the risk:
  i. slippery floors lead to more shearing forces on the feet (skidding);
  ii. abrasive floors (e.g. concrete with carborundum grit; sand on concrete; new concrete) lead to over-wear and thin soles; thin soles flex more causing greater forces at the white line junction;
  iii. rough floor surfaces (e.g. stones; tamped concrete; too closely spaced deep grooving) lead to greater pressure on the sole, which flexes more, leading to greater forces at the white line junction.

Complicated white line lesions

- secondary infection of deeper tissues, or an exposed corium with DD treponemes, is common, similar to a sole ulcer (see Figure 9.21)
- DD infection of the corium can lead to extensive under-running of the wall and/or sole, and a non-healing lesion
- sometimes verrucose lesions are seen

Treatment

- as for a sole ulcer: horn removal should extend to the point where the horn is firmly attached

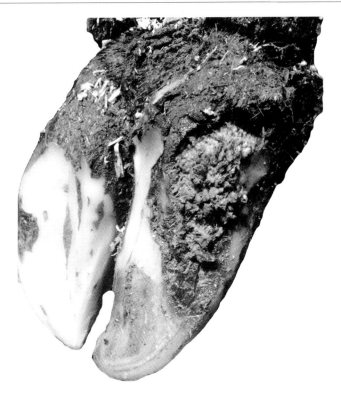

Figure 9.21   White line disease with a chronic secondary verrucose digital dermatitis infection on the underlying corium.

- wall removal, if the abscess has an under-run wall, is very difficult as the wall is hard horn; first thin the wall using a cutting disc or knife, then carefully pare the thinned wall with the knife to remove all unattached wall whilst avoiding bleeding (and damaging the germinal layer below) (see Figure 9.22)
- IVRA, a tourniquet to reduce bleeding and cotton-wool to swab blood will all allow a better job to be done, and permit careful removal of all unattached horn; local anaesthesia is essential for extensive horn removal
- wall deficits take longer to heal than sole deficits, but new horn will be formed from the underlying germinal laminar corium as long as infection is controlled; topical antibiotics are warranted
- bandaging may keep the wound clean until the first signs of re-keratinisation are seen; very regular bandage changes are necessary (every 2 or 3 days)
- a complete new wall can grow from the coronary band in about 12 months

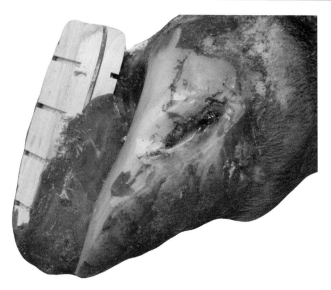

Figure 9.22 A white line lesion that has under-run the wall, pared correctly to the full extent of the lesion.

- lesions extending to the coronary band cause damage to the coronary corium, which is responsible for new wall production, so a deformed horn is likely
- apply a block to the partner claw; NSAIDs; house the cow in a clean environment; avoid bandaging if possible
- deep sepsis and non-responsive cases require digit amputation or culling; conservative treatment is useless, causing chronic pain, and is unacceptable from a cow welfare perspective

Prevention

- attention to risk factors (see aetiology)
- biotin supplementation 20 mg/head/day, all year round
- early detection and prompt effective treatment of early MS 1 and MS 2 cows
- avoidance of over-trimming/thin soles

9.12 Toe necrosis

Synonyms

- rotten toe; hollow toe; *apicalis necrotica*

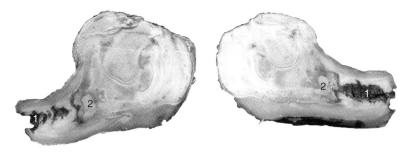

Figure 9.23 Bisected digit with necrotic toe showing sinus (1) at the apical horn and osteomyelitis of the apical pedal bone (2).

Definition

- non-healing infection of the toe extending to the pedal bone (see Figure 9.23)
- pedal bone osteomyelitis is a feature
- infection rarely extends beyond the digit (or into the distal interphalangeal joint), so many cases remain chronically infected for months or years
- two predominant routes of infection are recognised:
  i. infected toe ulcer (over-wear or over-trimming)
  ii. infection tracking distally under the wall from the coronary band (usually DD treponemes)

Signs

- affected animals stand with a characteristic toe-extended position and walk back on their heels
- can appear short-toed (after trimming) or long-toed ('Turkish slipper feet') due to chronic walking on the heel
- affected animals are lame – usually MS 3
- can present as acute severe lameness, particularly when infection stems from an infected toe ulcer or over-trimmed toe
- **Incidence:** common in US dairies (after DD, SU, WLD and interdigital necrobacillosis) though its long duration probably reflects a high prevalence and not true new incidence; in UK dairies, the estimated prevalence is 2–4%

Aetiology

- formerly, toe necrosis was always considered a sequel to infected toe ulcers; over-wear (e.g. long walking distances on abrasive floor systems; transport with steel checker-plate floors; mixing of large groups of beef animals on concrete flooring) and over-trimming are implicated

- more usual aetiology in adult cows is infection tracking under the dorsal or axial wall towards the apex of the pedal bone (proximal to distal direction) to cause a focal infection and an abscess cavity; usually, this extends to the apex of the hoof horn once a trim has been conducted, giving rise to the typical 'hollow toe' appearance
- DD treponeme infection has been found in necrotic toe and pedal bone osteomyelitis; where infection originates from the coronary band, many arise due to a primary DD skin lesion at this point, followed by distal tracking of DD infection under the dorsal wall following the line of the laminae
- poorly controlled DD infection in the herd is implicated, particularly DD on the dorsal and axial aspects of the foot (e.g. shallow footbaths; automated footbath designs that fail to control DD at the front of the foot).

Treatment

- conservative treatment not effective; due to chronic pain, cows should be treated surgically or culled
- many cows mistakenly remain in the herd with chronic necrotic toe infections for months or years, managed by repeated trimming of the over-grown digit and blocking of the paired digit. Surgical treatment necessarily means veterinary care, which professional foot trimmers and herdsmen are unable to perform legally, ethically or practically
- surgical treatment includes digit amputation, with a particularly good prognosis due to the localised nature of infection; often the most pragmatic (and quickest) option
- **digit-conserving radical resection technique:**
  - local anaesthesia (IVRA) followed by radical horn removal, ensuring that the small sinus under the dorsal and/or axial wall is followed all the way to the coronary band (not easy to see, especially once the digit bleeds)
  - this alternative surgical intervention is particularly useful for early cases
  - curettage of the necrotic bone, followed by control of the infection using a systemic and topical antibiotic leads to underlying germinal layers producing new horn to gradually fill the defect over 4–6 weeks
  - infection must be controlled for this time; Figure 9.24 shows a healing lesion four weeks after surgery
  - bandaging is necessary initially for haemostasis; change the dressings every 2–3 days, with reapplication of topical antibiotics until re-keratinisation begins (after 2 weeks)
  - any untreated DD infection will result in a non-healing lesion
  - extensive infections make some cases unsuitable for digit-conserving surgical treatment

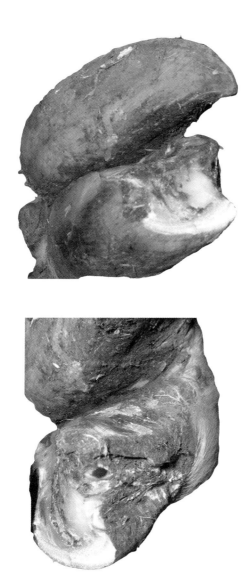

Figure 9.24   Surgically resected necrotic toe 4 weeks post-surgery showing considerable shortening of the toe length together with dorsal wall resection to the coronary band. Keratinisation has begun in the wall defect and the exposed apex of the pedal bone can no longer be seen.

- **amputation of distal claw:**
  - cases **without** a sinus to the coronary band (either dorsal or axial) may respond to amputation of the distal part of the digit to remove all infected tissue in the digit apex using embryotomy wire or a saw (see Figure 9.25)
  - re-keratinisation of the stump will occur only if infection is controlled and will begin after approximately 2 weeks. **Very carefully check for a sinus under the hoof wall extending proximal to the amputation level**
  - for either digit-sparing technique, the partner digit should be blocked; 4–5 days of systemic antibiotics; NSAIDs

Prevention

- attention to the risk factors for a toe ulcer (if this is the cause of a necrotic toe): over-wear/over-trimming
- good herd control of DD
- deep footbaths (>12 cm depth) to control DD on the skin of the dorsal aspect
- early detection of lame cows and prompt effective treatment, especially identifying DD infections on the skin of the dorsal aspect of a foot and above the axial wall

9.13 Vertical (longitudinal) or horizontal (transverse) wall fissures

Synonyms

- vertical fissure originating from the coronary band: sand crack
- vertical fissure originating from the distal wall: grass crack
- horizontal wall fissures: hardship cracks
- *fissura ungulae longitudinalis et transversalis*

Definition

- fissure of the horny wall parallel to the dorsal wall or parallel to the coronary band
- axial wall fissures can also occur

Signs

- sometimes asymptomatic
- single claw (local stress) or multiple claws (e.g. all eight) indicating a previous systemic insult, e.g. parturition; diet change; systemic disease

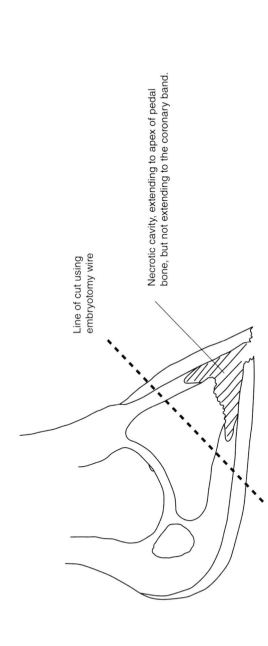

Line of cut using
embryotomy wire

Necrotic cavity, extending to apex of pedal
bone, but not extending to the coronary band.

Figure 9.25 Amputation of the distal portion of the digit may be used successfully for cases where infection is confined to the apex of the digit.

- vertical fissures may involve an entire wall from the coronary band to the weight-bearing surface
- usually only painful when secondary infection occurs on the underlying corium, most commonly at the coronary band with sometimes a granulomatous inflammatory reaction.
- **Incidence:** low in dairy herds but a high prevalence in some beef herds (e.g. reported up to 37% in Canadian Hereford herds)
- **Predisposition:** vertical fissures occur mainly in dry conditions: dehydrated horn or possibly trauma at the coronary band. Horizontal fissures can result from overgrown horn, previous episodes of systemic illness or true laminitis (hardship lines), where horn growth was temporarily interrupted

Treatment

- **horizontal wall fissures:**
  - pare the distal section of the wall horn, especially when it forms a hinge with a more proximal portion, causing pain when flexed upwards
  - shorten the toe and bearing surface to avoid movement of the fractured portion
- **vertical fissures:**
  - no action if non-painful
  - if painful, clean the fissure with a knife, Dremel drill or grinder, and follow any under-run fissures to the point of firm horn attachment; IVRA and tourniquet (to reduce bleeding); cut a horizontal groove in the wall at the distal end of the crack and block the partner digit
  - do not fill the defect with resin or glue but leave open and control infection with repeated topical application of antibiotic (e.g. oxytetracycline aerosol)
  - where granulation tissue protrudes, the tissue should be trimmed back and thorough resection of the surrounding wall should be done to avoid pockets of infection remaining
  - prognosis is more guarded for large granulomatous lesions at the coronary band where digit amputation may be required

9.14 Fractured pedal bone

Pedal bone fractures are almost invariably intra-articular, unless secondary to an osteomyelitis/necrotic toe.

Signs

- sudden onset lameness (usually medial claw) in the fore limb (MS 3) and occasionally in the hind limb

- rarely bilateral
- medial digit of the fore limb is commonly involved; the limb is typically carried across the midline of the body to minimise weight-bearing; occasionally a cross-legged stance or leg held forward in the stall or cubicle
- **no** digital swelling, possibly slight heat
- pain on percussion, or pincer pressure and extension; an acute pain response when twisting the affected digit in the absence of any overt lesions is the best way to diagnose the condition
- flexion of digit resented
- definitive diagnosis on a mediolateral radiograph of the affected digit (plate inserted interdigitally)
- **Incidence:** uncommon, usually in one to five year olds, no breed prevalence; associated with trauma such as bulling activity in a concrete yard or following a first turnout into a rock-hard (dry) pasture, broken slatted floors, fluorosis, subclinical osteoporosis and pathological fractures in osteomyelitis
- **Differential diagnosis:** most likely is an acute white line abscess with an undetected minute tract; an infected vertical fissure of the hoof wall may similarly go undetected.

Treatment

- blocking the partner digit results in immediate improvement and clinical healing within 4–6 weeks; full repair of the fracture gap may take up to 6 months
- untreated animals remain lame for many weeks as intra-articular fractures heal very slowly; may heal as a fibrous union

9.15 Punctured sole

Synonyms

- 'stone'; penetration injury

Definition

- penetration of the sole by a sharp object in the absence of a primary claw horn lesion
- a true punctured sole is uncommon, although reported more frequently in grazing dairy herds with a high prevalence of thin soles
- may be confused with white line disease or sole ulcer, particularly where a stone/grit becomes lodged in a sole ulcer site

Signs

- acute onset sudden lameness (MS 2 or 3)
- examination of the digit will reveal a puncture site, with an object possibly still in place
- a deep abscess may be present; if synovial structures are penetrated, deep sepsis results

Treatment

- unless synovial spaces are penetrated or deep sepsis is present, paring of the puncture site is followed by systemic and topical antibiotics; blocking of partner digit; NSAIDs
- where synovial spaces are punctured or deep sepsis is present, surgical treatment is indicated, e.g. amputation

9.16 Heel bulb haematoma/abscess

Definition

- retroarticular haematoma of the heel bulb possibly with haematogenous secondary infection and abscessation

Signs

- acute onset lameness (MS 2 or 3)
- swollen, painful heel bulb without another claw horn lesion or penetration injury
- sporadic incidence, single digit affected
- confirmation by aseptic needle aspiration (particularly to differentiate a haematoma from an abscess) or by ultrasound
- **Differential diagnosis:** deep sepsis; distal interphalangeal joint infection; navicular bursitis; infected flexor tendon sheath. Unlike deep sepsis, there will be no sinus or tract of infection from a primary claw horn lesion or penetration injury

Aetiology

- traumatic
- possibly prolonged standing times
- may be a sequel to traumatic (as opposed to septic) enthesiopathy of the flexor tendon at insertion on the pedal bone

Treatment

- **haematoma**: conservative treatment with NSAIDs; block partner digit; systemic prophylactic antibiotics **may** reduce the risk of abscessation
- **abscess**: drain and rinse with copious water, NSAIDs, systemic antibiotics and block partner digit. Leave the lesion open (no bandage) unless required for haemostasis

Possible complications

- if the injury includes mechanical disruption of the deep flexor tendon or an avulsion fracture of the distal phalanx, there is a risk of involvement of the navicular bone or bursa causing deeper sepsis. The toe is likely to be hyperextended. Digit amputation or more aggressive resection may still be required

9.17 Deep digital sepsis

Definition

- any infection beneath the superficial structures of the digit
- the bacteria of greatest importance is *Trueperella pyogenes*
- infection into synovial and joint spaces is progressive: the ascending infection usually travels primarily via synovial fluid along the digital flexor sheath, eventually infecting the fetlock joint by bursting through the sheath. The fetlock joint capsule, common to all the fetlock articular surfaces, is large and mobile. The pastern joint capsule has limited capacity and is relatively less mobile, with no connection between the two digits

Signs

- progressively severe lameness (MS 3), possibly leading to recumbency, pyaemia, weight loss, poor appetite, swelling and erythema around the coronet and pastern, later involving the flexor tendon sheath and extensive distal limb oedema
- most cases have a fistulous track
- cases have in common severe pain that is only slightly alleviated by foot blocks or NSAIDs
- **Diagnosis:** infections involving the DIP joint have a characteristic discharging fistula. Diagnosis may be further aided by radiography and ultrasonography, by using blunt probes to investigate fistula or by inserting

14G or 16G needles into synovial sheaths or joint spaces (high-risk iatrogenic infection)

Aetiology

Deep sepsis is a secondary condition and there are several routes of infection other than a penetration injury:

1. Sole ulcer:
   * necrosis of the deep flexor tendon (digit hyperextended/tilting upwards)
   * osteomyelitis of the pedal bone (distal phalanx) and the navicular bone (distal sesamoid)
   * septic navicular bursitis
   * distal interphalangeal septic arthritis
   * ascending septic tenosynovitis of the common digital flexor sheath
2. White line sepsis/punctured sole:
   * osteomyelitis of the pedal bone and septic navicular bursitis
   * distal interphalangeal septic arthritis
   * septic spread to the coronary band, possibly partial or complete secondary exungulation
3. Toe ulcer:
   * distal pedal bone osteomyelitis (necrotic toe)
4. Interdigital necrobacillosis (phlegmon):
   * distal interphalangeal septic arthritis
   * septic tenosynovitis of the digital flexor tendon sheath
   * retroarticular abscess of the bulb
5. Infected vertical wall fissure (sandcrack) at the coronary band:
   * distal interphalangeal joint septic arthritis
   * navicular bursitis
   * common digital flexor tendon sheath
   * surrounding soft tissues including the retroarticular heel bulb

Treatment

* animals suffering from deep sepsis are truly suffering; a decision must be made in the first instance whether to treat, euthanase or slaughter for human consumption
* bony changes are severe in chronic cases
* surgical treatment options are described in Sections 9.18 to 9.20
* some options allow preservation of the digit but amputation is often the most pragmatic surgical option

---

Warning

Conservative treatment/systemic antibiotics alone will not resolve deep sepsis, which is secondary to claw horn lesions, without prolonged and inhumane chronic pain. The blood supply does not extend to septic foci in the osteomyelitic bone or tendon sheath so systemic antibiotics fail to penetrate these infected areas.

9.18 Digit amputation

Indications

- in descending order of frequency, the indications include:
  - osteomyelitis of the distal pedal bone (advanced necrotic toe)
  - septic arthritis of the distal interphalangeal (DIP) joint (sequel to an infected sole ulcer or less frequently white line disease)
  - septic tenosynovitis of the deep flexor tendon (usually accompanying a septic DIP joint)
  - osteomyelitis of the navicular (distal sesamoid) bone (often sequel to the above)
  - severe digital trauma, e.g. exungulation; coronary band trauma
  - septic vertical wall fissure with protruding granulation tissue
  - sepsis of the coronary band
- common procedure with an excellent prognosis following careful case selection
- deep sepsis that extends proximal to the digit (e.g. ascending infections of the flexor tendon) has a poorer prognosis
- necrotic toes (due to a localised infection) have the best prognosis
- can be safely considered for any digit (medial; lateral; front; hind) and many cows survive for several lactations afterwards, with only a slightly reduced long-term survivability compared with herd mates without digit amputation; subsequent lactation yields tend to be largely unaffected

Preparation

- preferable to work with the cow standing in a foot crush
- access for the rear limb digit amputation is usually straightforward
- front foot medial claw amputation is more difficult, but can be done by working the embryotomy wire from the opposite side of the crush; the contralateral rear leg should also be lifted in this case to avoid being kicked whilst positioning oneself under the cow; alternatively, consider the disarticulation technique
- sedation with xylazine (0.1–0.2 mg/kg i.m.) may be used to cast the cow on her side with the affected digit uppermost; good restraint is required (multiple assistants) where casting is being used

- regional anaesthesia: IVRA; regional nerve block or local infiltration (see Section 1.9)
- digit surgery in the field is clean but not sterile; clipping the hair may be beneficial
- surgical spirit/surgical scrub can be used to clean the area around the amputation after dry wiping with a stiff brush; scrubbing with water/wet solutions of disinfectant may be counterproductive; certainly, the leg needs drying very well after cleaning if water is used. Running a bandage through the interdigital space is the most effective way to clean this area
- analgesia (NSAIDs) and systemic antibiotics should be administered prior to surgery
- a foot block can be applied to the partner digit but usually this is unnecessary and in fact may destabilise the digit

Possible techniques

There are three broad techniques of amputation above the coronary band (see Figure 9.26):

   i. Amputation at the distal third of the proximal phalanx (P1) (with or without a skin flap)
   ii. Amputation at the proximal third of the middle phalanx (P2)
   iii. Disarticulation at the proximal interphalageal (P1/P2) joint

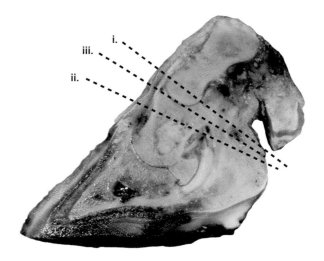

Figure 9.26   Sites for digital amputation or disarticulation relative to the position of the accessory digit, coronary band and heel bulb/skin junction.
i. distal third of proximal phalanx (P1); ii. oblique cut through second phalanx (P2); iii. exarticulation through proximal interphalangeal joint.

Discussion

- Amputation at distal P1 is our recommended technique, without a skin flap.
- Amputation at P2 can result in sequestrum formation and delayed healing.
- Disarticulation can be unnecessarily awkward and the articular cartilage requires curettage to allow healing.
- Skin flaps, though possible, rarely give any advantage on healing time.

Recommended method, amputation at distal P1:

- apply tourniquet above the fetlock or hock to reduce haemorrhage
- incise with a scalpel the interdigital space close to the affected digit along the whole length, continuing proximally 3 cm dorsally and 2.5 cm at the plantar aspect
- insert embryotomy (obstetrical) wire into the incision and adjust to a level 1–2 cm above the axial aspect of the proximal interphalangeal joint, level with the accessory digit (see Figure 9.27)
- with an assistant firmly applying a counterforce (holding the digit down towards the ground if the cow is recumbent or pulling on a strap/rope above the fetlock if upright in a crush), saw rapidly at an oblique angle until the wire cuts into the proximal phalangeal bone; then straighten up slightly so that the cut emerges 1–2 cm above the abaxial joint level, continuing through the skin (use a scalpel if necessary)

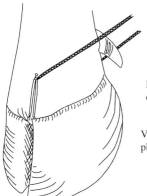

Embryotomy wire at level of accessory digit at an oblique angle

Vertical incision between digits 3cm dorsally and 2.5cm at plantar aspect

Figure 9.27   Correct position of the embryotomy wire during the recommended site of amputation (distal third of proximal phalanx).

- trim off the protruding interdigital fat pad
- twist off any major vessels, e.g. the dorsal digital artery lying axially (optional)
- examine the cut surface for signs of abscessation and necrosis, peritendinous infection and septic tenosynovitis; scrape (with a scalpel) bone dust from the wound
- check the accuracy of the amputation level: it should be possible to wobble the distal part of P1 in the amputated digit
- massage distally along the deep flexor tendon sheath to check the synovial appearance
- purulent synovia should be irrigated out of the tendon sheath (male dog catheter, 50 ml syringe and saline) and consider the need for resection of part of the deep flexor tendon (see Section 9.19)
- dress the wound with topical oxytetracycline aerosol (not essential); apply non-adherent dressing (e.g. Melolin®) followed by cotton-wool and hold in place with a pressure bandage (e.g. 3 layers: Sofban®; cohesive self-adherent bandage; adhesive fabric bandage)
- remove the tourniquet and release the limb (if the cow is upright)
- apply a further bandage layer if excessive bleeding is apparent
- give a 4 day course of systemic antibiotics (e.g. amoxycillin); NSAIDs

Tip

- In order to apply adequate pressure for haemostasis whilst avoiding the risk of pressure necrosis on the remaining digit caused by the bandage, fill the dead space left by the amputated digit with a fist-sized wad of cotton wool.
- Using a good quality self-adherent bandage (e.g. Vetwrap®) to apply pressure reduces the risk of the bandage slipping and forming a tight tourniquet around the remaining digit.

Aftercare

- Change the dressing after 2–4 days and check for residual infection
- apply a second dressing (as the first) for 8–10 days
- the surface may then safely be left exposed for granulation and epithelialisation
- keep the animal in dry surroundings (housed or outdoors) during a three week recovery period, but avoid deep straw yards or loose boxes to reduce the risk of stump irritation
- if lameness worsens during the recovery period, it is likely the stump is infected and a 4 day course of systemic antibiotics plus NSAIDs should be

given; occasionally excessive granulation tissue needs trimming back and the stump re-dressing
- epithelialisation should be complete after 6 weeks

Possible complications

- secondary infection on the stump (see above)
- infection and severe swelling proximal to the amputation site (advanced sepsis): requires a prolonged (10 day) course of systemic antibiotics and possible flexor tendon resection (Section 9.19)
- very rarely, dislocation of the proximal interphalangeal joint of the remaining digit due to loss of lateral stability (requires immediate slaughter)
- pressure necrosis (tourniquet effect) of the remaining digit due to poor bandaging (see Tip Text box)

Advantages of digit amputation

- pain relief
- immediate removal of the focus of infection (reducing the risk of pyaemic spread)
- simple surgical procedure
- excellent prognosis with sensible case selection; best with early decision making

Disadvantages of digit amputation

- potential failure if the case selection is poor and infection is present above the amputation site (e.g. procrastination over treatment in cases of deep sepsis)
- persisting poor gait in some heavy cows and bulls due to the altered stance and strain on the remaining digit, especially in difficult terrain
- lowered market value

Alternative amputation techniques

1. Disarticulation at the proximal interphalangeal joint.

   Advantages:
   - end result of surgery is a hollow cavity ideal for pressure packing by bandage or swabs
   - avoids exposure of medullary cavity (marrow) of the proximal phalanx which could potentially become the focus of a post-operative infection

Disadvantages:
- longer procedure
- difficult to locate the joint level axially for the initial incision
- risk of a scalpel blade breakage and personal injury
- preferable to use a 'sage knife' (a curved solid two-edged instrument) and a small curette
- failure to heal/delayed healing if the articular cartilage is not sufficiently curetted

2. Amputation through the mid/proximal P2.
   Advantages:
   - very easy: no prior incision required between the digits
   - possibly better lateral stability of the remaining digit
   - easy wound to bandage (not 'L' shaped)

   Disadvantages:
   - delayed wound healing due to sequestrum formation of the bone stump (proximal P2)
   - poorer long-term prognosis due to wound failure and prolonged pain

3. Skin flap preservation. The skin flap may be preserved and placed over the amputation surface, following removal of the digit through the distal one third of the proximal phalanx. The flap is created initially by a semi-circular incision from 5–6 cm above the interdigital space on the dorsal and plantar aspects, passing down to the coronary band. Ensure the flap is large and thick, and is then reflected proximally. Amputation is done in a conventional way and the skin flap, trimmed as needed, is then sutured over the stump.
   Advantage:
   - potentially cosmetic improvement and faster healing

   Disadvantages:
   - longer procedure
   - inability to inspect the amputation site when the dressing is changed; risk of retaining infection in a blood clot; therefore leave unsutured distally
   - sutures may tear out due to post-operative swelling
   - good case selection is essential (e.g. clean facilities; no interdigital hyperplasia)

9.19 Resection of flexor tendon

Indication

- technique can be an immediate sequel to digit amputation if sepsis extends proximal to the amputation site along the flexor tendon sheath and if drainage of the infected synovia is poor

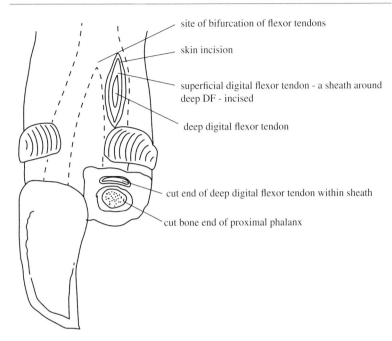

site of bifurcation of flexor tendons

skin incision

superficial digital flexor tendon - a sheath around deep DF - incised

deep digital flexor tendon

cut end of deep digital flexor tendon within sheath

cut bone end of proximal phalanx

Figure 9.28 Landmarks for incision to resect the deep digital flexor tendon.

Technique

- make a 3 cm long skin incision parallel to the path of the tendon over the affected branch of the flexor tendon, immediately proximal to the accessory digit (see Figure 9.28)
- strong fascia surrounds the sheath of the deep and superficial flexor tendons; the superficial tendon forms a sheath around the deep flexor tendon
- sharply dissect to reveal the deep flexor tendon and grasp with forceps or slide curved scissors under the tendon to pull the free end clear; traction is required if extensive adhesions are present between the deep and superficial flexor tendons, or it may be necessary to dissect away adhesions
- cut the exposed tendon proximally (the flexor tendons of the medial and lateral digits fuse to form single tendon 5–7 cm proximal to the accessory digits, which limits the transection level)
- place a Penrose drain in the tendon sheath fixed with a single suture proximally
- suture the skin incision
- leave the drain in place (exposed distally) and remove after 7 days
- extended (10 day) course of systemic antibiotics

9.20 Digit-sparing techniques: curettage and arthrodesis of distal interphalangeal joint

Indications

- alternative (to amputation) method of surgical treatment for deep sepsis involving the DIP joint, for example after a sole ulcer infection

Techniques

Curettage of the DIP joint may be achieved by several methods, including:

   i. 'coring' with a hoof knife via the original sole ulcer lesion to effect drainage from the DIP joint and flush with copious water

  ii. 'coring' with a hoof knife at the heel bulbs to dissect on to and remove the navicular bone, gaining access to the DIP joint and flushing with copious water

 iii. drilling across the joint beginning at the sole ulcer site and ending just proximal to the coronary band on the dorsal aspect

 iv. dissecting down on to the navicular bone, removing the navicular bone and affected parts of the deep digital flexor tendon, followed by drilling through the DIP joint to remove articular cartilage, exiting at the dorsal aspect just distal to the coronary band

The technique that gives the best chance of complete removal of necrotic material, drainage of the joint and most removal of articular cartilage for rapid arthrodesis is likely to achieve the best results (i.e. technique iv, followed by iii, ii and then i). Figure 9.29 illustrates the four techniques and Table 9.7 compares advantages and disadvantages.

Recommended procedure (technique iv)

- tourniquet at mid-metatarsal (-carpal) region
- intravenous regional analgesia
- skin preparation as for digit amputation
- carefully probe the fistula after removing all visible granulation tissue
- 4 cm horizontal incision just proximal to the sole–heel junction; then remove a wedge of tissue to include the corium, digital cushion and distal part of the deep digital flexor tendon, to visualise the navicular bone (see Figure 9.30)
- remove the navicular bone: this is relatively easy if very necrotic; to facilitate removal, ensure the flexor tendon at insertion on the pedal bone is fully excised and split the navicular bone in two using a drill bit
- resect any remains of insertion of the deep flexor tendon with a 'sage' knife (double-sided, slightly curved solid scalpel)
- drill from the plantar incision infected cartilage and subchondral bone of the distal interphalangeal joint surfaces ('apple core procedure') using a

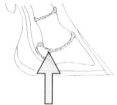

Technique i.: coring sole ulcer site to gain access to joint space, and removing as much necrotic material as possible.

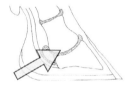

Technique ii.: coring heel to gain access to navicular bone, which is removed to access joint space, and removing as much necrotic material as possible.

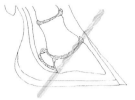

Technique iii.: drilling via sole ulcer site through DIP joint to exit just above or below coronary band at dorsal aspect.

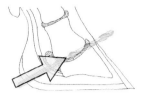

Technique iv.: incising through heel to expose navicular bone; drilling through navicular bone to aid excision; finally, drilling through DIP joint to exit at dorsal horn wall distal to coronary band.

Figure 9.29 Digit-sparing surgical techniques for deep sepsis.

10 mm drill bit, exiting just distal to the coronary band through the dorsal wall horn
- flush the joint space with copious water (e.g. using a hose pipe)
- place rubber tubing (e.g. from flutter tube) through the plantar incision to emerge at the dorsal hole and tie the ends of the tubing together. Optional: insert a second piece of tubing via the plantar incision to exit at the sole ulcer fistula and tie the ends together
- pack the wound with antibiotic powder (optional) and suture the plantar skin incision
- bandage for 3 days, then remove
- remove the drain tubes after 10–14 days
- put a block on sound partner digit; NSAIDs
- give a high dosage of systemic antibiotics for ten days (e.g. amoxycillin)
- remove the block at six to twelve weeks by which time arthrodesis should be complete

Variations
- instead of the elliptical skin incision above the heel horn/skin junction, a larger circular (5 cm diameter) incision can be made to include the heel horn, centred around the fistula of the sole ulcer (if present). In this case,

Table 9.7   Comparative advantages and disadvantages of four digit sparing techniques.

Technique	Advantages	Disadvantages
Method i	• quick; easy	• poor access to DIP joint • granulation tissue likely to quickly block and impede drainage • does not remove articular cartilage – arthrodesis ineffective
Method ii	• does not require drill • good access to DIP joint • removes distal part of deep digital flexor tendon	• difficult to remove navicular bone (unless very necrotic) • granulation tissue likely to quickly impede drainage • does not remove articular cartilage
Method iii	• quick • removes some articular cartilage to speed arthrodesis	• navicular bone left in place • does not remove distal deep flexor tendon • granulation tissue likely to quickly occlude drainage – inserting tubing will keep open longer
Method iv	• removes articular cartilage most effectively to speed arthrodesis • good access to joint spaces and for drainage • allows insertion of tube (optional) • allows removal of distal part of deep digital flexor tendon	• requires long drill bit • complete removal of navicular bone can be difficult • obliterates insertion of deep flexor tendon resulting in very unstable digit until arthrodesis develops

the incision is left open and not sutured. This is a combination of techniques ii and iv and may facilitate removal of the navicular bone, as well as ensuring a large drainage hole, which means the tubing may be superfluous
- toes can be wired together to prevent over-extension of the digit; this may not assist healing and may in fact delay arthrodesis
- an irrigation tube can be placed into the cavity and fixed along the metatarsus to allow repeated (daily) flushing of wound, e.g. a 5 mm perforated tube tied or wired at the end

After-care and possible complications

- the period of convalescence is usually longer than for digit amputation
- cows require sympathetic housing and daily inspection for premature occlusion of drainage and thorough cleansing of the foot

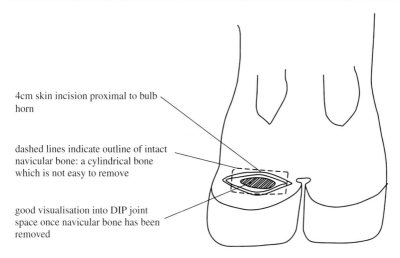

4cm skin incision proximal to bulb horn

dashed lines indicate outline of intact navicular bone: a cylindrical bone which is not easy to remove

good visualisation into DIP joint space once navicular bone has been removed

Figure 9.30   Illustration of initial incision for technique iv.

- infection may nevertheless spread proximally and the cow may still require a digit amputation
- the functional use of the preserved arthrodesed digit at the end of the recovery phase may be poor: the digit is likely to be hyperextended and require regular trimming
- extensive exostoses along the arthrodesis site may give chronic pain

Discussion

- One USA study suggested that cows with septic DIP joints treated with arthrodesis using technique iv outperformed cows with digit amputation (survivability and subsequent milk yield) but the method used for amputation was not the one recommended in this text.
- A German study found no significant differences in long-term survival between cows treated with digit amputation or joint resection, but the recovery time for the amputation patients was significantly shorter.

9.21 Osteomyelitis

Introduction

- may occur subsequent to open wounds, but haematogenous osteomyelitis is more usual, particularly in calves

Signs

- osteomyelitis following wounds or foreign bodies is usually obvious
- chronic bony proliferation may occur
- haematogenous osteomyelitis of the pedal bone presents as acute lameness often isolated to one digit, but with no apparent swelling or lesion; almost always occurs in calves less than 12 weeks old and *Salmonella dublin* infection is usually implicated
- less commonly, fore limb or hind limb ataxia progressing to paralysis is associated with osteomyelitis of one or more thoracic or cervical vertebrae; pain response may be elicited with manipulation of the spine or neck
- **Diagnosis:** clinical signs and thorough examination to rule out other causes of lameness, such as white line disease

Treatment and prognosis

- prolonged course of antibiotics and NSAIDs (14–21 days)
- pedal bone osteomyelitis in young calves carries a reasonable prognosis but recovery may take 6–10 weeks
- vertebral osteomyelitis has a guarded prognosis: early recognition and commencement of treatment is important; euthanasia may be the most humane approach

9.22 Infectious arthritis ('joint ill') of calves

Introduction

- joint ill (neonatal polyarthritis) is usually caused by the haematogenous spread of septic infection from the umbilicus, less commonly the lungs or liver
- organisms may be *Escherichia coli*, *Salmonella* spp., *Streptococcus* spp. and *Trueperella pyogenes*
- major factors contributing to disease include the environmental pathogen load (i.e. cleanliness of the parturition area) and the immune status of the calf, including passive transfer of colostral immunoglobulin.

Signs

- depression, lameness or recumbency, anorexia, dehydration
- joint swelling and pain within 24 hours of onset of infection
- common sites include hock, stifle, carpus and fetlock (hip, shoulder rarely)
- umbilicus may show obvious signs of infection, with pain on deep palpation
- later nervous signs (e.g. head tremors, opisthotonus) develop in some calves

- **Diagnosis:** swelling and pain in one or several joints (rarely with symmetrical involvement) in depressed calf are usually diagnostic. Arthrocentesis (cytology, culture), radiography and ultrasound may help confirm the diagnosis

Treatment and prognosis

- cleanse the umbilicus and consider removal later of the septic umbilical focus
- systemic antibiotics for a prolonged period, e.g. potentiated amoxycillin for 7–21 days; NSAIDs
- improve the immune status with a whole blood transfusion
- immediate joint lavage (see Section 9.23)
- valuable calves with severe joint destruction may benefit from radical surgery via arthroscopy or arthrotomy with the aim of joint ankylosis
- prognosis guarded or poor without intensive nursing

Discussion

- Meningitis occurs in a minority of neonatal calves, usually in the first week, and is rapidly fatal
- In slightly older calves septic physitis (e.g. of the distal radius or distal tibia) may complicate the initial signs and radiography is then valuable
- 'Joint ill' is an emergency requiring rapid diagnosis and good nursing, as well as a prompt review of the possible predisposing factors

---

9.23 Antibiotic therapy of bone and joint infections

Management

- treatment of osteomyelitis, bone abscess and septic arthritis with systemic antibiotics presents major problems due to difficulties of penetration, especially of discrete foci of a purulent infection walled off from vascularised tissues
- appropriate antibiotic selection should be based on culture and sensitivity, but suggested choices are as follows:
  - streptococci: penicillin G, ceftiofur
  - salmonellae: oxacillin ampicillin amoxycillin
  - penicillinase-producing staphylococci: cephalosporin and trimethoprim and sulpha, ceftiofur

- gram-negative organisms: aminoglycosides (streptomycin, kanamycin, neomycin, gentamicin)
  - *Trueperella*: amoxycillin
- treatment of acute osteomyelitis should be continued for two to three weeks after signs of lameness have disappeared
- intra-articular or locoregional (e.g. IVRA for a distal limb) antibiotic therapy (e.g. oxytetracycline) may increase regional drug concentration at lower doses; limitations of the technique include the practicalities of giving multiple injections
- intra-articular injection of antimicrobials is controversial as there is little data on the benefits in cattle and chemical synovitis may develop, though not with lincomycin, penicillin, doxycycline and gentamicin. To avoid repeated injections, slow release delivery using gentamicin-impregnated polymethylmethacrylate beads has been used, but gentamicin is not licensed for use in cattle in North America or Europe, and there is little evidence of their benefit in cattle

Surgery

- joint drainage procedures for cattle include:
  - needle aspiration (usually inadequate)
  - joint lavage through separate entry and exit portals (14 gauge needles)
  - distension irrigation
  - arthrotomy with and without synovectomy
  - arthroscopy
- surgery is more effective than medical treatment alone for septic arthritis in cattle
- in chronic conditions of bones and joints specific indications for surgery include abscessation with a fistulous track into bone marrow or subperiosteal sequestrum formation
- delay in treatment reduces the chance of success by allowing further periarticular fibrosis and articular damage
- antibiotic therapy should be used alongside surgery and start before sensitivity results are available; ceftiofur is often the selected drug and should be given systemically for two weeks after the joint has returned to normal function
- in cases where the primary source of infection is the umbilicus, surgical resection is indicated.

Joint lavage:

- insert two or more 14 gauge needles aseptically into different joint pouches with the animal under deep sedation or light anaesthesia (e.g. ketamine) before intra-articular fibrin has developed (very acute cases)

- infuse lavage solution (polyionic) under pressure to distend the joint synovial membrane and break down adhesions
- periodically block the outflow needle to promote distension
- one to four litres is usually indicated in a septic joint
- arthroscopy permits large ingress and egress portals, larger volumes of solution (8–12 litres per session), removal of fibrin and visual inspection of the articular cartilage
- when the inflammatory process becomes chronic, remove the fibrin clots and abnormal synovial membrane by arthroscopy
- alternatively, perform arthrotomy and protect the open joint from environmental contamination by a sterile bandage until the incision heals by secondary intention

---

Tip

Prompt action is required for successful outcomes: begin joint lavage immediately septic arthritis is diagnosed. Arthrotomy or euthanasia are indicated if there is no improvement after 36 hours.

9.24 Contracted flexor tendons

Introduction

- most frequently observed congenital anomaly in dairy breeds and rarely acquired
- congenital flexed tendons (CFTs) are usually primarily in the forelegs and generally bilateral

Signs

- mild cases have slight carpal flexion and intermittent knuckling of the fore fetlocks, then bearing weight on the dorsum of the fetlock
- more severe cases can bear weight only on the flexed fetlocks
- advanced cases, with severe contracture, are often recumbent and, when encouraged to stand, tend to fall down immediately
- calves may be colostrum deficient, dehydrated and very weak, having failed to suck since birth
- palpation reveals excessive tension and tautness in both the superficial (SFT) and/or deep flexor tendons (DFT), when attempts are made to straighten the leg
- no pain is evident on extension and joint swelling is absent (compare 'joint ill'; Section 9.22)

Treatment

- in mild congenital cases, check the immune status and general condition (give colostrum in the first 12 hours post-partum) if doubt exists as to whether the calf has taken maternal milk
- observation for the initial 24–48 hours in a well-bedded loose box or at pasture, as exercise encourages progressive correction of the milder cases of flexion of the carpus and fetlock joint; most cases correct with conservative treatment
- in a mild case consider elongation of the claw toes with a piece of wood glued to the sole
- in a more severe case initially correct any systemic problem and consider applying a splint on palmar aspect of the limb: from the pastern to midmetacarpus (fetlock flexion) or up to the proximal radius (in carpal flexion)
- select a lightweight splint material, e.g. a split PVC piping; pad the limb (bandage) meticulously before fitting the splint; lift the calf if it is unable to stand up initially
- alternatively, consider fibreglass casting of the limb over padding, ensuring its easy removal for examination of flexion status after one to two weeks

---

Tip

There is anecdotal evidence that oxytetracycline (4 mg/kg i.v. repeated every 1 or 2 days for 1 or 2 treatments) aids conservative treatment. However, as most cases do in fact resolve spontaneously it is uncertain how beneficial this treatment is.

Surgery

In severe cases of fetlock and carpal flexion (CFT) surgical correction may be attempted (see Figure 9.31).

- perform surgery in the sedated calf (xylazine 0.2 mg/kg i.m.) restrained in lateral recumbency and after either IVRA or local infiltration of local anaesthetic
- make a routine skin preparation along the entire length and circumference of the metacarpus
- make a 10 cm longitudinal incision laterally over the SFT and DFT in the midmetacarpal region
- carefully dissect through the fascia, identifying and avoiding trauma to the lateral palmar digital nerve and adjacent vessels lying plantar to the metacarpus, both medially and laterally

distal

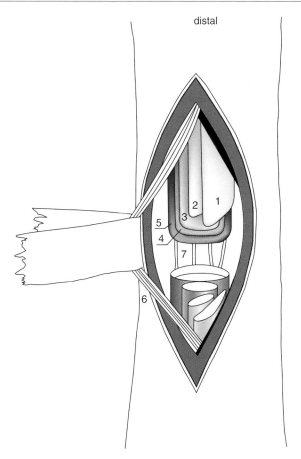

Figure 9.31 Tenotomy of superficial and deep flexor tendons and suspensory ligament over left metacarpus (palmar view).
1. superficial part of superficial flexor; 2. deep part of superficial flexor; 3. deep flexor; 4. superficial part of suspensory ligament (interosseus muscle); 5. deep part of suspensory ligament; 6. medial vein, artery and nerve; 7. palmar metacarpal veins. (From Dirksen, Gründer and Stöber, 2002.)

- elevate the SDF by inserting slightly curved Mayo scissors transversely between the SDF and DFT and transect the SDF
- check the degree of fetlock extension again and if inadequate elevate the DFT and section similarly
- finally, if necessary, section the suspensory ligament (interosseus muscle) in the proximal third of the metacarpus
- close the peritendinous fascia in a continuous pattern with non-absorbable material and the skin with interrupted sutures

- apply a light bandage and use a splint if flexion is still inadequately corrected by surgery and additional extension is needed, and also in the event of iatrogenic secondary over-extension of the fetlock
- in congenital carpal flexion, section of the *ulnaris lateralis* and *flexor carpi ulnaris* tendons is performed through a 7–8 cm incision, the distal commissure of which lies over the accessory carpal bone
- lightly bandage the limb
- prophylactic antibiotics are not needed, but NSAIDs are advisable for several days
- remove the splint and/or cast after 7–10 days to assess improvement

---

Discussion

- The prognosis for CFT is good in calves with a mild deformity, i.e. sporadic knuckling of fetlocks.
- Severe fetlock and carpal deformities often fail to be corrected despite the tenotomy procedures described above; flexion persists and locomotion is impossible.
- Scrupulous management of splints in neonatal calves avoids skin necrosis at potential pressure points.

9.25 Tarsal and carpal hygroma

Synonyms

- tarsal cellulitis, carpal/tarsal 'bursitis', swollen hock

Definition

- firm or fluctuating swelling involving pre-carpal bursa and acquired subcutaneous bursa over the lateral aspect of the hock

Signs

- often no lameness, no pain, and presents purely as a large swelling
- asymmetrical swelling (versus symmetrical joint distension)
- sometimes skin contusion, break in integument, with seropurulent discharge and invasion by *Trueperella pyogenes*
- distension of joint capsule, heat, pain and lameness indicate a further localised septic spread
- **Incidence:** high in housed cattle on hard floors with little bedding and/or poorly designed cubicles (free stalls)

- **Differential diagnosis:** precarpal abscessation, septic carpitis, septic tarsitis.

Treatment and prophylaxis

- transfer to soft bedding or turn outside
- broad spectrum antibiotics in cases with lameness and systemic signs
- do not open the cavity or inject local corticosteroids (risk of gross contamination)
- check the stall dimensions relative to the breed and any behavioural abnormalities that can be corrected
- check for and treat concurrent foot lameness
- surgical excision of a large non-infected carpal bursa with primary wound closure and a pressure bandage is a possible and surgically hazardous procedure in a clinic (not on-farm) situation, as wound breakdown commonly occurs despite good after-care

9.26 Patellar luxation

Three types can occur:

- dorsal patellar luxation or fixation in adults; sporadic incidence
- lateral patellar luxation; congenital, uncommon
- medial patellar luxation; congenital, rare

Dorsal patellar luxation or fixation

Temporary or permanent fixation of patella on the upper part of the medial femoral trochlear ridge.

Signs

- stiffness, later jerky action with leg extended caudally for longer than normal, followed by a forward jerk (temporary fixation)
- action sometimes intermittent and the limb may become fixed in rigid extension, dragging claws (permanent fixation)
- position evident on patellar palpation; manual reposition possible
- **Differential diagnosis:** displacement of the *biceps femoris* muscle; spastic paresis; acute gonitis

Treatment

Spontaneous recovery occurs in some individuals, especially cattle at grass.
  Complete recovery should immediately follow medial patellar desmotomy:

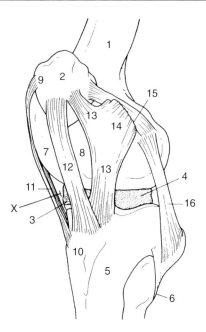

Figure 9.32 Lateral view of the left stifle joint of the cow.
1. femur; 2. patella; 3 and 4. medial and lateral menisci; 5. tibia; 6. fibula; 7 and 8. medial and lateral trochlear ridge; 9. patellar fibrocartilage; 10. tibial tuberosity; 11. medial straight patellar ligament (sectioned distally in patellar desmotomy); 12 and 13. middle and lateral straight patellar ligaments; 14. tendon of biceps femoris muscle; 15. lateral femoropatellar ligament; 16. lateral collateral ligament. X indicates site for femorotibial arthrocentesis.

- sedate the patient and produce local analgesia over the lowest palpable point of the medial straight patellar ligament (see Figure 9.32 (11)), just proximal to insertion into tibial tuberosity
- clip and disinfect a circular area 15 cm in diameter
- make a 3 cm vertical incision just cranial to the cranial edge of the medial patellar ligament
- insert a curved tenotome or bistoury (Hey-Groves pattern) through the incision in a vertical manner and into the triangular space bounded by the middle and medial ligaments and tibia
- turn the tenotome through 90° and section the medial ligament by a short sawing movement and percutaneous pressure with a finger
- after snapping and separation of the ligament is appreciated, withdraw the tenotome in a vertical position
- appose the skin edges with two simple sutures
- check the success of the surgery immediately by observing gait; recurrence has not been reported

- surgery is best performed in a standing position, though access to the site may be more difficult in a heavy lactating cow than when in lateral recumbency

Warning
Do **not** use a disposable scalpel blade and handle in place of a tenotome, due to risk of accidental breakage and loss of the blade into the wound or joint.

Possible complications

- accidental entry into the femoropatellar joint (rare)
- accidental section of the middle straight patellar ligament (disastrous)
- gross iatrogenic infection of the site
- severe haemorrhage

Lateral patellar luxation

Complete or incomplete lateral displacement of the patella, typically in new-born calves, usually accompanied by femoral nerve paralysis caused by dystocia (oversized foetus in anterior presentation, possibly 'hip-lock'). Therefore check skin sensation over the medial thigh. A hypoplastic lateral trochlear ridge has been postulated but remains unproven.

Signs

- gross uni- or bilateral flexion of stifles and hocks
- limb collapses when weight is taken
- patella forms an obvious bulge on the lateral aspect of the stifle joint and the lateral femoral trochlear ridge is clearly palpable
- obvious atrophy of quadriceps in cases of femoral nerve paralysis
- manipulative replacement usually possible (short-lived)
- **Differential diagnosis:** *quadriceps femoris* muscle rupture, which is rare and accompanied by swelling; gonitis, with evidence of increased synovial fluid and other joint signs; distal femoral epiphyseal (supracondylar) separation with limb malalignment and crepitus

Treatment

- general anaesthesia or heavy sedation and local anaesthesia
- in dorsal recumbency, with the affected limb extended, incise the skin over the medial femoral patellar ligament (7–8 cm)

- place the patella in the trochlear groove and create a new medial patellar ligament by suturing the patellar cartilage and femoral periosteum and fascia using several strands of non-absorbable heavy gauge synthetic suture material, followed by imbrication of the joint capsule medially by simple interrupted absorbable sutures
- check joint flexibility and movement of the patella in the groove before suturing the skin
- if the patella fails to remain in the trochlear groove, split the fascia of the thigh dorsally from the patella.

Discussion

Surgical correction allows continued physiotherapy, which is necessary to successfully treat femoral nerve paralysis. Following successful recovery from femoral nerve paralysis, expect gradual recovery and increased quadriceps muscle mass over 2–3 months.

Medial patellar luxation

Signs

- rare congenital condition
- complete or incomplete, permanent or intermittent
- limb flexed with the patella freely movable
- manual reposition sometimes possible

Treatment

- lateral capsular overlap procedure (see above)
- prognosis is poor.

9.27 Spastic paresis

Introduction

- progressive condition characterised by contraction of gastrocnemius and related calcanean tendons and muscle bellies, leading to severe over-extension of the hock
- certain breeds (e.g. Friesian, Aberdeen Angus) have a hereditary predisposition

Signs

- first seen typically at two to nine months old, rarely congenital or in older animals
- initially unilateral, later often bilateral hind limb stiffness and increasing rigidity with heel bulbs raised off the ground
- intermittent backward jerking of the limb, later over-extension of the hock
- raised tail head with an occasional upward movement
- leg is readily and painlessly flexed manually, but immediately resumes the over-extended position
- weight increasingly transferred to the forequarters with progressive atrophy of the hindquarters
- radiographic tarsal joint changes after several months are characteristic of chronic over-extension
- **Differential diagnosis:** dorsal luxation of the patella; septic or aseptic gonitis or tarsitis; fracture dislocation of calcaneus; joint ill; luxation of *biceps femoris* muscle

Aetiology

- an over-active stretch reflex is present in the gastrocnemius, with over-stimulation or lack of inhibition of motor neurons
- electromyogram (EMG) studies indicate increased electrical activity in the gastrocnemius muscle, and to a lesser extent in other muscles
- CSF studies have suggested an extra-pyramidal dopaminergic central disorder

Treatment

- tenotomy of gastrocnemius tendon or tibial neurectomy
- tenotomy often only temporarily successful in young calves (<9 months).

Tenotomy (see Figure 9.33)

- operate on the standing calf under local analgesia
- shave and disinfect the area over the calcanean tendon 10 cm proximal to the point of the hock
- incise the skin 6 cm long vertically over the caudal aspect of the tendon
- identify the gastrocnemius tendon and either section transversely or remove a 2 cm portion
- section through half of the transverse diameter of the adjacent superficial digital flexor tendon
- suture the skin
- the effect is an immediate marked dropping of hock on weight-bearing

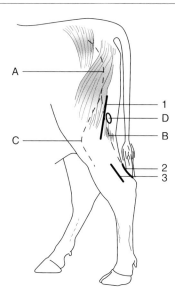

Figure 9.33 Neurectomy and tenotomy sites for alleviation of spastic paresis. 1. incision site for tibial neurectomy; 2. incision for caudal approach for gastrocnemius tenectomy; 3. incision for lateral approach for gastrocnemius tenectomy; A. sciatic nerve; B. tibial nerve; C. peroneal nerve; D. popliteal lymph node.

- some operated calves develop fibrous union in the operated area, leading to recurrence 1.5–3 months later
- guarded prognosis

Neurectomy of tibial nerve (see Figure 9.33)

- tibial nerve supplies the gastrocnemius muscle
- identify and mark on the skin the groove between two heads of biceps femoris in the standing calf
- operate in lateral recumbency under epidural or GA
- make an aseptic surgical approach between two heads of the *biceps femoris* muscle; the popliteal lymph node is a useful landmark adjacent to both the tibial and peroneal nerves
- insert a wound retractor
- identify the two nerves by an electrical nerve stimulator (e.g. ram electro-ejaculator) or (less reliably) by touching with forceps; the tibial nerve stimulates digital flexion and hock extension, while the peroneal stimulates digital extension and hock flexion
- remove a 2 cm length of the main trunk of the tibial nerve, as precise identification of gastrocnemius branches is difficult or impossible
- suture subcutaneous tissues and skin

- encourage limited exercise for two weeks
- good prognosis follows neurectomy

Possible complications

- continuing muscle atrophy
- temporary or persistent peroneal paralysis
- wound breakdown
- gastrocnemius rupture in heavy cattle one to five days after neurectomy, possibly due to over-stretching of the denervated muscle

Warning
This is a heritable condition and animals should not be used for breeding after surgery.

9.28 Hip luxation

Introduction

- relatively common condition in younger cows (two to five years)
- femoral head usually moves in a cranial and dorsal direction

Signs

- standing animal is obviously lame
- limb appears shortened (in dorsal dislocation)
- characteristic asymmetry of the greater femoral trochanters
- possible rotation of the femoral shaft is appreciable
- crepitus on femoral abduction and rotation
- rectal examination may reveal a femoral head in the obturator formen (caudal ventral dislocation) or cranial to the pubic brim (cranial and ventral) (see Figure 9.34)
- **Aetiology:** severe trauma (e.g. fall, knock, slipping); possibly secondary to obturator paralysis postpartum or to hypocalcaemia
- **Differential diagnosis:** obturator paralysis, pelvic fracture, fracture of the femoral neck, fracture of the femoral greater trochanter. Dislocation accompanied by an acetabular fracture is not uncommon and a thorough clinical examination should be performed before attempting treatment

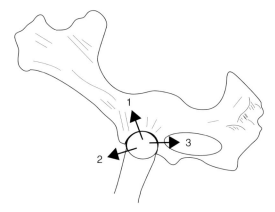

Figure 9.34 Lateral view of the left half of the bony pelvis showing directions of hip (femoral head) dislocation or luxation.
1. craniodorsal (frequent); 2. cranioventral; 3. caudoventral into obturator foramen (palpable).

Treatment

- manipulative or surgical reduction within 24 hours has a reasonable prognosis, particularly in lighter animals that are able to stand up. The method varies with the direction of dislocation.

Craniodorsal dislocation

- attempt reduction under deep sedation and muscle relaxation (guaifenesin 5%; i.v. chloral hydrate)
- cast with the dislocated limb uppermost
- fix the cow's pelvis with rope to an immovable object (e.g. stanchion, tree trunk)
- place a heavy block between the ground and medial femoral region to act as a fulcrum
- simultaneously exert force in three directions: longitudinally by rope on the metatarsus of an affected limb, medially by pressure on the lateral aspect of the stifle whilst lifting up the hock and caudally on the greater trochanter by an operator's hands. The longitudinal force required is considerable, particularly in larger animals; continuous smooth traction using a block and pulley is better than jerky movements
- relaxation improves with duration of anaesthesia and prolonged manipulation. Reduction into acetabulum is usually accompanied by an audible 'clunk'
- closed reduction in uncomplicated cases is successful in around 75% of cases treated within 12 hours of injury, reducing rapidly thereafter, probably due to a blood clot in the acetabulum and muscle contracture

- after successful reduction, hobbles should be applied to prevent the legs splaying and left in place for 2–3 weeks
- open reduction with reinforcement of the acetabular joint capsule has been described with a success rate of 75% (requiring clinic facilities)

Dislocation in other directions (see Figure 9.34)

- difficult or impossible reduction
- success rate of 30% is claimed for ventral luxation
- after successful reduction keep the cow recumbent for one to two days by hobbling the hind limbs above the hock to avoid the likelihood of immediate recurrence, and keep in a box for two months
- surgical methods of reduction and fixation are often unsuccessful

9.29 Stifle lameness

Introduction

- the stifle is often the site of non-digital joint problems in adult cattle, specifically degenerative arthritis
- bilateral spontaneous osteoarthritis may sometimes be inherited in Holstein and Guernsey cattle, possibly through a single autosomal recessive gene
- patellar abnormalities are discussed elsewhere (see Section 9.26)
- injuries may primarily affect:
  - cranial, and rarely also the caudal cruciate ligament (rupture)
  - menisci, usually medial (tear)
  - articular cartilage of femoral condyle, especially medial (erosion)

Signs and gross pathology of traumatic gonitis

- sudden onset of relatively severe lameness
- increased synovial fluid (joint capsule distension easily appreciated) and periarticular swelling
- pain and crepitus in the stifle on manual flexion, extension, rotation, abduction and adduction
- instability possibly evident in the stifle on medial to lateral movement of *os calcis* with the limb elevated
- synovial fluid (sterile puncture between the medial and middle straight patellar ligaments) blood-tinged, some debris, no evidence of sepsis
- rapid development of secondary damage following primary injury: severe erosion of cartilage, eburnation of bone, meniscal cartilaginous erosion,

tearing and displacement, extensive periarticular fibrosis, secondary cruciate rupture, muscle atrophy

---

Warning

The intimate relationship of cruciate ligaments, articular cartilage and menisci in this major weight-bearing joint leads to very quick, irreversible secondary changes following damage to any part of the stifle. Prognosis following stifle lameness is always very guarded.

Treatment

- cull those cases with a cranial cruciate rupture except for valuable cattle, where surgery may be attempted in a surgical clinic
- in other conditions ensure absolute rest and NSAIDs for seven to ten days
- prognosis is poor

9.30 Nerve paralysis of limbs

Five different nerves may occasionally be paralysed. The aetiology, signs, diagnosis, treatment and prognosis of obturator, peroneal, femoral, sciatic and radial paralysis are summarised in Table 9.8.

Crushed tail head syndrome

- sacrococcygeal injury seen in high-producing dairy herds is caused by mounting injury of cows in oestrus
- characterised by a depressed tail head and flaccid paralysis of the tail
- possibly over-flexed hocks and knuckling of fetlocks are caused by injury to the spinal nerve roots that contribute to the tibial nerve
- possibly also bladder paralysis
- treatment is symptomatic: NSAIDs may be beneficial
- in all but severe cases, there is usually a slow spontaneous recovery from hind limb weakness but tail paralysis often persists and tail amputation may be necessary due to secondary trauma (see Section 9.31).

9.31 Tail amputation

Indications

- severe trauma; soiling following tail paralysis; septic fracture of the tail

Table 9.8 Common paralyses of cattle.

	Obturator	Peroneal	Femoral	Sciatic	Radial
Aetiology	Dystocia	Falls, post-partum recumbency	Large neonatal calves unique stretch injury (dystocia)	Pelvic fractures; poor injection technique in hind leg	Prolonged lateral recumbency in GA; some humeral fractures; bearing weight over point of shoulder in some cattle crushes
Signs	Often bilateral Hind limbs abducted	Knuckling of fetlock	Partial weight-bearing possible, lateral patellar luxation, discrete quadriceps atrophy in one week	Non-weight-bearing	Dropped elbow, knuckled fetlock, inability to advance limb. Collapse after release from cattle crush
Diagnosis	Confirmatory signs of pelvic injury	Loss of skin sensation dorsally	Specific neurogenic atrophy, possibly limited skin analgesia	Loss of all distal skin sensation	Signs and some sensory loss over elbow laterally

(continued)

Table 9.8 (*Continued*)

	Obturator	Peroneal	Femoral	Sciatic	Radial
Differential	Adductor rupture, separated pubic symphysis	Dorsal patellar luxation	Femoral, pelvic fractures hip dislocation (dystocia) muscle tendon rupture	Femoral fracture	Humeral fracture, elbow infection
Treatment	In all five forms of paralysis only supportive treatment can be given: soft bedding, non-slip surfaces, analgesics, NSAIDs and physiotherapy (calves)				
Prognosis	Good, but risk of a secondary hip dislocation in struggling (keep hocks together with shackles until able to stand)	Good	Guarded, particularly if unable to stand/bilateral	Guarded	Moderate if not sectioned (humeral fracture ends). Guarded if unable to stand after 12 hours

---

> **Warning**
>
> - Routine tail docking of dairy cows was once practised in some countries including New Zealand and the USA.
> - Tail docking has never been accepted as ethical in EU countries and it is no longer practised in New Zealand.
> - In the USA, tail docking is now also considered an unethical routine procedure providing no benefit to the animal (AABP view expressed in 2010) and should only be performed under exceptional circumstances (indications above).

Treatment

- perform in a standing cow
- epidural anaesthesia, e.g. 5 ml lignocaine HCl
- select a site about 10 cm distal to the point of attachment of the tail where faecal passage will not be impeded, or 10–20 cm proximal to the injury
- close clip and surgically scrub the area
- apply a tourniquet proximally
- identify the site for transection (an intercoccygeal joint space)
- make V-shaped incisions in the dorsal and ventral skin about 4–5 cm distal to the transection site. Undermine both flaps with a scalpel proximally to the level of the coccygeal transection
- transect the intercoccygeal joint space; this can be done by firmly kinking the tail manually and by a blunt dissection; not normally necessary to ligate the exposed coccygeal artery and vein
- appose the skin edges with several simple interrupted sutures or cruciate sutures (e.g. monofilament polypropylene (PDS) or Vicryl™); this will also effect haemostasis
- topical antibiotic spray on site; systemic antibiotics or NSAIDs unnecessary
- anticipate the wound to be healed in 2 weeks
- surgical problems relate to lack of provision for adequate skin to cover the bone stump, leading to localised infection; then section the tail through the next more proximal joint space

9.32 Limb fractures

Introduction

- fractures can affect many bones in cattle including:
  - ribs: most common bovine fracture, often linked to foot lameness and secondary difficulty rising and lying in cubicles/free stalls

- tail: likewise common, and high prevalence may indicate poor stock-manship (twisting of tails)
- vertebrae: potentially fatal
- pelvis: dystocia, involving separation of pubic symphysis in heifers; trauma (e.g. during oestrus or passing through a narrow gateway) resulting in fracture of the *tuber coxae*

Limb fractures involving the appendicular skeleton, including epiphyseal separation in growing stock, are relatively common.
Specific features in cattle include:

- economic considerations: often salvage may be preferable to a prolonged recovery period
- humane handling and recovery facilities are often sparse compared to those for other species and may affect the proposed treatment

Long bone fractures

- common sites in descending order of incidence: metatarsus, metacarpus, tibia, femur, radius/ulna, humerus
- occasional cases are in neonates, traumatised by the dam, and others are in growing cattle; less common in mature cows and bulls

Tip
Where the incidence of fracture is high in groups of growing animals, check nutrition. Fracture epidemics have been associated with Vitamin A or Vitamin D deficiency (e.g. incorrect vitamin inclusion or expired date).

Signs

- metatarsal and metacarpal fractures are very obvious
- most tibial fractures are in the proximal or mid-diaphyseal region of the tibial shaft, oblique and comminuted, with over-riding of the fracture ends
- most tibial fractures are closed; compound fractures (open) tend to have a wound on medial aspect
- lameness is severe, with obvious mobility of the distal limb and marked crepitus at the fracture site

Treatment

Immediate immobilisation on-farm if transported to a clinic: it is imperative to minimise movement at the fracture site during transport, as a simple fracture can so easily be converted into a compound disaster. A Robert Jones bandage, with lateral support proximally to the level of the *tuber coxae* in tibial fractures, is a good insurance policy against further iatrogenic injury.

1. Casts:
   - treatment of choice for closed fractures of the lower limb
   - plaster of Paris (least cost but heavy and not waterproof: usually not practical) or fibreglass and resin (stronger, waterproof, lighter: always preferable)
   - only suitable if the joint above and below the fracture can be immobilised (so not for a tibial fracture)
   - sedate the animal (e.g. xylazine) before applying the cast
   - pad well: e.g. a Softban® layer followed by cotton-wool held in place with a coloured flexible bandage (e.g. Vet-wrap®), followed by a fibreglass layer; the coloured bandage is easier to see when removing the cast with an oscillating saw
   - in neonates, rapid growth can soon lead to a cast becoming outgrown, leading to pressure necrosis of the skin; remove or replace after 3 weeks
   - a walking bar can be incorporated in the cast to transfer weight from the ground to above the fracture; maintain a 1 cm space between the bottom of the foot and the walking bar; the feet should always be enclosed in a cast
   - Thomas splint casts can be used for fractures of the tibia or radius/ulner. These incorporate a purpose-built external frame that transfers weight to the inguinal area or axilla by means of a loop welded to a walking bar and padded well with bandages. These need careful management and are more suitable for lighter animals (<350 kg)

Tip

- Pre-placing a length of embryotomy wire beneath the full length of fibreglass can be useful for sawing through the cast for removal.
- Placing wire through a plastic uterine/AI pipette on either side of the cast minimises the wire sticking to the cast material.

Tip

Placing rubber or Technovit™ glue on the bottom of a limb cast may reduce the risk of eroding through the foot of the cast.

---

2. External skeleton fixation:
   - preferred treatment for tibial and radial/ulner fractures, but requires referral to a specialist clinic where controlled traction, sterile facilities, general anaesthesia and radiology are available

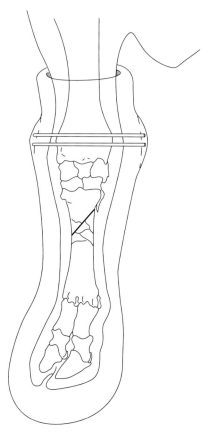

Figure 9.35 Walking cast for stabilisation of a comminuted metacarpal (MCIII/IV) fracture with two pins inserted into the distal radius.

- transfixation pins (3 proximal, 3 distal), connected externally by methylmethacrylate side bars or fibreglass. Pins are removed after six to eight weeks, ideally after a radiographic check to confirm that fracture healing is appropriate. Minor complications include suppuration around the pin holes. Major problems are continuing inability to bear weight, leading to severe lateral bowing of the contralateral hind leg and failure of adequate callus formation. Suitable for calves only
- only option for open fractures, but very guarded prognosis
- walking casts using external fixation pins can be used to transfer weight to above the fracture site (see Figure 9.35)
3. Internal fixation:
    - good option in valuable animals but requires full hospitalisation and specialist facilities

- best option for femoral and humeral fractures
- limited to young animals due to weight
- screws and pins may loosen in soft bones of neonates

Common problems of bovine long bone fractures

- high incidence of comminuted fractures, often grossly displaced
- frequently compound with gross contamination
- often severe muscular contraction, increasing difficulty in manipulative reduction

Physeal separation (Salter-Harris fracture)

Introduction

- affected tissue is the cartilage of the growth plate, so separation is a more accurate term than fracture
- majority occur at 0–12 months old
- common sites include proximal and distal femur, proximal tibia, and distal metatarsus and metacarpus
- the last two forms usually result from forced traction during dystocia and have a poor prognosis due to severe bruising and failure of blood to reach the separated epiphysis, which has no nutrient artery; osteomyelitis is a common sequel

Signs and treatment

- slight or no displacement causes mild lameness, slight crepitus, swelling and little or no abnormal mobility
- marked displacement causes considerable movement and crepitus at the fracture site and little weight-bearing, though pain may not be marked
- prognosis is good following reduction and immobilisation of the fracture under sedation or anaesthesia of the lower limb
- poor prognosis for external coaptation in the proximal tibial and any femoral epiphyseal separation with marked displacement, due to the difficulty of adequate immobilisation
- if external immobilisation is impossible, the choice is referral to a specialist clinic or immediate slaughter

Appendix

1 Further Reading

Anderson, D.E., & Desrochers, A. (2014) Bovine orthopedics, *Vet. Clin. N. Amer.*, **30**, 1.

Andrews, A.H. (ed.) (2000) The health of dairy cattle, Chapter 10, in *Internal Cattle Building Design and Cow Tracks* (J. Hughes), Oxford: Blackwell Scientific.

Blowey, R.W., & Weaver, A.D. (2011) *Color Atlas of Diseases and Disorders of Cattle*, 3rd edn, London: Mosby.

Cox, J.E. (1987) *Surgery of the Reproductive Tract in Large Animals*, 3rd edition, University of Liverpool Veterinary Field Station, Neston, Wirral.

Dirksen, G., Gründer, H.D., & Stöber, M. (2002) *Innere Medizin und Chirurgie des Rindes*, 4th edn (German 'bible', formerly Rosenberger), Berlin: Blackwell.

Dyce, K.M., & Wensing, C.J. (1971) *Essentials of Bovine Anatomy*, Philadelphia: Lea and Febiger.

Dyce, K.M., Sack, W.O., & Wensing C.J. (1987) *Textbook of Veterinary Anatomy*, Philadelphia: W.B. Saunders.

Fubini, S.L., & Ducharme, N.G. (eds) (2017). *Farm Animal Surgery*, 2nd edition, Philadelphia: W.B. Saunders.

Green, M. (ed.) (2012) *Dairy Herd Health*, Wallingford, UK: CABI.

Greenough, P.R., & Weaver, A.D. (1997) *Lameness in Cattle*, 3rd edn, Philadelphia: W.B. Saunders.

Hall, L.W., & Clarke, K.W. (1991) *Veterinary Anaesthesia*, 9th edn, London: Bailliere Tindall.

Hickman, J., Houlton, J., & Edwards, G.B. (1997) *Atlas of Veterinary Surgery*, 3rd edn, Oxford: Blackwell.

International Committee for Animal Recording (ICAR) (2015) *Claw Health Atlas 2015*.

Kersjes, A.W., Nemeth, F., & Rutgers, I.J.E. (1985) *Atlas of Large Animal Surgery*, Baltimore: Williams and Wilkins (excellent colour photos).

Bovine Surgery and Lameness, Third Edition. A. David Weaver, Owen Atkinson, Guy St. Jean and Adrian Steiner.
© 2018 John Wiley & Sons Ltd. Published 2018 by John Wiley & Sons Ltd.
Companion website: www.wiley.com/go/weaver/bovine-surgery

NOAH (National Office of Animal Health) (2015) Compendium of Data Sheets for Animal Medicines, NOAH, Enfield, England.

Noakes, D.E. (1997) *Fertility and Obstetrics in Cattle*, 2nd edn, Oxford: Blackwell Science.

Noakes, D.E., Parkinson, T.S., & England, G.C.W. (2001) *Arthur's Veterinary Reproduction and Obstetrics*, 8th edn, London and Philadelphia: W.B. Saunders.

Noordsy, J. (2014) *Noordsy's Food Animal Surgery*, edited by N. Ames, Kent, Iowa: W.B. Saunders.

Pavaux, C. (1983) *A Colour Atlas of Bovine Visceral Anatomy*, London: Wolfe.

St. Jean, G. (ed.) (1996) *Advances in Ruminant Orthopedics Vet. Clin. N. Am.: Food Animal Practice*, **12**, 1–298.

Toussaint Raven, E. (1985) *Foot Care and Claw Trimming*, Ipswich: U.K. Farming Press.

Tyagi, R.P.S., & Singh, J. (1993) *Ruminant Surgery*, Delhi: CBS Publishers (includes camel and buffalo).

Westhues, M., & Fritsch R. (1964) *Animal Anaesthesia*, Vol. 1 *Local Anaesthesia*, Bristol: Wright (details of nerve blocks, e.g. retrobulbar and pudic).

Wolfe, D.F., & Moll, H.D. (1999) *Large Animal Urogenital Surgery*, Baltimore and London: Williams and Wilkins (penile surgery, ovariectomy)

Youngquist, R.S. (ed.) (1997) *Current Therapy in Large Animal Theriogenology*, Philadelphia: W.B. Saunders (ovariectomy).

2 Abbreviations

ACP	acepromazine
AHDB	Agriculture and Horticulture Development Board
AHVLA	Animal Health and Veterinary Laboratories Agency (known since 2015 as APHA)
AI	artificial insemination
AMR	antimicrobial resistance
ALT/SGPT	alanine aminotransferase/serum glutamin-pyruvic transaminase
APHA	Animal and Plant Health Agency
AST/SGOT	aspartate aminotransferase/serum glutamic-oxaloacetic transaminase
BAL	bronchoalveolar lavage
BRSV	bovine respiratory syncytial virus
BPV-1	bovine papillomavirus type 1
BVD/MD	bovine viral diarrhoea/mucosal disease
CCF	congestive cardiac failure
CCP	corpus cavernosum penis
CFT	congenital flexed tendons
CNS	central nervous system
Co	coccygeal
CSF	cerebrospinal fluid

DA	displaced abomasum (see also LDA, RDA)
DD	digital dermatitis
DEFRA	Department for Environment, Food and Rural Affairs
DFT	deep flexor tendon
DIP	distal interphalangeal (joint)
DNA	desoxyribonucleic acid
EDTA	ethylene diamine-tetra-acetic acid
EMG	electromyogram
EU	European Union
FARAD	Food Animal Residue Avoidance Databank
FAT	fluorescent antibody test
FB	foreign body
FMD	foot and mouth disease
G	gauge
GA	general anaesthesia
HCl	hydrogen chloride
IBR	infectious bovine rhinotracheitis
ICAR	International Committee for Animal Recording
IgG	immunoglobulin G
i.m.	intramuscular
i.v.	intravenous
IVRA	intravenous regional anaesthesia
L	lumbar
l.a.	local anaesthetic
LDA	left displaced abomasum
LDH	lactate dehydrogenase
mEq	milliequivalent
mmHg	mm of mercury (unit of pressure)
MRL	maximum residue limit
MS	mobility score
NA	not applicable
NI	Northern Ireland
NOAH	National Office of Animal Health
NS	not suitable
NSAID	non-steroidal anti-inflammatory drug
NZ	New Zealand
ORT	oral rehydration therapy
P	phalanx
PCR	polymerase chain reaction
PCV	packed cell volume
PDS	(monofilament) dioxanone
PGA	polyglycolic acid
PM	postmortem
PVC	polyvinylchloride
RDA	right displaced abomasum

S	sacral
SARA	sub-acute ruminal acidosis
s.c.	subcutaneous
SCC	squamous cell carcinoma
SD	standard deviation
SFT	superficial flexor tendon
SGOT	see AST
SGPT	see ALT
SI (units)	International System of Units
SU	sole ulcer
T	thoracic
TA	tunica albuginea
TMR	total mixed ration
UK	United Kingdom
USA	United States of America
vCJD	variant Creutzfeldt-Jakob disease
VMD	Veterinary Medicines Directorate (UK)
WLD	white line disease

3 Conversion factors for old and SI units

	Old units	Multiplication factors		SI units
		Old units to SI units	SI units to old units	
RBC	millions/mm^3	10^6	10^{-6}	$\times 10^{12}$/l
PCV	%	0.01	100	1/l
Hb	g/100 ml	None	None	g/dl
WBC	thousands/mm^3	10^6	10^{-6}	$\times 10^9$/l
Total serum protein	g/100 ml	10	0.1	g/l
Albumin	g/100 ml	10	0.1	g/l
Bilirubin	mg/100 ml	17.1	0.0585	μmol/l
Calcium	mg/100 ml	0.25	4.008	mmol/l
Chloride	mEq/l	None	None	mmol/l
Creatinine	mg/100 ml	88.4	0.0113	μmol/l
Globulin	g/100 ml	10	0.1	g/l
Glucose	mg/100 ml	0.0555	18.02	mmol/l
Inorganic phosphate	mg/100 ml	0.323	3.1	mmol/l
Magnesium	mg/100 ml	0.411	2.43	mmol/l
Potassium	mEq/l	None	None	mmol/l
Sodium	mEq/l	None	None	mmol/l
Urea	mg/100 ml	0.166	6.01	mmol/l

Index

Page numbers in *italic* refer to figures, those in **bold** to tables

Bovine Surgery and Lameness, Third Edition. A. David Weaver, Owen Atkinson, Guy St. Jean
and Adrian Steiner.
© 2018 John Wiley & Sons Ltd. Published 2018 by John Wiley & Sons Ltd.
Companion website: www.wiley.com/go/weaver/bovine-surgery